DEMCO

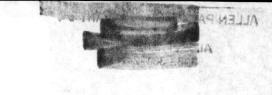

The Family Guide to
SYMPTOMS

Notice to the Reader

MANUSCRIPT WRITERS
Colette Pellerin
Caroline Baril
Véronique Robert

Mylène Paradis
Suzanne Champoux
Aline Charest
Lucie Chartrand
Marc Thibodeau

EDITOR
Annika Parance

SCIENTIFIC DIRECTORS
Dr. André-H. Dandavino
Dr. William Hogg

SCIENTIFIC COMMITTEE
Dr. Jacques E. Des Marchais
Dr. Wilhem B. Pellemans
Dr. André G. Trahan

Thanks are due to the AMLFC, and particularly
to its General Director, André de Sève, and to Ms Diane Bircher,
administrative assistant, for their close cooperation.

The Family Guide to
SYMPTOMS

Under the supervision of Dr. A.-H. Dandavino

With the collaboration of Dr. William Hogg, Director of Research,
Department of Family Medicine, Institute of Population Health,
University of Ottawa

Rogers Media Publishing

National Library of Canada cataloguing in publication

Main entry under title:
    The family guide to symptoms: 130 symptoms: their causes and treatments

    Translation of: Guide familial des symptômes.
    Includes index.

    ISBN 2-922260-12-7

    1. Symptoms – Popular works. 2. Diseases – Popular works. 3. Diagnosis – Popular works. 4. Therapeutics – Popular works. I. Dandavino, André-H., 1950-.

RC69.G8413 2003   616'.047   C2003-941833-2

Translation: Vera Roy
Revision: Anna Griffiths
Cover photo: Superstock
Back cover photo: Pierre Longtin
Graphic Design: Dino Peressini

© Rogers Media, 2003
1200 McGill College Avenue, suite 800
Montreal, QC, H3B 4G7
Tel.: (514) 845-5141
Fax: (514) 843-2183

Legal deposit: 4th 2003
Bibliothèque nationale du Québec, 2003
National Library of Canada, 2003

The publication of this work was made possible through an unrestricted educational grant from Pfizer Canada Inc.

Printed in Canada

Preface

Is it really necessary to see a doctor for every little health worry? No, certainly not, since so many small problems can be effectively treated at home. But when is a minor nuisance actually a sign of a more serious problem? The answer to this question can only be found by consulting a doctor—or this book. A number of doctors have collaborated to create this "pocket doctor", a handy reference guide to help you interpret symptoms that are worrying you or your family members.

The Family Guide to Symptoms presents 130 of the most common symptoms, providing descriptions, lists of causes, and effective home remedies. Valuable tips for prevention and emergencies are also included, as well as guidance about whether or not medical attention is required, what happens during a visit to the doctor's office, and any treatments that may be prescribed.

The aim of this book is to make clear and accessible information available at your fingertips. All the chapters are presented in a standardized format for handy consultation, with the detailed index at the back of the book making finding what you need as easy as flipping a page.

While numerous sources of information on diseases can be found on the internet, for example (among other places), it is very hard to tell which ones to trust. As doctors, we know that the best medical treatment results from a healthy relationship between patient and doctor, and believe that reading this book is the closest thing to a medical visit a person can have without actually going to the doctor's office.

The authors

FROM THE SAME PUBLISHER

Dr. Michael McCormack et al.
Male Sexual Health
(2003)

Dr. André-H. Dandavino et al.
The Family Guide to Health Problems
(2001)

Dr. Jean-Louis Chiasson et al.
Understand your Diabetes... and Live a Healthier Life!
3rd edition (2001)

Dr. Jacques Boulay
Bilingual Guide to Medical Abbreviations
3rd edition (1998)

Table of contents

Abdominal Bloating and Flatulence

The digestive tract is a flexible canal made up of smooth muscles that, from one end to the other, receives food, digests it, and expels the left-over waste.

Chewed food remains in the stomach for an average of two to three hours in preparation for digestion in the small intestine. Food matter then passes into the large intestine (colon), where normal bacterial fermentation produces gases (primarily hydrogen and methane).

Abdominal bloating (swelling) and flatulence (anal gas expulsion) is usually caused by an accumulation of intestinal gas, although other phenomena may be responsible.

WHAT ARE THE CAUSES?

- *Type of food consumed.* Once consumed, all food goes through a stage of bacterial fermentation. Some foods—particularly those containing sugar (either natural or artificial), carbohydrates or fibre—cause more bloating and gas than others. Large amounts of dairy products consumed in a short period of time (two or three glasses of milk at breakfast, for example) also produce excess gas.

- *Lactose intolerance* occurs when there is a deficiency of lactase, the enzyme responsible for the digestion of lactose (the natural sugar contained in dairy products). The lactose consumed with dairy products reaches the large intestine undigested and ferments even further, causing bloating, flatulence, and sometimes diarrhea or intestinal cramps. The condition is usually hereditary, although it can also develop if a severe case of gastroenteritis (stomach flu) washes away all the lactase from the intestine and damages the cells that produce it. In this case, the condition that results is permanent. It also arises if a person refrains from consuming dairy products for a few months and causes the intestine to stop producing the enzyme.

► *Constipation.* After a few days of constipation, stool accumulates in the large intestine; as the fermentation process continues, a greater amount of gas is produced.

► *Slowing of intestinal movement.* Heavy, rich meals are difficult to digest and slow down the intestinal mechanism. While this may cause discomfort, it does not necessarily indicate an increase of intestinal gas.

► *Aerophagia* describes the tendency to swallow too much air while eating or drinking. Excess air in the intestine leads to a bloated sensation, gas and burping.

► *Intestinal or liver disease.* Certain diseases cause bloating. Blockage caused by a cancerous tumour or Crohn's disease (chronic condition causing intestinal ulcers) can lead to swelling of the intestine, and as a result, the abdomen. Liver cirrhosis can cause water retention in the abdomen.

PRACTICAL ADVICE

Keep a journal. If your bloating and flatulence problems are very bothersome, keep a journal of your diet to help determine which foods are responsible and adjust your consumption of these items accordingly.

Take a walk after dinner. A fifteen-minute walk stimulates digestion and prevents bloating and the development of intestinal gas.

Watch what you drink. Avoid soft drinks and beer. Herbal teas like chamomile, mint or fennel help prevent bloating and flatulence, and are recommended instead of coffee or black tea after dinner. A glass of water with a few drops of mint, cinnamon or ginger extract has the same effect.

Consume less fat. Avoiding heavy and fatty meals eases digestion and prevents bloating. Don't forget to chew your food well.

Eat several small meals. Large meals may cause a bloating sensation. Four or five small meals a day keep the digestive system working continuously.

Take medication. Over-the-counter medications such as simethicone-based or activated carbon products help reduce bloating and intestinal gas with virtually no side effects. Take one pill before eating, as needed. Ask your pharmacist for advice.

Treat lactose intolerance. Some dairy products contain less lactose than others. Milk, ice cream, yogurt and white cheeses (cottage, ricotta) should be avoided, while cheeses such as cheddar, gruyere, brie, camembert, mozzarella, and brick, can be consumed without negative consequences. If you don't want to give up dairy products, take Lactaid (an artificial enzyme to aid lactose digestion) before consumption to prevent reactions. Take supplements to ensure you have a sufficient amount of calcium in your diet.

FOODS TO WATCH OUT FOR

Here is a list of the most common foods responsible for bloating and flatulence:

- ► Fatty foods (bacon, chips, fried food, chocolate, etc.)
- ► Beer and soft drinks
- ► Pretzels (large quantities)
- ► Whole wheat cereals, rice, oats, refined and sweet corn (Rice Krispies, Corn Flakes, Corn Pops, etc.)
- ► Raw vegetables
- ► Fruit (particularly apricots and bananas)
- ► Vegetables from the cabbage family (broccoli, green cabbage, cauliflower, Chinese cabbage, Brussels sprouts)
- ► Legumes (dried beans, lentils, chickpeas, etc.)
- ► Onions
- ► White bread
- ► Potatoes
- ► Peas
- ► Dairy products (large quantities consumed quickly)

Prevent or treat constipation. Instead of using over-the-counter laxatives, increase your consumption of dietary fibre. Because fibre can also cause flatulence, increase consumption gradually to facilitate the intestinal adjustment.

Avoid swallowing too much air as you eat. Excess air in the digestive tract causes bloating, gas and belching. If you have a tendency to swallow air while eating, avoid chewing gum or eating food that is either too hot or too cold (this makes you eat faster and consequently swallow more air). Take time to chew.

Neutralize gas caused by legumes. If you love baked beans but hate their after-effects, a solution is available. Soaking the beans in water overnight and cooking them on low heat reduces their gas-producing properties. Taking Beano (an over-the-counter liquid enzyme) with your first bite also prevents flatulence. Follow instructions carefully.

WHEN TO CONSULT?

► Bloating is accompanied by weight loss, diarrhea, or abdominal cramps, particularly after meals.
► Bloating is accompanied by swelling in the legs and weight gain.
► You find a lump in your stomach.

WHAT HAPPENS DURING THE EXAM?

The doctor will take a thorough history, administer an assessment questionnaire and perform a complete physical examination. Blood tests may be required, as well as an abdominal ultrasound, intestinal X-rays, axial tomography scans or magnetic resonance imaging.

WHAT IS THE TREATMENT?
Type of food consumed, lactose intolerance, constipation, slowing of intestinal movement, aerophagia

No medical treatment will definitively eliminate the problem, although symptoms can be controlled and quality of life improved. In cases of constipation, the doctor may prescribe emollient stool softeners or laxatives. Lactaid is recommended to prevent reactions to dairy products in cases of lactose intolerance. Drugs are available to regulate bowel movements and control aerophagia.

Intestinal or liver disease

Intestinal cancer requires surgical ablation and chemotherapy.

Crohn's disease is treated with medication to prevent ulcers, or surgery to remove the affected portion of the intestine.

Cirrhosis of the liver may be treated with diuretics that reduce water retention in the abdomen. If the condition is caused by alcohol, the sufferer must reduce or eliminate consumption.

Abdominal Pain

Abdominal pain is a symptom of a number of different conditions. People of all ages are familiar with cramps, as well as burning, nagging, or stabbing pains in the abdomen. Depending on the cause, the pain can be progressive, intermittent, constant, shooting, dull, mild, intense, recurring, acute, chronic...and the list goes on.

Abdominal pain may be diffused or concentrated in one area. In some circumstances, it radiates from another part of the body. It is frequently accompanied by symptoms such as nausea, vomiting, fever, diarrhea, bloating, or difficulty urinating. There are various possible causes, the most common of which are listed below.

Biliary colic (gallstones)
► Pain in the right side, below the lower ribs, radiating like a belt around the torso to the back.
► Usually accompanied by nausea and vomiting.
► Occurs most often after excessively large or fatty meals.
► May be accompanied by icterus (jaundice), pale stools, and dark urine.

Acute appendicitis
► Pain intensifies over a twenty-four-hour period.
► Usually begins around the navel and moves down to the lower right side of the abdomen.
► Accompanied by fever, nausea, vomiting, loss of energy and appetite, and very rarely, diarrhea.

Gynecological problems
► Frequently causes acute pain in the lower abdomen, either in the centre or sides.
► Sometimes accompanied by fever and, in rare cases, nausea and vomiting.
► In cases of ectopic pregnancy, usually accompanied by swelling of the breasts, cessation of menstruation, nausea, and vomiting.

Urinary infection
- ► Progressive pain in the centre of the lower abdomen.
- ► Difficulty passing urine accompanied by a burning sensation when the sufferer can urinate.
- ► Frequent need to urinate, even during the night.
- ► Cloudy foul-smelling urine.
- ► Sometimes accompanied by back pain, fever, and blood in the urine.

Intestinal problems
- ► Cramps in the central or lower abdomen.
- ► In cases of gastroenteritis (the most common intestinal problem), the pain is usually accompanied by nausea, vomiting, and diarrhea.
- ► Frequently accompanied by constipation, the pain is chronic, evolving over several days, and accompanied by abdominal bloating and discomfort. Evacuation of stools may be difficult, but generally brings relief.
- ► Peptic ulcers cause pyrosis (heartburn) and pain above the navel that may radiate around to the back and throughout the entire abdomen.
- ► The pain caused by diverticulitis is initially diffused, then builds and eventually becomes concentrated in the lower left side of the abdomen. It is accompanied by fever, abdominal bloating, and a change in the appearance of the stool (smaller, jagged pieces). It may cause gas build-up and constipation. In some cases, the colon becomes perforated and peritonitis can develop.
- ► An intestinal obstruction that prevents the movement and release of gas and stool causes cramps and severe abdominal bloating that lead to nausea, vomiting and, possibly, an intestinal perforation.

WHAT ARE THE CAUSES?
Biliary colic (gallstones)
- ► *Accumulation of bile.* Stones in the gallbladder or a blocked bile duct (linking the liver and the small intestine) prevent the evacuation of bile.
- ► *Family history,* in most cases.

Acute appendicitis

► *Blockage of the appendix* by stools, followed by bacterial infection.

Gynecological problems

► *Menstrual pain* is usually caused by uterine contractions as a result of an otherwise benign chemical imbalance. Only rarely is it a result of a medical condition such as endometriosis.

► *Ovarian cysts* may be congenital or acquired.

► *Salpingitis* (infection of the fallopian tubes) is generally spread through sexual contact.

► *Ectopic pregnancy* (development of the foetus outside the uterus) can be caused by previous surgery, endometriosis (abnormal growth of uterine mucous membrane), infection, or congenital abnormality of the fallopian tubes.

Urinary tract infection

► *Bacteria.*

► *Poor hygiene,* such as moving the toilet tissue from back to front after a bowel movement.

► *Not caused by "getting a chill",* contrary to popular belief.

Intestinal problems

► *Gastroenteritis* is caused by a viral or bacterial infection.

► *Constipation* can be caused by opiate drugs (morphine, codeine) and certain other medications, as well as diets that are low in fibre and liquids.

► *Peptic ulcer* can be caused by medications such as aspirin, anti-inflammatories, or cortisone.

► *Diverticulitis* is an infection of the intestinal wall that can lead to an abscess.

► *Intestinal obstructions* are frequently caused by hernias (either abdominal or inguinal), whereby a segment of the intestine protrudes from the abdominal cavity due to a weakness in the abdominal wall. An intestinal obstruction may be congenital or acquired; i.e., directly caused by abdominal surgery, for example, or postoperative adhesions (intra-abdominal scarring).

PRACTICAL ADVICE

Avoid spicy or acidic foods. This will to ease the symptoms of a peptic ulcer (heartburn).

Improve your eating habits. Chew your food well, drink plenty of liquids (prune juice is especially good), and eat more natural fibre to encourage regularity. Avoid binding diets that can cause constipation (for example, the BRAT diet: Bananas, Rice, Apples and Toast).

Never take laxatives without a prescription. This can aggravate your problem.

Go to the bathroom when you feel the urge. Follow your own rhythm. It is perfectly normal if you do not have a bowel movement every day.

Gallstones: liquid diet. All kinds of liquids are fine, except those containing fat, such as milk.

Take antispasmodic drugs. Available over-the-counter, antispasmodics (such as Bentylol) can help ease intestinal cramps or spasms.

Recurrent gallstones: watch what you eat and see a doctor. As you wait for surgery, control the frequency of attacks by limiting your consumption of fatty foods.

If you suspect acute appendicitis, go to the emergency room. The longer you wait, the higher the risk of serious complications, such as a perforated appendix and peritonitis.

For menstrual pain. Take painkillers, rest, and place a heating pad on the abdomen.

Use a condom. Unprotected sexual intercourse can lead to sexually transmitted infections, such as salpingitis.

Drink plenty of water. This can sometimes clear up a urinary tract infection as it is developing. Consult a doctor if the pain persists and your condition gets worse. Good hydration also helps flush out most other viral infections of the intestine. Avoid drinking alcohol, coffee and tea.

Be careful in the bathroom. Use a short, front-to-back movement with the toilet tissue in order to avoid contamination with intestinal bacteria. Wash your hands thoroughly after using the toilet. Good hygiene stops the proliferation of bacteria.

WHEN TO CONSULT?

► The pain persists for more than six hours.
► The pain intensifies or becomes generalized and constant.
► The pain prevents you from performing your usual activities.
► Abdominal pain is accompanied by fever, jaundice, or back pain.
► You feel pain on the right side of the abdomen, below the ribs, which becomes more intense after fatty or large meals. You have had gallstones in the past.
► You have recurring gallstones.
► Vomiting persists for a prolonged period of time (more than 24 hours). The vomit is bloody or has a fecal smell.
► There is blood in your urine or stools.
► You are pregnant.
► You have been unable to pass wind or have a bowel movement for 24 hours.
► You are very dehydrated (your skin is creased and the inside of your mouth is very dry).
► Your hernia protrudes persistently or causes you a great deal of pain.

WHAT HAPPENS DURING THE EXAM?

The doctor briefly interviews the patient and performs a physical examination, which may include a digital exam of the rectum or vagina. He or she may order blood and urine tests, as well as abdominal X-rays. An abdominal or pelvic ultrasound may also be necessary. Women of childbearing age may be asked to take a pregnancy test.

WHAT IS THE TREATMENT?
Biliary colic (gallstones)
The gallbladder is surgically removed.

Acute appendicitis
Surgery to remove the appendix is necessary. Patients may require antibiotics.

Gynecological problems
Menstrual pain
Oral contraceptives, painkillers, rest, and some home care (*see Practical Advice*) can help bring relief.

Ectopic pregnancy
Surgical removal is necessary.

Ovarian cyst
Cysts often disappear on their own, although surgical removal is also often necessary.

Salpingitis
This condition is treated with antibiotics.

Urinary tract infections
The cause determines which antibiotic treatment is used. Antibiotics are delivered orally or intravenously.

Intestinal problems
Gastroenteritis
Allowing the intestines to rest is the best treatment. Eliminate solid foods from your diet and drink plenty of liquids. Slowly resume eating solid foods a little at a time.

Constipation

Constipation can be eased with a fibre-rich diet and good hydration. In some cases, the patient is required to have an enema, take mineral oils, or undergo a digital removal of a fecaloma (stool obstruction).

Peptic ulcers

These are treated with anti-ulcer medications and antibiotics (if the presence of the *Helicobacter pylori* bacteria is suspected). The doctor may also prescribe a diet.

Diverticulitis

A strict diet is imposed to ensure the intestine has a chance to rest. A liquid and low-residue diet must be followed for three to four weeks. The doctor will prescribe oral or intravenous antibiotics, depending on the severity of the infection. Oral antibiotics are taken for 7 to 14 days. Recurrent diverticulitis is treated with surgery.

Intestinal obstruction

The stomach and intestine are cleared using a tube inserted through the nose. If the occlusion persists, surgery is necessary.

Hernias

They often require surgery.

Persistent intestinal obstruction and perforated intestine due to complications from an intestinal obstruction

Surgery is necessary.

Abnormal Vaginal Bleeding (Premenopausal)

In general, there should be no vaginal bleeding other than during the menstrual period, except perhaps for a few drops during ovulation. Bleeding between periods can be benign, but may also indicate one of a number of underlying problems requiring medical treatment.

WHAT ARE THE CAUSES?

- *Low-dose contraceptives ("minipill").* In some women, low doses of estrogen lead to a thinning of the endometrium (inner lining of the uterus).
- *Forgetting a pill.* If a woman forgets to take her birth control pill for more than 24 hours, light bleeding can occur. While harmless, it does increase the risk of unwanted pregnancy.
- *Bleeding during ovulation.* About 5% of women experience spotting during ovulation. It may be accompanied by mild pain in the left or right side of the abdomen.
- *Ovarian dysfunction.* The ovary may begin to function irregularly at least ten years before menopause, leading to a thickened endometrium and the elimination of fragments or bleeding.
- *Complications linked to pregnancy.* Bleeding may be a sign of a miscarriage or ectopic pregnancy (egg fertilized outside the uterus in the fallopian tube).
- *Polyps.* These benign tumours on the cervix bleed easily if touched.
- *Fibroma.* Also benign, these tumours are located in the uterine wall and may cause irregular bleeding and, in some cases, pain, depending on their location.
- *Atypical cells (cervical dysplasia).* Abnormal cells on the cervix are not dangerous in themselves, although they have the potential to become cancerous.
- *Infection of the cervix (cervicitis).* Bleeding may occur with or without sexual intercourse. Chlamydia, a sexually transmitted infection, is often the cause.

► *Infection of the inner uterine lining (endometritis)* is most commonly caused by bacteria. It is accompanied by fever, pain and foul-smelling, yellowish vaginal discharge.

► *Cervical, uterine or vaginal cancer.*

► *Sexual intercourse* may cause micro-abrasions or even lacerations on the vaginal wall or cervix. Vigorous sexual activity or insufficient vaginal lubrication can render the mucous membranes more fragile, aggravating the problem. Inadequate lubrication may be due to psychological factors like stress, or hormonal factors such as menopause.

► *Foreign body.* Intra-uterine devices (IUDs) may cause bleeding between periods. In children, a foreign body in the vagina (eraser or Lego brick, for example) may be the cause.

► *Trauma.* Violent sexual intercourse, rape, or a fall (onto a fence or bicycle crossbar, for example) can cause heavy bleeding.

► *Medications.* Certain medications cause heavier bleeding, such as aspirin or anticoagulants.

► *Systemic diseases,* such as thyroid disease, blood disorders, and coagulation problems.

► *Bleeding from another area* (such as the bladder or rectum). The origin of the blood is not always clear, due to the proximity of the vagina, urethra (urination duct) and anus. A medical examination may be necessary.

PRACTICAL ADVICE

Do not ignore bleeding. Consult a doctor.

Do not use a vaginal douche after bleeding. This is not helpful. In fact, the use of vaginal douches is generally not recommended, because they alter the pH (acidity levels) of the vagina.

Take a pregnancy test. Any woman in her child-bearing years who notices abnormal bleeding (even if she has used contraception) should take a pregnancy test.

Have a regular Pap test. This routine test will detect abnormal cells at an early stage and may save your life. Many women are advised to have the test done once a year, although more or less frequent testing may be required, depending on a variety of factors. The doctor will perform a complete gynecological exam at the same time.

Be gentle. Sexual intercourse that is violent or causes excessive friction can lead to bleeding.

Use a lubricant. If the vagina is inadequately lubricated for sexual intercourse, use a sterile gel available in pharmacies (such as K-Y Jelly).

WHEN TO CONSULT?
- You notice bleeding between your periods.
- You notice bleeding during pregnancy.
- Your menstrual cycle is irregular.
- Your bleeding is abnormally heavy (requiring one pad or more every hour).

WHAT HAPPENS DURING THE EXAM?
The doctor examines the vagina and cervix, taking a cervical cell sample in a Papanicolaou (Pap) test. This routine test is used to screen for potential cervical dysplasia or cancer. If an inflammation or infection is suspected, the doctor will take secretion samples for lab analysis. Ultrasound may be used for more in-depth examinations. After a trauma, examinations generally take place under general anesthesia.

WHAT IS THE TREATMENT?
Contraceptives, bleeding during ovulation, ovarian dysfunction
If the cause is low-dose contraceptives ("minipill"), the prescription will be modified. If caused by ovarian dysfunction, a gynecological assessment is ordered. An endometrial biopsy (removal of tissue for analysis) may be performed, using a curettage. The doctor may also prescribe hormonal treatment or low-dose contraceptives.

Complications linked to pregnancy
If pregnancy is suspected or has already been confirmed, a medical examination is required. This is an emergency.

Polyps
A biopsy is performed or the polyps removed in a surgical procedure in the doctor's office.

Fibroma
It is not always necessary to remove fibroma, as hormone treatment may be sufficient. In many cases, the fibroma shrink and disappear after menopause.

Atypical cells (cervical dysplasia)
This is a common and benign problem, although it may be a warning sign of potential cancer and therefore requires medical attention. Abnormal cells are destroyed using cryotherapy (cold treatment) or laser therapy. These treatments are simple and can be performed in a colposcopy clinic. The doctor may also perform a small surgical procedure on the cervix known as a "conization" to confirm the diagnosis or if suspicious lesions are present.

Cervical infection (cervicitis) and infection of the inner uterine lining (endometritis)
Antibiotics will be prescribed to the patient and, if necessary, her partner.

Cancer
The prognosis is excellent if this type of cancer is detected early, with a 95% cure rate. It requires immediate surgical intervention followed by chemotherapy or radiation therapy.

Sexual intercourse
If the bleeding is due to inadequate lubrication and the gels available in pharmacies are not satisfactory, the doctor may prescribe hormonal treatment in the form of a pill (hormone replacement therapy) or

topical cream. If the problem has psychological origins, the appropriate treatment will be advised.

Foreign body
If an IUD is causing irregular bleeding, it should be removed. In most cases, the presence of a foreign body in the vagina requires examination under general anesthesia.

Trauma
This requires an in-depth examination, usually under general anesthesia. Any lacerations will be repaired.

Medications
Lab tests to identify the precise cause are required before treatment is prescribed.

Aches

The word "ache" generally refers to diffuse muscular pain. Aches are usually not serious and may be accompanied by fever or fatigue.

Everyone has experienced aches at some point in their life. They may be brought on by trauma, infection, inflammation, or a metabolic disorder in the muscle fibre.

WHAT ARE THE CAUSES?

► *Physical over-exertion.* Muscles may develop aches in the 72 hours after intense physical activity.
► *Viral infections,* such as colds, hepatitis, pneumonia, or septicemia.
► *Rheumatic disorders,* such as arthritis or myositis. Aches are generally experienced in the early stages of the disease.
► *Endocrine disorders and cancer.* These are very rare causes.

PRACTICAL ADVICE

Get some rest. If your aches are due to overwork or infection, rest is essential. Even if you cannot stay in bed all day, try to reduce or slow the pace of your daily activities.

Take a hot bath. This is an excellent way to relieve benign aches. While hot water bottles, hot compresses and medicated balms are effective for specific areas, hot baths soothe the entire body. Be careful: if you have a high fever (starting at 39 °C if taken orally, or 39.5 °C if taken with a rectal thermometer), avoid hot baths and try to find ways to lower your body temperature.

Avoid hot baths if suffering from cardiovascular disease. Hot baths may cause vasodilation, low blood pressure (leading to generalized weakness), and increased heart rate (to compensate for the decreased pressure).

Take painkillers. Taking acetaminophen or aspirin every four hours will help reduce discomfort and any fever you might have. Non-prescription anti-inflammatories can also provide relief. Be careful, though: aspirin and anti-inflammatory drugs can cause complications in the elderly and children, as well as in those suffering from stomach ulcers or digestive bleeding. These medications must also be avoided by people taking anticoagulants, in which case acetaminophen is the recommended alternative.

Be patient. Aches due to overwork or infection usually disappear within 48 hours.

Stay in shape. People in poor physical shape who engage in intense exercise often develop muscle aches. Make sure to work out steadily, build your exercise routine up slowly, and always warm up beforehand. If you lead a sedentary lifestyle, consult your doctor before beginning an exercise programme.

WHEN TO CONSULT?

► Your aches have lasted more than four or five days.
► You have a high and persistent fever.

Side cramps

Side cramps are light pains felt in the muscle wall. They develop after certain movements or during physical activity (such as running).
The best cure is to stop the activity and wait. The cramp will disappear after a few minutes without medication.

Consult a doctor in any of the following situations:
- **The pain persists or intensifies.**
- **You have difficulty breathing.**
- **You feel chest pain that radiates out towards the arm or the neck.**
- **You feel faint.**
- **You have heart palpitations.**
- **You experience abdominal pain along with nausea or vomiting.**

► Your joints are swollen.
► Your muscles feel weak.
► You feel generally under the weather.

WHAT HAPPENS DURING THE EXAM?

If the patient's symptoms are worrying, the doctor takes a thorough history, administers an assessment questionnaire, and performs a complete physical examination. Depending on the results, he or she may order laboratory analyses, cultures, X-rays, or any other appropriate test.

WHAT IS THE TREATMENT?

If there is an underlying illness, the doctor will begin appropriate treatment immediately.

Antibiotics may be prescribed in the case of infection. A rheumatic disease requires anti-inflammatories or possibly physiotherapy.

Acute Lower Abdominal Pain (Women)

Acute lower abdominal pain appears suddenly, is intense and constant, and shoots through the lower abdominal (pelvic) area.

WHAT ARE THE CAUSES?

► *Infection.* Infections causing acute lower abdominal pain are usually due to sexually transmitted infections or bacteria associated with intrauterine devices (IUDs). They may also cause fever and vaginal discharge.

► *Torsion of the ovary.* Women who have had several children are particularly at risk, due to decreased muscle elasticity after childbirth.

► *Ovulation.* For some women, ovulation is accompanied by pain in the side of the abdomen. The discomfort lasts anywhere from five minutes to an hour before gradually subsiding.

► *Tubal rupture due to ectopic pregnancy* causes very sharp pain and sometimes loss of consciousness. This is an emergency situation.

► *Rupture of an ovarian cyst.* The ovaries can develop two types of cysts. Physiological cysts develop when the corpus luteum does not disintegrate after ovulation. They are generally under 7 centimetres in diameter and disappear after a few months. Non-physiological cysts are bigger and permanent. Large cysts can be painful if disturbed by a gynecological exam, sexual intercourse, or intestinal swelling, for example.

► *Non-gynecological ailments.* Infections of the bladder or sigmoid colon, appendicitis, diverticulitis, and gallstones can cause acute lower abdominal pain.

PRACTICAL ADVICE

Protect yourself against sexually transmitted infections. They can have long-term negative effects, including infertility and adhesions. The latter are web-like growths of inflammatory tissue that cover the ovaries, fallopian tubes and abdominal wall, impeding the mobility of the organs. They are caused by improperly treated infections or abdominal surgery.

Avoid vaginal douches. The vagina is a natural organ of the body with flora to protect against the intrusion of other micro-organisms. It does not need to be disinfected. Douches run the risk of transporting bacteria from the vagina to the uterus or disturbing vaginal flora.

WHEN TO CONSULT?

► You have been experiencing sharp pain in the abdomen for the last few hours.
► Abdominal pain is preventing you from carrying out normal activities.
► The pain has spread to the entire abdomen.
► The pain is accompanied by other symptoms (fever or somewhat foul-smelling vaginal discharge), or its recent appearance coincides with the arrival of a new sexual partner in your life.

WHAT HAPPENS DURING THE EXAM?

A history of the illness assessment questionnaire, and gynecological exam are the first steps towards reaching diagnosis. In the latter, the doctor can determine the presence of infection and the state of the cervix, and manipulate the organs to determine their relative size and location. This information is generally enough to make diagnosis possible, but if the results are inconclusive, the doctor will order an ultrasound, laparoscopy (internal exam using fibre optics), blood tests, or urinalysis to screen for infection.

WHAT IS THE TREATMENT?

Infection

Infections are treated with antibiotics. Treatment must begin early and continue to its prescribed end. This will ensure full recovery and prevent long-term damage such as adhesions or infertility resulting from tissue deterioration in the fallopian tubes.

Torsion of the ovary
Painful ovarian torsion requires surgery.

Ovulation
If the pain is intense, the doctor will prescribe oral contraceptives. There is no treatment for less severe cases.

Tubal rupture due to ectopic pregnancy
This requires emergency consultation and surgery. Every effort will be made to repair the fallopian tube so the woman's fertility is not compromised.

Rupture of an ovarian cyst
The patient will be kept under observation for a few hours. If there is no improvement, surgery to remove the cyst may be required. This operation does not affect the woman's fertility.

Non-gynecological ailments
Infections of the bladder and the sigmoid colon, as well as diverticulitis, are treated with antibiotics. Appendicitis usually calls for removal of the appendix. If the body does not expel gallstones naturally, the doctor may choose to break them up with ultrasound waves, extract them through an existing orifice, or surgically remove them.

Anal Incontinence

Anal continence (the ability to control the passage of stool) is learned between the ages of two and three. This complex activity requires the participation of the brain, spinal cord, nerves of the anus and rectum, rectal muscles (sphincters), and the small and large intestines.

The sphincter apparatus (the internal and external sphincter muscles) plays a primary role in continence. The internal sphincter is almost continually contracted and differentiates between feces and gas to prevent the escape of small amounts of fecal matter during the release of gas. The external sphincter and puborectal muscles are also contracted to control defecation. Hemorrhoids (dilated veins of the anus and rectum) act as small vascular cushions, also playing an important role in the prevention of fecal incontinence.

Anal incontinence can be difficult to treat because the anal continence mechanism is so complex and a disturbance can occur at any one of a number of levels. Although not life-threatening, the affliction is traumatizing and, because sufferers are often too embarrassed to seek help, exact statistics are unavailable. Some individuals limit their social contact because they fear a humiliating situation may arise, or, in rare cases, are hospitalized in a chronic care facility. Fecal incontinence is frequently associated with urinary incontinence, causing the sufferer even greater distress.

There are four classes of anal incontinence:

True incontinence
► Involuntary evacuation of stool.
► In some cases, accompanied by urinary incontinence.

Overflow incontinence
► Liquid stool, difficult to control.

Stress incontinence
► Urgent need to defecate.
► More or less liquid stool.

Partial incontinence

► Involuntary passage of mucus (transparent, viscous and thready liquid) or gas; in rare cases, passage of stool.
► Blood- or mucus-stained underwear.

WHAT ARE THE CAUSES?

Common causes of the four classes of anal incontinence:

► *Neurological disorders* such as multiple sclerosis, spina bifida and chronic diabetes can all provoke anal incontinence. Chronic diabetes diminishes anal sensitivity, thereby weakening the muscle contractions necessary to control the passage of stool. Diabetes also irritates the bowels, changing the consistency of stool (often making it liquid or loose).
► *Intestinal disorders,* such as Crohn's disease (an inflammatory digestive tract illness) and irritable bowel syndrome (causing digestive problems, pain, bloating, and transit disturbances, without organic cause) can also cause anal incontinence.
► *Laxative abuse.*

True incontinence

► *Weakening of the pelvic floor.* The pelvic floor is comprised of three muscles supporting the bladder and intestines. In women, the muscles are subjected to the additional strain of supporting the uterus. For this reason, women are more likely to experience a weakening of the pelvic floor muscles than men. Vaginal childbirth, episiotomies, perineal tears and decreased hormone levels during menopause can also adversely affect pelvic floor muscle tone. If the pelvic floor loses the strength to resist the pressure of a full, dilated intestine, stool cannot be retained.
► *Aging* diminishes an individual's ability to coordinate the mechanisms of continence.
► *Cerebral vascular accidents (CVA)* can deregulate the control of urinary and fecal elimination.
► *Anal tear.* Vaginal delivery or anal penetration (either sexual or by a foreign body) can tear the perineum as far as the anus.

► *Deterioration of the sphincter mechanism.* Anal penetration can damage the anal sphincter mechanism. An infected episiotomy wound can also compromise sphincter competence.

► *Rectal prolapse.* In older individuals, particularly women with a relaxed pelvic floor, the muscles may be so weak that the rectum or anus protrude outside the body (rectal prolapse). Round red masses (often as large as a grapefruit) appear when defecating or simply crouching. This problem is not usually painful and the organs generally return to their natural position on their own. However, because the condition is recurrent, the rectal sphincter eventually becomes dilated to the point that the sufferer is unable to retain stool. There is also the possibility that the rectum and anus will protrude permanently.

Overflow incontinence
► *Constipation.* Lack of fluid slows intestinal activity. Fecaliths (hard impacted stool in the colon or rectum) can form, blocking the passage of solid stool, while overflowing liquid stool (diarrhea) cannot be controlled.

Stress incontinence
► *Traveller's diarrhea* **(turista).** Travellers frequently suffer from this form of diarrhea after ingesting contaminated food. Fatigue, jet lag, and change of diet contribute to the problem.

► *Gastroenteritis* is diarrhea occurring secondary to a viral or bacterial infection and is often accompanied by nausea, vomiting and fever

► *Rectal surgery.* Surgery for rectal cancer, proctitis (inflammation of the rectum) or anastomosis (joining two parts of the intestine) may result in fecal incontinence.

► *Radiation x-rays* of the genital area (in cases of prostate, anal, rectal, or uterine cancer) can dilate the rectum and sphincters, causing incontinence.

Partial incontinence
- *Aging.*
- *Hemorrhoidectomy*, the surgical excision of hemorrhoids, can also lead to incontinence.

PRACTICAL ADVICE

Eat well. Loose or liquid stool is difficult to control. If you have diarrhea, reduce your consumption of fibre (bran cereals, whole wheat bread, vegetables, fruit and legumes), reintroducing it into your diet gradually. Sufferers of overflow incontinence should maintain fibre intake to encourage regular intestinal activity and proper stool consistency.

Drink plenty of water. Adequate hydration prevents constipation. Drink at least six glasses of water a day.

Avoid certain foods. Coffee, tea, chocolate, soft drinks and certain spices can cause anal pruritus (itching). The repeated scratching that results produces small ulcers or lesions that may become infected and decrease the sensitivity of the anus, which makes it harder for the sphincters to detect the presence of stool, leading to progressive incontinence. If you suffer from anal itching, avoid caffeine.

Strengthen the pelvic floor. Episiotomies can weaken the pelvic floor muscles, leading to true incontinence. Regular perineal massage can help develop the required elasticity to avoid vaginal tears and episiotomies during delivery. Regular Kegel exercises effectively strengthen the pelvic floor muscles and are simple to perform: contract the muscles that control urination, holding for several seconds. Perform once or twice during urination, or repeatedly at any other time.

Modify sexual activities. Avoid anal penetration.

Avoid laxatives. If you are constipated, eat more fruit, vegetables and drink more water. Over-the-counter laxatives cause intestinal contractions. In cases of intestinal blockage, this does not help the sufferer eliminate stool and only increases the pain. Also avoid strong herbal laxatives (such as senna), found in a number of herbal teas.

Avoid sitting on the toilet for prolonged periods. Spending too much time on the toilet stretches and lowers the pelvic floor, eventually weakening the muscles. It can also cause vein congestion (veins filling with blood) and hemorrhoids. Do not read on the toilet!

WHEN TO CONSULT?
► You are having trouble controlling the passage of stool.

WHAT HAPPENS DURING THE EXAM
Your physician performs a physical exam (including a digital rectal exam) and ask you about how much time you spend on the toilet, whether defecation is a strain, and whether you practice passive anal penetration.

Medical diagnosis may also require tests such as an anuscopy or rectoscopy (involving the inspection of the anus and rectum with a lighted speculum or tube), and a barium enema (colon X-ray following the infusion of a radiopaque contrast liquid). In some cases, the physician will prescribe more in-depth exams.

WHAT IS THE TREATMENT?
True and partial incontinence
The best treatment involves physiotherapy and biofeedback (relaxation techniques). Physiotherapy provides the patient with a series of exercises to reinforce pelvic floor muscles and improve the sphincter apparatus function. Biofeedback techniques stimulate the nerves of the rectum and anus to help them recover their sensitivity and improve continence.

Overflow incontinence
An enema and rectal suppositories are often required to evacuate the fecalith. The patient is then encouraged to drink plenty of liquids. The doctor may also recommend fibre supplements that absorb water and increase the size of the stool, triggering the defecation reflex.

Stress incontinence

Stress incontinence is often treated with antidiarrheal medications. In cases of irritable bowel syndrome, Crohn's disease or rectal surgery, a dietary fibre supplement may be prescribed.

Corrective surgery for anal incontinence

Five surgical techniques are available to treat persistent problems, particularly in cases of true incontinence. The type of surgery recommended depends on the patient's condition and the physician's expertise.

Surgical correction of rectal prolapse involves fixing the rectum or anus in its natural position to prevent recurrence upon exertion or defecation. The procedure can be performed through the abdomen or perineum.

Sphincters are repaired by tightening the puborectal muscle. Although this has immediate effects, the procedure may need to be repeated in three to four years, since there is a risk of relaxation. This surgery is also an effective means of repairing tears due to trauma (postpartum or anal penetration). Once again, however, while short and intermediate term results are favourable, the chance of recurrence remains.

A recently-developed technique, practiced only in highly specialized centres, involves transposing a portion of the thigh muscle to the perianal region.

Implantation of an artificial sphincter involves a patient-controlled pump that contracts and deflates the anal canal to facilitate the passage of stool. The treatment is experimental.

Colostomy is a surgical procedure creating an artificial excretory opening from the colon on the abdomen (in the form of a plastic bag). This is a radical and permanent treatment for anal incontinence in most cases.

Angina Pectoris

The heart muscle pumps blood throughout the entire body. To do so, it requires blood and oxygen, which are provided by three main arteries. If one of these vessels becomes partially obstructed, the heart cannot do its job properly, resulting in chest pain known as angina pectoris.

Angina pectoris manifests within the following symptoms:
- Pain or tightness in the chest during physical exertion.
- Pain radiating outwards to the arms, neck and shoulders.
- General breathlessness or unusual breathlessness upon exertion.
- Disappearance of symptoms when at rest.

WHAT ARE THE CAUSES?

- *Arteriosclerosis.* High cholesterol levels may lead to cholesterol deposits in the coronary arteries, causing partial or complete obstruction.
- *Smoking and diabetes* increase the risk of arteriosclerosis.
- *High blood pressure and obesity.* Reduced elasticity of the blood vessels (high blood pressure), or excess weight (obesity) requires extra effort from the heart muscle.
- *Genetic factors.* The risk of angina pectoris is higher if there is a family history of the disease developing in relatives under the age of sixty.
- *Post-menopause* causes a drop in the production of hormones (estrogen) that protect against heart disease.

PRACTICAL ADVICE

Avoid going out in cold, windy weather. The cold makes the heart and lungs work harder. Many sufferers find it brings on angina attacks, particularly if the weather is windy.

Avoid intense physical exertion. An angina attack can be brought on by activities such as shovelling snow or playing squash.

Quit smoking. Smoking causes progressive obstruction of the arteries. Furthermore, each cigarette smoked triggers an immediate contraction of the arteries, diminishing their capacity to transport blood and reducing the flow of oxygen to the heart. Quitting smoking significantly reduces the risk of dying from a heart attack (myocardial infarction). A long-time smoker's risk decreases to the level of a non-smoker's only two years after quitting.

Reduce fat consumption. Excessive consumption of fat (particularly animal fat) causes the levels of "bad" cholesterol to climb and accumulate along the walls of the arteries that lead to the cardiac muscle, eventually blocking blood flow to the heart. Eating a balanced diet and eliminating as much fat as possible will not only help prevent hypercholesterolemia, but also obesity, diabetes and high blood pressure, which also cause angina pectoris.

Get informed. For information on appropriate diets, consult reliable sources such as the Fondation québécoise des maladies du coeur and the Canada Food Guide, or speak to a dietician or doctor.

Get moving. Angina pectoris sufferers are not advised to engage in aerobic exercise or go running, but they are encouraged to take part in milder forms of exercise, such as walking, bicycling or swimming to reduce bad cholesterol levels and get back in shape. Exercise also plays a role in diabetes management as it makes the tissues more receptive to the action of insulin. To get the full benefits, you need to exercise for at least 45 minutes, three times a week.

Relax. Reducing stress and anxiety helps control angina pectoris. There are a variety of ways to reduce stress, including yoga, meditation, listening to soft music, and taking hot baths.

WHEN TO CONSULT?
► You feel pain or tightness in your chest.
► You are increasingly out of breath in general, or suffer from excessive breathlessness upon physical exertion.

WHAT HAPPENS DURING THE EXAM?

The diagnosis is based on a physical examination, electrocardiogram, consideration of the clinical history and risk factors, and, if necessary, more specialized tests. For example, the patient may undergo an exercise electrocardiogram (the "treadmill test"), or myocardial radioisotope scanning, which is administered while the patient exercises or is on medication that mimics the effects of exercise (this is a type of nuclear medicine testing used to determine whether the heart lacks oxygen during physical exertion). Coronary arteriography may also be necessary, which determines the state of the arteries through an injection of dyeliquids directly into the coronary arteries. In most cases, however, the doctor can arrive at a precise diagnosis without resorting to advanced technology.

WHAT IS THE TREATMENT?

The medications available for angina pectoris aim to improve a sufferer's quality of life and prevent heart attacks.

Nitroglycerine (in sublingual, inhaler or pill form), long action nitrates, and calcium inhibitors dilate the arteries to allow a greater flow of oxygen. The doctor may also prescribe beta-blockers to decrease oxygen consumption and slow the heart rhythm.

The doctor may also recommend a daily dose of 80 mg to 325 mg of aspirin, the cheapest and most effective treatment against heart

---

BEWARE OF HEART ATTACKS

Angina can remain stable for many years if properly treated. In some cases, however, the condition deteriorates and manifests in unprovoked chest pain even when the sufferer is at rest. This indicates the development of a blood clot that will eventually block the artery completely.

This symptom may be a warning sign of an impending heart attack or unstable angina (the most serious form of angina pectoris). See a doctor immediately.

attack. It is important to note, however, that this treatment should only be followed under a doctor's orders, since aspirin increases the risk of brain or stomach hemorrhage.

If the prescribed treatment fails or the angina worsens, the patient has two surgical options for revascularization: angioplasty, and coronary bypass. In angioplasty, the doctor remodels the shrunken blood vessel, inserting and opening a balloon catheter to dilate the artery. In a coronary bypass, blood circulation is restored by circumventing the cholesterol build-up obstructing the artery.

Ankle Pain

The ankle is an especially vulnerable joint, as it provides support for the body while also acting as a hinge to enable movement. Walking, running and jumping put pressure on the joint and injuries are common. Athletes are particularly at risk.

Ankle pain can occur with or without injury, although the symptoms are different in either case.

- Pain due to injury.
- Inability to stand on the toes.
- Limping.
- Swelling and sensitivity of the ankle.
- Bluish tint to the skin due to an effusion of blood.
- Bone sensitivity.
- Swelling of the back of the ankle.
- Bone deformation.

Pain without injury
Sensation of heat, redness, swelling, and tenderness.

WHAT ARE THE CAUSES?

Pain due to injury

- *Exercise without warm-up,* or inappropriate playing surface for sports.
- *Sprain.* Partially or completely torn ligament.
- *Chipped or wrenched bone.* An injury may cause the tendon to tear, removing a small piece of bone in the process. This is frequently caused by a sprain.
- *Strained muscle.* Partially torn muscle.
- *Fractures.* One or more bones break or chip, possibly causing deformity of the ankle. The area next to the bone is painful.
- *Ruptured achilles tendon.* The ankle swells and the patient cannot stand on his or her toes. Without appropriate treatment, the tendon will stretch and develop scar tissue, limiting foot mobility.

Without injury

- ► **Infection.** If bacteria penetrates the ankle area, usually through a wound, there is a risk that the infection will spread to the rest of the leg.
- ► **Rheumatoid arthritis.** This inflammatory disease goes in and out of remission and can affect one or numerous joints in the body. In advanced cases where the joints are severely damaged, it may cause permanent deformities that leave the ankle crooked and misshapen, much like arthritic fingers.
- ► **Osteoarthritis.** An old fracture, sprain or infection may weaken the cartilage.
- ► **Gout.** This is a form of arthritis caused by an accumulation of uric acid crystals in the joints. While some small nodules or bumps may become permanent, highly painful attacks causing deformity (ankle swelling) are followed by remissions where the joint regains its normal shape.

PRACTICAL ADVICE

Pain due to injury

Raise the injured limb to reduce swelling and promote better blood circulation. As soon as possible after the injury, elevate the ankle by 5 to 10 cm (using cushions, for example), or raise the foot of the bed by placing blocks of wood under the legs. Putting the wood between the mattress and the box spring is not recommended, as this creates an uneven surface and provides little or no elevation.

Apply ice. Place ice cubes in a plastic bag and wrap in a towel (or use a bag of frozen vegetables). Apply to the ankle for 15 to 20 minutes, three to four times a day.

Take an analgesic. For the first few days, analgesics are recommended to soothe intense pain. Take moderate doses: one or two tablets (325 mg to 500 mg) of acetaminophen four times a day, up to a maximum of 4 grams daily. Nonsteroidal anti-inflammatories like aspirin or ibuprofen can have side effects (bleeding in the joints; stomach ulcers) and should be avoided. While pain relief is important, it is also crucial to be aware of discomfort so that care is taken to avoid any further injury that might impede the healing process.

Move your ankle as soon as you can. The day after the injury, raise your leg and move the foot and toes in every direction possible (unless the movement causes or increases pain). Avoid painkillers for this exercise so you can judge how extensive your movements should be. After the injury begins to heal, exercises like internal and external rotations, walking without limping, and standing on your toes will help recovery.

Wear a brace during high-risk activities. Better safe than sorry. A good quality brace is much more effective than an elastic bandage and is worth the investment. Braces are also highly recommended as a preventive measure for people with weak ankles and a tendency to sprain.

Go for rehabilitation before resuming sports. Consult a physiotherapist or sports therapist to help prepare your ankle for physical activity.

Infection
Clean any cuts or wounds on the ankle thoroughly, no matter how small. After washing with soap and water, apply a disinfectant and bandage, if necessary.

See a doctor. If the pain continues, consult a doctor as soon as possible. Early treatment will help avoid the risk of complications.

Rheumatoid arthritis or gout
Ease the pain. Use home remedies as well as medication. Apply cold compresses during acute attacks, and hot compresses for chronic pain. Elevate the injured limb (*see above*). Rest, and use crutches to walk.

Change your diet. Modify your eating habits to help control the frequency of gout attacks.

See your doctor regularly. Proper, medically-supervised treatment will help prevent incapacitating deformities.

Osteoarthritis
Apply hot or cold compresses. Choose the temperature that works best for you and apply the compress to the painful area for 15 minute periods. Swallow your pride and use a cane to walk if the pain is intense.

Prevention
Watch your weight. Excess weight puts pressure on the ankles, making them more vulnerable to injury.

Wear the proper shoes for each of your different sports activities. Every sport requires a different type of shoe. It is worth the investment.

Don't forget to warm up. If you play sports that require you to run and jump, always be sure to warm up beforehand. Most injuries are caused by lack of flexibility and strength in the ankle.

Use only well-maintained sports facilities. Badly-maintained facilities put people at risk of injury.

Avoid running on uneven surfaces. Stepping in a hole causes all your weight to fall on one ankle. You may trip and injure yourself.

WHEN TO CONSULT?
▶ You have suffered an injury and cannot stand on your toes. You have a bad limp when you walk.
▶ You have suffered an injury and can no longer walk. Your ankle is misshapen or your foot is in an abnormal position.
▶ You have not suffered an injury, but your ankle is painful, red, hot and swollen.
▶ The pain increases after three or four days.

WHAT HAPPENS DURING THE EXAM?

The doctor performs a clinical exam to confirm a sprain or muscle strain. X-rays are required to diagnose fractures, a wrenched chipped bone, or osteoarthritis. Removing joint fluid from the affected joint with a needle tap is necessary to determine the type of arthritis. Blood tests are ordered in cases of infection or to assess uric acid levels.

WHAT IS THE TREATMENT?

Injury
Sprain, wrenched chipped bone and strained muscle
The ankle is immobilized with elastic bandages and the patient uses crutches or a cane to move around. In most cases, doctors avoid placing the ankle in a cast, except when the patient requires a higher level of mobility. Ankle rehabilitation begins as soon as possible with rotation and reinforcement exercises (among others). Surgery is very rarely necessary unless you are a high level athlete.

Fractures
In some cases, a fractured ankle is put immediately into a cast; in others, surgery is necessary. Patients with minor fractures may simply require crutches for a few days.

Ruptured Achilles tendon
In many cases, surgery is necessary. Casts are generally less effective, but are sometimes preferred when, for example, the patient is suffering from multiple injuries.

Without injury
Infection
Antibiotics are administered orally or intravenously, depending on the severity of the infection.

Rheumatoid arthritis
Pain is treated with anti-inflammatories and locally-administrated cortisone injections. Controlling the inflammation helps avoid deformities.

Osteoarthritis

The usual treatment consists of rehabilitation exercises to regain strength and flexibility in the ankle and, if necessary, prescription painkillers. If rehabilitation exercises do not lead to improvement, surgery may be required.

Gout

Pain is controlled with analgesics. Some medications can lower the rate of recurrence of attacks. Diet is particularly important: limit the consumption of animal proteins, such as those found in seafood, offal, cold cuts and dairy products.

Aphasia

Understanding aphasia requires a general familiarity with the structure of the human brain. The brain is divided into two parts, the dominant and the minor hemispheres. The speech centre, responsible for linguistic expression and comprehension, is located in the dominant hemisphere. The functions of perception and spatial orientation are headquartered in the minor hemisphere, with each hemisphere containing centres for vision, sense perception and motor skills.

Aphasia is a neurological phenomenon caused by a problem in the dominant hemisphere. Depending on the type of aphasia, sufferers are unable to understand and/or produce speech, and may also have trouble reading and writing.

The onset of aphasia can be sudden or progressive. Of the different types, the following are the primary forms:

Broca's aphasia (or motor aphasia)
► Linguistic expression is affected.
► Excellent language comprehension.
► Impeded or no access to appropriate vocabulary.
► Truncation of sentences (for example, "I went to the hospital," becomes "Go hospital.").

Wernicke's aphasia (or sensory aphasia)
► Comprehension is affected.
► Ability to produce speech is retained.
► Long, sometimes meaningless sentences.
► Addition of inappropriate words (for example, "The dog is chewing paper I will go tomorrow.").
► Substitution of one word for another or of one syllable for another (paraphasia).

Global aphasia
► Both expression and comprehension are affected.

WHAT ARE THE CAUSES?

▶ *Cerebrovascular accident (stroke)* is the most common cause. When a clot or thrombus obstructs the arteries leading to the dominant hemisphere of the brain, the resulting aphasia is frequently accompanied by complete or partial paralysis of one side of the body. If the obstruction blocks nourishment to the minor hemisphere, the stroke may cause diction problems due to paralysis of the mouth and phonation muscles. The ability to speak and comprehend are not affected in these cases.

▶ *Trauma,* such as a head injury.

▶ *Brain tumour.* The growth of a tumour may cause progressive compression of the brain's language centre.

▶ *Demetia (for example, Alzheimer's disease).* This type of illness slowly destroys the brain cells responsible for language.

PRACTICAL ADVICE

Take symptoms of aphasia seriously. Losing your train of thought or being unable to find the appropriate word is a normal consequence of being worried or extremely tired, and is no cause for alarm. However, if there is no apparent reason for these symptoms, see a doctor as soon as possible. Early detection means a better chance of recovery.

Prevent stroke. Smoking, a heart condition, high blood pressure, diabetes, arteriosclerosis, and aging are all risk factors for cerebrovascular accidents. Maintain a healthy body weight, be physically active, eat well, check your blood pressure regularly, and above all, quit smoking.

If a loved one suffers from aphasia. Be patient: recovery can be a long and difficult process. Let the sufferer finish his or her own sentences and encourage all attempts at speech and communication. Use simple language and short sentences (but never "baby talk") in conversation.

Ask for help. Organizations like the Heart and Stroke Foundation of Canada are there to provide support and information to aphasics and their families. For a list of resources in your area, contact your local clinic.

WHEN TO CONSULT?

▶ You believe you are suffering from aphasia.
▶ You believe a person close to you is suffering from aphasia.
▶ People around you have pointed out that you have problems with diction.

WHAT HAPPENS DURING THE EXAM?

The doctor will perform a complete medical examination, including a history and neurological exam. He or she may also order an electroencephalogram (EEG) test, cerebral tomodensitometry (CT) scan, isotopic tomography of the brain (brain SPECT), or a magnetic resonance imaging scan (MRI). An examination by a speech pathologist or a neurophysiological exam may also be required.

WHAT IS THE TREATMENT?

There is no medical or surgical treatment for any type of aphasia. Only time and speech therapy can help, although the condition cannot be improved if caused by a brain tumour or dementia.

If aphasia results from stroke or trauma, severe disability will probably improve, but recovery is limited. In most cases, significant recovery of linguistic ability occurs, despite lingering aphasia (the patient still stumbles over certain words, for example). The earlier the rehabilitation process begins, the greater the chances are for success, since the brain is most responsive shortly after the event.

Speech therapy often begins in the hospital in the days following diagnosis and the rehabilitation period usually lasts about three months. If the aphasic is depressed, he or she should receive professional psychological support. If possible, therapy takes place in a rehabilitation centre on an outpatient basis. Close family and friends are encouraged to provide support and help the sufferer with the exercises.

The speed of improvement will vary according to the severity of the lesions, the general health of the patient, as well as his or her motivation and level of education. In general, recovery is most pronounced in the first six weeks, but the patient can continue to make significant progress over a full year.

Bad Posture

Proper posture is defined by the normal curve of the spine when seen in profile. The graceful and elongated "S" shape curves in at the neck, gently out at the upper back, then back in at the lower back or lumbar region. Bad posture generally begins in adolescence and is not only unattractive, but also causes pain, deformities and functional disturbances.

Bad posture exaggerates the normal spinal curves and generally develops out of carelessness, although disease is sometimes responsible.

Lordosis, kyphosis and scoliosis are the three types of spinal deformities that develop from bad standing, sitting, or lying posture. Over time, they can cause the abdominal muscles (among others) to weaken. Two of the three deformities often co-exist, as, for example, in the fictional case of the Hunchback of Notre-Dame, who seems to have suffered from thoracic kyphosis and scoliosis. Teenagers who are careless about their posture may develop mild lordosis or kyphosis.

Lordosis
- Exaggeration of the curve of the cervical spine (neck), causing the head to bend backward.
- Exaggeration of the lumbar curve and arch of the back.
- Often accompanied by knock-knees, flat feet, and pigeon toes.
- Pain in the cervical and lumbar regions.

Kyphosis
- Exaggeration of the outward curve of the upper back, causing the head and shoulders to hunch forwards.
- Pain in the upper back, shoulder blades and sides.

Scoliosis
- Lateral (sideways) deviation of part of the spine (in the form of a snake). Unlike lordosis and kyphosis, this is not an exaggeration of normal curves.

► May be accompanied by unequal length of the legs.
► In many cases, scoliosis does not cause discomfort or pain.

WHAT ARE THE CAUSES?

Lordosis

► *Hereditary predisposition.*
► *Abdominal obesity* changes the body's centre of gravity and forces the individual to bend backwards in compensation, which exerts undue pressure on the muscles supporting the spine, causing lordosis.
► *Bad postural habits.* People who tend to arch their back while standing may develop lordosis.
► *Weak abdominal muscles.*
► *Excessive muscle contraction* in the back of the body.
► *Arthritis.* This inflammatory disease of the joints may affect the spinal column, causing swelling around and between the vertebrae. Over time, this can alter the curve of the spine and displace the muscles attached to it.
► *Cushing's syndrome.* This rare disease describes an exaggeration of the lumbar spine's curvature and is caused by abdominal obesity.

Kyphosis

► *Hereditary predisposition.*
► *Osteoporosis* in elderly women causes kyphosis where the cervical and dorsal sections of the spine meet ("widow's hump" or "buffalo hump").
► *Habitually hunched posture.* For example, adolescent girls who are self-conscious about their developing breasts may try to camouflage them by hunching their shoulders forward. Other teenagers may find growth spurts embarrassing and try to make themselves appear smaller.
► *Extreme contraction* of the anterior muscles of the spine causes the back to arch and is usually due to a predisposition that manifests during adolescence.
► *Arthritis.*

▶ *Scheurmann's disease* usually appears during adolescence. As the individual grows, the vertebrae compress, causing hyperkyphosis (exaggerated arch).

▶ *Scoliosis.*

▶ *Incorrect posture,* such as slouching or always leaning on one elbow.

▶ *Unequal leg length* is an aggravating factor.

▶ *Predisposition* (possibly hereditary) that manifests during growth spurts at adolescence.

▶ *Trauma* to the spinal column (from a fall, for example).

PRACTICAL ADVICE

Avoid sleeping on your stomach. This position exaggerates the cervical and lumbar curves (lordosis).

Avoid high heels. Heels more than five centimetres high will aggravate lordosis.

Adopt good postural habits. When standing, keep the back straight and abdominal muscles contracted. Wear comfortable shoes and be sure you can balance easily. If you have to stand for a prolonged period of time, place one foot on a slightly raised step, alternating feet. When lifting heavy objects, hold the weight as close to the body as possible and bend your knees instead of stooping from the waist. When sitting, place a flat, hard cushion or rolled up towel behind the lower back to keep your back straight and use a footrest to keep the knees bent at a level slightly higher than the pelvis. In bed, lie in the foetal position and tuck a firm yet malleable pillow in the crook of your neck to support the head. When lying on your back, use a slimmer pillow and place another under your knees. Sleeping half on your stomach and half on your side with one knee bent is another comfortable position. Always roll onto your side before getting up.

Change positions frequently. If you work in an office, avoid sitting in one position for an extended period of time. Move slowly and avoid twisting the torso.

Teach young children good posture. Children who learn good posture at the age of three or four will benefit for the rest of their lives.

Read Bob Anderson's book on stretching. This has been considered the stretching bible for over fifteen years. It describes strengthening exercises for the abdominal muscles, as well as stretches for various posture problems.

Control your weight. Obesity aggravates lumbar lordosis.

Use appropriate furniture. A good desk chair, stuffed armchairs, and firm mattresses and pillows are essential.

WHEN TO CONSULT?
► You have chronic back or neck pain.
► You notice a deformity in the curve of the spine (in yourself or another person).

WHAT HAPPENS DURING THE EXAM?
An X-ray is always necessary. In some cases, the doctor will order orthodiagraphy to measure the length of the legs and flexibility tests for the affected muscles.

WHAT IS THE TREATMENT?
Lordosis
Plantar orthoses (special orthopedic soles worn inside the shoes) can help correct posture, while certain stretching exercises will loosen contracted muscles at the back of the spine. The doctor may also recommend exercises to strengthen the abdominal muscles. The patient may be required to lose weight. In cases of Cushing's syndrome, the underlying disease is treated.

Kyphosis
The doctor will recommend stretching exercises for the anterior muscles of the spine. Hormone replacement therapy is occasionally used to help prevent osteoporosis in menopausal women. If this

treatment is contra-indicated, the doctor will prescribe another pharmacological treatments are also available.

Scheuermann's disease is treated with physiotherapy or global
posture rehabilitation (GPR), which prescribes exercises to reinforce
different muscle groups. In severe cases, the patient may be required
to wear a spinal support corset.

Scoliosis

In mild cases, observation is recommended until the individual
grows to his or her full height and the scoliosis stabilizes, at which
time, posture rehabilitation may be recommended. Orthopedic soles
can help correct the unequal length of the legs. In serious cases, surgery or a spinal support corset may be necessary.

Pain

The treatment for pain is the same for all three conditions. In acute
stages, muscle relaxants, analgesics or anti-inflammatories are prescribed. The doctor or physiotherapist may recommend particular
exercises to prevent pain.

Changes in stool colour from normal to bright red or black (melena) is generally caused by bleeding from the gastrointestinal tract. There could be bleeding directly from the anus or blood mixed with the stool. The rate of bleeding will also affect stool colour. Bright red blood indicates rapid bleeding (or that the hemorrhage is located near the anus) because the blood has not been "digested" in the intestines. Dark red or black stools mean a slow bleeding rate. The stool turns black as a result of a chemical change caused by a prolonged stay in the digestive tract.

Black or red stools may be accompanied by other symptoms including abdominal pain, heartburn, fatigue, general weakness, rapid heart beat, dizzy spells, fainting and significant unexplained weight loss. The stool can also sometimes become smaller than usual, possibly reducing to the size of a pencil. If this is the case, it could be a tumour of the rectum or colon, or an inflammatory lesion that causes the inside of the intestine to shrink (Crohn's disease, for example).

WHAT ARE THE CAUSES?

► *Swallowed blood* as a result of a nosebleed.
► *Ruptured esophageal varices.* Esophageal varices are dilated (varicose) veins in the esophagus. Diseases (such as cirrhosis of the liver) that increase blood pressure in the liver cause the veins in the esophagus to dilate, leading to varicose veins. In general, they do not cause any problems and do not bleed unless ruptured. If they do, however, blood will appear in the stool and the patient may feel weak, particularly if there is significant blood loss. This requires emergency medical attention. If left untreated, a ruptured esophageal varicose vein can be fatal.
► *Stomach or duodenal ulcer.*
► *Intestinal cancer.* As the cancer progresses, intestinal tissue becomes more fragile and susceptible to tearing.
► *Eroded colonic diverticulum.* Diverticula are hernias resembling small, grape-like sacs that run along the external wall of the colon containing

blood vessels. Erosion of a diverticulum leads to bleeding. Although in most cases benign, you should see a doctor for a diagnosis.

► *Inflammatory diseases of the intestine,* such as Crohn's disease and ulcerative colitis. These diseases are often accompanied by diarrhea and abdominal pain.

► *Hemorrhoids or anal fissure.*

PRACTICAL ADVICE

Do not wait to consult a doctor. Hesitating runs the risk of aggravating the situation.

Do a "prediagnostic" review. Ask yourself whether you have recently started a new iron treatment or eaten any beets or blood pudding. In the case of menopausal women, occasional vaginal bleeding could be the source. If you cannot come up with a logical, harmless explanation, consult a doctor.

WHEN TO CONSULT?

► There is blood in your stools.

► Bleeding is accompanied by loss of consciousness, dizzy spells, extreme fatigue or abdominal pain. Such symptoms warrant an emergency consultation.

► You are vomiting blood. This is an emergency.

Exercise good judgement!

Because red stools are often a sign of hemorrhoids, some people avoid seeking a medical opinion. This error in judgement can entail serious consequences. Hemorrhoids leave traces of blood on toilet paper or in the toilet bowl. Sometimes, however, the blood becomes mixed with the stool. Before drawing any hasty conclusions, see a doctor to rule out other possible causes of bleeding. "False" red or black stools can also occur: ingesting beets, blood pudding or iron tablets stains the stool and simulates bleeding.

WHAT HAPPENS DURING THE EXAM?

The doctor will take a thorough history and try to determine whether there has been any recent weight loss. He or she will then perform a complete physical examination including an abdominal and digital rectal exam and may order a blood work to verify the extent of bleeding. Depending on the bleeding rate and patient's condition, the patient may also be given a gastroscopy, colonoscopy or barium enema (X-ray examination of the colon).

WHAT IS THE TREATMENT?

Ruptured esophageal varicose vein

The doctor will check the state of the esophagus with a tiny camera. He or she may apply a product to stop the bleeding and form a scar on the vein, or insert a balloon catheter (which is later removed) to compress the vein against the esophageal wall.

Stomach or duodenal ulcer

Different types of drugs are available to prevent the secretion of gastric acid, including proton pump inhibitors (Prevacid, Pentaloc, Losec, Pariet, or Nexium) and H2 blockers such as Zantac (ranitidine).

Intestinal cancer

Surgical intervention will be required.

Eroded diverticulum

Sometimes, the problem resolves without treatment. In the event of a recurrence, a surgical resection may be required.

Inflammatory bowel disease, Crohn's disease and ulcerative colitis

These diseases are managed with cortisone or anti-inflammatories. If drug treatment does not produce the desired results, the doctor may recommend surgery.

Hemorrhoids or anal fissures

Treatment consists primarily of avoiding constipation by increasing dietary fibre consumption and drinking plenty of water. In some cases, surgery will be required to remove the hemorrhoids.

Black Spots and Flashes in the Visual Field

Black spots, or flashes of dark or light in the visual field that cause vision problems, are known as scotoma.

There are four types of scotoma and each can affect one or both eyes simultaneously.

Central scotoma
- Black spot.
- Loss of vision in the centre of the visual field.

Hemianopia
- Loss of vision in the left, right, bottom, or top half of the visual field. Central vision remains intact.

Vitreous floaters
- Small black spots.
- Change location with every eye or head movement
- Affects nearly everyone at some point. The phenomenon is completely normal and no cause for concern.

Scintillating scotoma
- Flashes of light (similar to the after-effects of a flashbulb).
- Lasts for 20 to 40 minutes.
- May occur several times a day.
- May be accompanied by a headache.

WHAT ARE THE CAUSES?
Central scotoma
- *Macular degeneration* describes the gradual loss of vision due to the drying of the retina. It is generally caused by aging and primarily affects people over the age of 60. In some cases, it is

caused by heredity, poor retinal circulation, or overexposure to the sun's rays.

► *Sudden optic nerve disorder* caused by a viral infection, inflammatory disease, hereditary condition, or multiple sclerosis. It most commonly occurs around 30 years of age, affects only one eye, and is accompanied by pain.

► *Pressure on the optic chiasma.* The optic chiasma is the point at which the optic nerves cross behind the eye. A lesion (caused by a cerebrovascular accident, hemorrhage, brain tumour or tumour on the chiasma itself) can put pressure on the chiasma, causing central scotoma (along with other symptoms). In serious cases, the pressure may cause total loss of vision.

Hemianopia

► *Cerebrovascular accident.* Both eyes are affected symmetrically. Smoking, diabetes, high blood pressure, high cholesterol, and a personal or family history of heart disease are all risk factors.

► *Thrombosis affecting the optic nerve or retina.* Only one eye is affected.

Vitreous floaters

► *Vitreous detachment.* The vitreous body (gelatinous mass inside the eyeball) can become detached due to aging, severe myopia, eye surgery (such as a cataract operation), head trauma, or a family history of retinal disease.

► *Internal eye hemorrhage* due to diabetes (diabetic retinopathy), head trauma, or high blood pressure.

Scintillating scotoma

► *Migraine* in people under 60 years of age.

► *Insufficient blood circulation to the brain* (transitory cerebral ischaemia). This abnormality is caused by diabetes, high blood pressure, or high cholesterol and affects people over the age of 60.

► *Vitreous detachment.* In this case, the light flashes last for a fraction of a second.

PRACTICAL ADVICE

Get a check-up. If you are over 40 years of age, be sure to have regular medical check-ups to ensure that any vascular or heart condition (frequently at the root of vision problems) are well-controlled.

Manage your diabetes. Diabetics should have a yearly ophthalmological examination to detect diabetic retinopathy that may cause vitreous floaters.

Wear sunglasses. The sun's ultraviolet rays damage the retina, eventually leading to macular degeneration. Sunglasses reduce the glare, accentuate contrasts, and protect the eyes.

Use a magnifying glass. Use a magnifying glass to compensate for the loss of vision caused by macular degeneration.

Add more antioxidants to your diet. Get into the habit of eating fruit, vegetables, and other foods rich in antioxidants (zinc, beta-carotene, vitamins C, E, and A) or add antioxidant supplements to your diet to combat the effects of aging on the retina.

Do not smoke. Tobacco consumption triggers a number of conditions that can lead to ocular or cerebral thrombosis and vision loss. Nicotine causes the blood vessels to contract and leads to cholesterol build up in the arteries.

WHEN TO CONSULT?

► You have suffered trauma to the head or eye and there are persistent black spots in your field of vision. This may indicate retinal damage. Consult immediately.

► You are diabetic and your vision has suddenly deteriorated due to the presence of small black spots. This may indicate an internal eye hemorrhage. Consult your ophthalmologist immediately.

► You see flashes of light for a few seconds or hours.

► You see floating black spots.

WHAT HAPPENS DURING THE EXAM?

A standard ophthalmological examination is performed to check visual acuity, the external appearance of the eye, and the inner eye (using a slit lamp). The patient is asked to read an eye chart. The doctor uses fixed and moving lights and screens to identify the affected area of the visual field and type of scotoma. An angiogram (an X-ray with contrasting colours) may also be used to examine the affected area.

In many cases, the doctor must dilate the pupils with eye drops to examine the retina and optic nerve. The drops also cause blurred vision for four to five hours and make the eyes more sensitive to light. It is therefore recommended that patients be accompanied to the doctor's office, refrain from driving a vehicle for this period of time, and wear dark glasses to protect the eyes.

WHAT IS THE TREATMENT?

Central scotoma
Macular degeneration

There is no specific treatment, although in some cases, laser surgery is effective.

Optic nerve disorder

Painkillers are prescribed. Recovery is spontaneous, does not require treatment, and there are no permanent after-effects. In the rare cases where both eyes are affected, the doctor may prescribe cortisone treatment.

Pressure on the optic chiasma

The underlying cause (cerebrovascular accident, hemorrhage, tumour) is immediately treated, generally relieving the central scotoma. However, if the pressure has caused complete loss of vision, no recovery is possible.

Hemianopia
Cerebrovascular accident or optic nerve vascular problems

The doctor prescribes long-term aspirin treatment (one tablet a day). Plavix (clopidogrel bisulfate) is an anti-platelet drug and may also be prescribed to prevent blood clotting. Specific pharmacological treatments are prescribed according to the underlying cause. The degree of recovery depends on the extent of damage suffered.

Vitreous floaters
Vitreous detachment
Whatever the cause of the detachment, there is no treatment. The patient must learn to adapt to seeing black spots.

Internal eye hemorrhage due to diabetes (diabetic retinopathy)
The doctor may perform surgery (vitrectomy) to remove or replace the vitreous body made opaque by a hemorrhage or use laser treatment to destroy the affected blood vessels. In most cases, vision returns to normal.

In some cases, blood gets in between the vitreous body and the retina (attached), leading to detachment. If this results in a torn retina, it can be repaired with laser treatment. Unless the vitreous body has become detached, patients generally regain normal vision in such cases.

Scintillating scotoma
Migraine
Treatment is adapted to the individual patient. Scotomas disappear with the migraine.

Insufficient circulation to the brain (transitory cerebral ischaemia)
The doctor prescribes long-term aspirin treatment. The aspirin is coated to reduce stomach problems. Plavix may also be prescribed. The degree of recovery depends on the extent of damage suffered.

Again, if the vitreous body has detached, no treatment is possible.

Bleeding After Menopause

Menopause is characterized by the permanent cessation of menstruation and the end of a woman's fertility. The process lasts a number of years, beginning with pre-menopause near the end of the woman's forties, when her periods may become irregular (occurring once every two, three, or even six months). Menopause is said to have occurred only after you have missed your period for an entire year, so there is no need for concern if you have not reached this stage.

Bleeding that occurs a year or more after the woman's last period is abnormal and as likely to happen to those undergoing hormone replacement therapy as to those who are not.

Bleeding may occur in a number of different ways:

► Blood loss lasting a day or more.
► Variable flow (light spotting to heavy flow).
► May occur only once or repeatedly, like menstruation.
► There are generally no other symptoms.

WHAT ARE THE CAUSES?

► *Hormone replacement therapy,* if the doses are not properly adjusted or the patient is intolerant to the medication.
► *Polyps* are small, fleshy growths on the endometrium (the mucous membrane lining the uterus). In most cases, they are benign.
► *Fibroma.* The myometrium (uterine muscle tissue) swells to create small lumps around or inside the uterus. This condition is usually benign.
► *Dryness or atrophy of the vaginal mucous membrane.* If the bleeding occurs after sexual intercourse (which may be painful), the mucous membranes are either dry or thinning.
► *Tumours.* Cervical or uterine tumours are rare, although postmenopausal women suffering from high blood pressure, diabetes or obesity are more at risk of developing this type of cancer.
► *Cystitis.* This infection sometimes causes bleeding from the bladder, which may be confused with vaginal bleeding. Cystitis

is frequently accompanied by a sensation of burning with urination.

► **Rectal problems.** Bleeding may be due to hemorrhoids or anal fissures.

PRACTICAL ADVICE

Take notes. Write down the date the bleeding began, how long it lasted, and the heaviness of the flow (heavy, medium or light). Give this information to your doctor.

Do not ignore bleeding. Many women do not see a doctor if there is very light or infrequent bleeding, chalking it up to stress. However, stress does not cause vaginal bleeding. It is always best to consult even though vaginal bleeding after menopause is only rarely caused by a serious problem.

WHEN TO CONSULT?

► You notice vaginal bleeding (even if it is light) one year or more after your last period.

► The bleeding is worrying you.

WHAT HAPPENS DURING THE EXAM?

The doctor takes a history and performs a physical and gynecological examination. Hormone levels are measured with a blood test to determine whether the woman really is menopausal. If necessary, an endometrial biopsy is performed (this technique is now used instead of curettage). An endovaginal ultrasound (an examination of the reproductive organs with an ultrasound probe) and hysteroscopy (an examination of the uterus using an optic tube equipped with a small light) may also be administered.

WHAT IS THE TREATMENT?

Hormone replacement therapy

If the doses are responsible for the bleeding, the prescription will be modified.

Polyps and fibroma

If the polyps or fibroma become very large and cause hemorrhaging, they may be removed by curettage or excision of the endometrium. Curettage involves scraping the surface of the uterine wall with a surgical instrument. Removal of the endometrium destroys the inner wall of the uterus and definitively removes any possibility of reproduction (although there are no other consequences). Polyps and certain fibroma may permanently disappear on their own.

Dryness or atrophy of the vaginal mucous membrane

Dryness or atrophy of the vaginal mucous membrane is treated with hormone-based medications in the form of a vaginal cream, pill, or intra-vaginal device (inserted into the vagina, this device releases hormones into the vaginal walls and must be changed periodically). This treatment may be combined with systemic hormone therapy if higher hormone doses are required.

Tumours

A hysterectomy, the complete removal of the uterus and ovaries, is recommended in cases of uterine cancer.

Cystitis

Cystitis is treated with antibiotics, sometimes in combination with hormone replacement therapy to reinforce the bladder or uterine mucous membranes.

Rectal problems

Hemorrhoids or anal fissures respond well to cortisone creams. The patient is also advised to eat a diet rich in fibre to avoid constipation. In some cases, surgery is required to remove hemorrhoids.

Other types of bleeding

If the bleeding persists and there is no trace of a tumour, polyp or fibroma, the doctor may recommend hormone replacement therapy. Complete removal of the endometrium is also becoming a more common treatment for abnormal bleeding and can be done in a number of ways: with a surgical cuff, cryotherapy, laser treatment, or microwave therapy. Each method causes the endometrial tissue to coagulate. These new, highly effective treatments are performed under local anesthesia and allow the patient to return to her regular routine in a short period of time. In 80% of cases, these treatments allow the woman to avoid a hysterectomy.

Hysterectomy is a last resort.

Blood in the Semen (Hematospermia)

Although it is a perfectly normal reaction for men to be concerned if they notice blood in their semen (known medically as hematospermia or hemospermia), they should rest assured that it rarely indicates a serious problem. Nevertheless, it is still a good idea to see a doctor.

The phenomenon is most worrisome for men who already have a prostate infection, blood coagulation disorder, or are taking blood-thinning medications (patients with phlebitis or heart disease), as the bleeding may be significant and difficult to control.

The symptoms of hematospermia manifest in the following manner:

► Light or dark (blackish) blood in the sperm.
► In some cases, pain with ejaculation.

WHAT ARE THE CAUSES?

► **Blood in the seminal vesicles** is the most common cause. The seminal vesicles are two reservoirs located behind the prostate gland containing seminal fluid. When they contract to expel semen, fragile blood vessels sometimes tear and cause bleeding. This is not serious and there are no other symptoms.

► **Infection of the prostate gland (prostatitis)** may be caused by bacteria from a urinary tract or sexually transmitted infection. Along with hematospermia, the man may also experience fever, shivering, lower abdominal and lower back pain, a frequent need to urinate, as well as burning with urination and ejaculation. If left untreated, acute prostatitis can become chronic, presenting a milder version of the same symptoms, minus the fever.

► **Coagulation disorders** can complicate bleeding from weakened blood vessels, making them susceptible to rupture. If this affects the blood vessels of the seminal vesicles, tearing can occur during ejaculation, leading to potentially heavy bleeding that is difficult to control.

▶ *Blood thinning medications.* Aspirin (taken over the long term), anti-platelet drugs, and anticoagulants can make weakened blood vessels weaker and more susceptible to rupture, potentially causing heavy bleeding.

▶ *Inflammation of the epididymis (epididymitis).* This condition leads to blood in the semen (in some cases), shooting pain, fever, redness of the genital area, and swollen testicles. In men under the age of 40, it is usually caused by a Chlamydia infection. In men over 40, it is generally associated with a bladder infection.

▶ *Prostate cancer,* in rare cases.

PRACTICAL ADVICE

Do not take aspirin or any other blood-thinning medication, unless it has been prescribed as a long-term treatment (for heart disease, for example). It can make the bleeding worse.

Speak to your doctor. Be sure the problem is your own (and the blood is not your partner's). Check for blood in your sperm when you masturbate or wear a condom. Don't panic. In the vast majority of cases, hematospermia is harmless and there is no need to abstain from sexual intercourse.

WHEN TO CONSULT?

▶ There is blood in your sperm.

▶ Along with blood in your sperm, there is pain when you ejaculate or urinate and pain in the genital and anal area. You feel an urgent need to urinate, have a fever, and there is redness in the genital area.

▶ You have one or more of these symptoms and are over 50 years of age.

WHAT HAPPENS DURING THE EXAM?

The doctor examines the genital organs and performs a digital rectal exam to check the prostate gland. A urine culture and analysis is performed and a blood test may be ordered to rule out prostate cancer. This is generally only done for men over the age of 50, as prostate cancer is extremely uncommon in younger men. Other tests (such as a sperm culture) may be required. In some cases, a prostate ultrasound (through the rectum) and a blood test called prostate-specific antigen (PSA) is used to rule out prostate cancer. This is generally only done for men over the age of 50, as prostate cancer is extremely uncommon in younger men.

In certain cases, the doctor will perform a cytoscopic exam, inserting a tiny camera into the urethra to view the inside of the urethra and prostate and bladder walls.

WHAT IS THE TREATMENT?

Hematospermia is usually benign. Most cases of prostate or epididymis infection can be effectively treated with antibiotics and anti-inflammatories.

In cases of coagulation disorders, the patient's anticoagulant medication is checked and the prescription modified if necessary. If blood-thinning drugs are responsible for the hematospermia, the doctor determines whether the dosage is appropriate and the patient is following the prescription. The medication is changed, if necessary.

Treatment for prostate cancer is undertaken immediately.

If there is no evidence of infection or prostate cancer, no treatment is necessary, since the condition should resolve on its own within a few weeks or a few months at the most. If the patient is very disturbed by the problem, he should abstain from sex for two weeks. In most cases, this is enough time for the blood vessels to heal.

Blood in the Urine

Red-tinted urine usually, but not always, means blood in the urine. If blood is indeed present in the urine (a condition known as hematuria), it may signal an abnormality of the urinary tract. The urinary tract consists of the kidneys, the ureters, the bladder and the urethra. The ureters are the two tubes through which urine is transported from the kidneys to the bladder; the urethra is the tube through which it is discharged from the body.

Hematuria can cause the urine to take on a range of hues, from red to brown, and may also cause pain, depending on the origin of the problem. (*See Changes to Urine for more information on what other factors can turn the urine red in the absence of hematuria.*)

WHAT ARE THE CAUSES?

► *Antiplatelet drugs (such as aspirin) or anticoagulants (drugs used to prevent blood clots).* These drugs are not a direct cause of bleeding themselves, but may be a contributing factor if the patient has an injury or lesion that is susceptible to bleeding.

► *Endurance sports or vigorous exercise.* Physical activity can cause a small blood vessel in the urinary tract to bleed or the muscle cells to break down. In the latter case, a substance known as myoglobin is released into the circulation, giving the urine a reddish or brownish tinge. Since muscle cells can regenerate, this breakdown is not a serious problem.

► *Urinary tract infection.* Bacterial or viral urinary tract infections cause inflammation and irritation of the bladder wall that leads to bleeding. The blood is discharged during urination, which is usually accompanied by pain or a burning sensation. Clots or small clumps of aggregated blood resembling skin fragments may also be visible in the urine. The infection may spread to the kidneys, causing fever, shivering, and back pain.

► *Kidney stones (renal calculi)* are calcium or uric acid deposits in the kidneys that form stone-like agglomerations. They tend

to occur when a person does not drink enough liquid to properly eliminate calcium and uric acid, or when there is too much of
one of these substances in a person's diet (enthusiastic meat eaters
absorb a lot of uric acid, for example). Kidney stones cause blood
in the urine, although the primary symptom is sharp pain radiating from the abdomen to the genital organs (often compared to
the pain of childbirth). When the stone passes through the urethra
during urination, the sufferer may experience pain and a burning
sensation.

▶ *Benign prostate hypertrophy.* This non-cancerous enlargement of
the prostate (occurring in 80% of men between the ages of 55
and 70) may cause small tears in the prostate tissue, leading to
bleeding. Other than hematuria, symptoms include difficulty
voiding and a diminished urinary stream.

▶ *Trauma.* The kidney may be injured in a fall or car accident, for
example.

▶ *Inflammation of the kidney (glomerulonephritis).* This rare ailment is generally caused by exposure to an antigen (bacteria or
virus, for example). The urine takes on a brownish colour (similar
to Coca-Cola) and accompanying symptoms include swelling,
a headache and discomfort. A medical consultation may also
reveal an increase in blood pressure. Generally speaking, blood
from the kidney does not form clots.

▶ *Tumour of the urinary tract.* This is also a rare occurrence.
Bleeding is usually intermittent.

PRACTICAL ADVICE

Consult a doctor. Although the appearance of blood in the urine is
alarming, it is not necessarily serious. Nevertheless, it is important to
see a doctor for a proper diagnosis. Take note of any clots, the colour
of the urine (bright red or brownish), and the point at which it
appears (start/end of urination, during urination).

Review your medications with the doctor. Ask him or her whether the
drugs you are taking may be causing blood in your urine. If the
answer is yes, he or she may either reassure you that there is no need

for concern or discontinue treatment and recommend an alternative drug. Remember: never stop taking a medication without speaking to your doctor first.

WHEN TO CONSULT?

► See the doctor if your urine is consistently tinged red. If you are also running a fever and experiencing pain, consult immediately.

WHAT HAPPENS DURING THE EXAM?

The doctor will take a history and conduct a thorough physical examination. He or she will take a urine sample to confirm or rule out the presence of blood, and possibly order a urography (kidney ultrasound), which is specifically designed to study the kidneys and urinary tract. The doctor may also examine the bladder with a scope (small flexible tube with a light at one end) inserted via the urethra.

WHAT IS THE TREATMENT?

Urinary tract infection

The doctor will generally prescribe oral antibiotics in pill form. In rare instances, intravenously administered antibiotics may be required, particularly if there is a danger of the infection spreading to the kidneys, or the patient has severe symptoms.

Kidney stones

If the stones are small, ingesting copious amounts of liquid may be enough to flush them from the system. Otherwise, they may have to be removed with a more specialized technique such as endoscopic extraction, pulverization by laser, or surgery.

Benign prostate hypertrophy

The doctor may recommend oral medications (pills) aimed at reducing the size of the prostate and managing the symptoms. In serious cases, surgery may be recommended.

Trauma

Depending on the type of injury, the doctor will prescribe supportive treatment (rest and pain relievers) until healing is complete, or recommend surgery.

Inflammation of the kidney (glomerulonephritis or nephritis)

In most instances, supportive therapy (rest and analgesics) is sufficient. Sometimes, a kidney biopsy will be recommended to determine the exact cause of the nephritis and the appropriate treatment.

Tumour of the urinary tract

The doctor will recommend ablation (removal) or excision surgery that varies according to the location of the tumour.

Body Odour

In some cases, body odour is a symptom of an underlying ailment. Otherwise, the phenomenon is a normal hereditary characteristic that serves the purposes of recognition and seduction. Nevertheless, in our current society, people are increasingly concerned with eliminating body odour.

Sweat is produced to regulate body temperature, and contrary to popular belief, does not have an odour. The secretions of the apocrine glands in the armpits, groin and, for women, under the breasts, are the only exception, producing an odour that becomes stronger if bacteria is present. Body odour appears at puberty along with the development of the apocrine glands and is primarily an adult concern.

Other types of (usually unpleasant) body odour are produced by bacteria, fungus, or the skin itself.

Primary body odour (not symptomatic of a disease)
► Underarm or foot odour varies in intensity according to the individual.
► Skin may exude a smell of garlic or spices.

Secondary body odour (symptomatic of a disease or caused by an external agent; exuded through the skin)
► Unusual odour (fruity, sweet, acidic or resembling rotten apples).
► Any unidentifiable odour.

WHAT ARE THE CAUSES?
Primary body odour
► **Genetic predisposition**
► **Poor foot hygiene** creates a breeding ground for bacteria and fungi, which, particularly when combined, give the feet an unpleasant odour.
► **Overactive apocrine glands** create a breeding ground for bacteria, particularly under the arms, where the hair retains secretions, causing a stronger odour.

► *Spicy food.* The odour of certain foods (in particular, garlic, curry, and cumin) can emanate through the skin for up to 24 hours after they are consumed.

Secondary body odour

► *Pitted keratolysis* is an infection characterized by whitish, macerated skin and small pits and craters on the soles of the feet. It causes strong foot odour and is particularly common in adolescents.

► *Diabetes or urinary tract infections* can cause a sweet or fruity body odour.

► *Certain infections or bedsores* can emit an odour of rotten apples.

► *Excessive alcohol consumption* can make body odour acidic.

► *Gastrointestinal problems (belching and flatulence) and kidney or liver disease* frequently cause unusual body odour. The body odour of people with kidney failure may be somewhat acidic, while people with liver failure may exude an odour resembling rotten apples.

PRACTICAL ADVICE

Use deodorant and antiperspirant. Deodorants mask odour produced by the apocrine glands, while antiperspirants reduce the amount of secretions from the exocrine glands. Be sure your antiperspirant contains aluminum chloride or zirconium (note, however, that these substances cause irritation in some individuals).

Use absorbent powder on the feet to soak up perspiration. Aerosol products for the feet are also effective. Fungus infections can be treated with cream, powder, or aerosol antifungal medications, depending on the area affected. All these products are available over-the-counter.

Use antibacterial soap. If mild soaps (like Dove or Ivory) are not effective, try an antibacterial soap, remembering that it may cause irritation. Products containing triclosan (Tersaseptic or Lever 2000) or chlorhexidine (Spectro Gram "2", pHisoHex, or Habitane) are recommended.

Do not wash too frequently. Compulsive washing three or four times a day can cause skin irritation.

Do not apply perfume directly on the skin. This can irritate the skin or cause contact allergies.

Shave. Hair is a breeding ground for bacteria. Both men and women should shave their armpits.

Change your socks frequently. This will slow down the proliferation of bacteria. Wear cotton socks to better absorb humidity and change them once or twice a day.

Take foot baths. Use the traditional preparation of lukewarm water and Biurow's solution, or put tea in your foot bath (tannic acid effectively controls odour).

Ask your doctor for a prescription. In stubborn cases of underarm or foot odour, the doctor can prescribe Drysol or aluminum chloride preparations. While these products do not prevent perspiration, they effectively neutralize odour.

Don't become obsessive about body odour. Some people have the mistaken impression that their body odour is unpleasant. Psychotherapy may be necessary.

WHEN TO CONSULT?

- Odour persists even though you have followed the advice listed above.
- Your body odour is unusual.
- You have strong foot odour and the skin on your feet is macerated, whitish and pitted, with small craters on the soles.
- A prepubescent child has underarm odour (this may indicate diabetes or kidney failure).

WHAT HAPPENS DURING THE EXAM?

The doctor assesses the skin of the affected areas and performs a complete physical exam. If an underlying ailment is suspected, he or she will order tests.

WHAT IS THE TREATMENT?

Primary odour

If your body odour resists the treatments listed here, the doctor may prescribe clindamycin, a non-irritating topical antibiotic to treat the underarms and feet. In extreme cases of underarm odour, the patient may undergo surgery (electrosurgery or superficial liposuction) to remove the apocrine glands or the attached nerves.

Secondary odours

Pitted keratolysis

In most cases, the infection disappears with a local antibiotic, although there may be recurrences.

Diabetes or urinary tract infections

Managing your diabetes will help control body odour. The problem will disappear as the urinary tract infection clears up.

Infections or bedsores

The doctor will apply creams and special bandages to heal the skin.

Gastrointestinal problems and kidney or liver disease

The underlying disorder must be treated.

Bruising, Hematomas and Petechiae

Bruising, hematomas and petechiae are all forms of subcutaneous bleeding.

The common bruise (ecchymotic purpura) is completely benign in 95% of cases. Women are particularly vulnerable to bruising because their skin is generally more delicate and hormonal changes make the blood vessels more fragile. The elderly also have thinner, more transparent skin.

A hematoma is an effusion of blood in an organ, muscle wall or the abdomen that gradually appears on the surface of the skin.

There are two types of petechiae (purpura petechial): those caused by a deficiency of blood platelets (necessary for coagulation), and those that occur with healthy platelets. Petechiae are rare and more serious than bruises or hematoma, since they almost always indicate a serious underlying problem.

The symptoms are the following:

Bruising and hematoma
- Spots of varying size, either bluish or reddish in colour.
- Possible swelling and pain if touched.
- Blanching (paling) when pressure is applied.
- Blue, green or yellow discoloration before fading.
- May take several days to appear after a trauma.
- In the case of hematoma, may be accompanied by a fever.

Petechiae
- Very small red lesions (less than 3 mm in diameter).
- Appear suddenly and in large number.
- Usually appear on the legs.
- Do not blanch when pressure is applied.
- Are not accompanied by pain, swelling or itching.
- Disappear after a few days, leaving brownish spots.

WHAT ARE THE CAUSES?

Bruising and hematoma

▶ *Trauma.* Physical trauma almost always leaves a bruise. Violent blows (for example, a baseball bat to the leg) can cause hemorrhaging on the surface of the skin and within the body at the same time (simultaneous bruising and hematoma).

▶ *Medications.* With time, cortisone thins the skin, making it more likely to bruise. People who take aspirin, anti-coagulants, anti-inflammatories, or oral or inhaler cortisone are more susceptible to bruising because these drugs impede the proper functioning of the blood platelets.

Petechiae

▶ *Blood platelet disorders* such as lymphoma, metastatic cancers, leukemia, Hodgkin's disease, AIDS, myelodysplasia, Bernard-Soulier disease, serious bacterial infections (such as the flesh-eating bacteria) can cause petechiae. Deficiency of vitamin K, C, or B_{12} also affects coagulation and serious alcohol or drug abuse weakens the platelets. In advanced stages, platelet disorders can lead to hematomas.

▶ *Medications.* The medications that cause bruising can also lead to the development of petechiae (*see above*).

▶ *Disorders that do not affect blood platelets,* such as rheumatoid arthritis, vasculitis, disseminated lupus erythematosus, and Werlhof's or Sjögren's disease (benign and rare skin disorders) can also be responsible.

PRACTICAL ADVICE

Apply ice as soon as possible after a trauma to avoid swelling and stop the hemorrhaging. Keep the ice on for fifteen minutes and repeat several times a day.

Keep the limb elevated to ensure that blood does not spread to the neighbouring tissues. Keep it in a raised position as often and for as long as possible. This will also help drain the blood and prevent bruising.

Do not bandage a bruise or a hematoma. This will only increase the pressure on the area, causing the blood to collect even more deeply under the skin.

Choose your medications carefully. If you are in pain, take one or two acetaminophen tablets (325 mg to 500 mg) four times a day, never exceeding 4 grams daily. Avoid aspirin and anti-inflammatories (such as ibuprofen) because they affect the function of the blood platelets and may delay healing.

Apply heat. Forty-eight hours after the trauma, apply lukewarm compresses to dilate the blood vessels and improve circulation. Do this several times a day for 20 minutes each time.

Cover up your bruise. A bit of foundation makeup can work wonders.

Vitamin C supplements. If you are vulnerable to bruising, take 500 mg of vitamin C, three times a day, to encourage the production of collagen (a protein that reinforces the skin tissues).

WHEN TO CONSULT?
- ► You have petechiae.
- ► Bruises or hematomas reappear for no reason.
- ► Bruises or hematomas spread all over the body.
- ► You have suffered a serious trauma and believe there may be a hematoma.

WHAT HAPPENS DURING THE EXAM?
The doctor inquires about the patient's personal and family medical history and dietary habits. Past experience with tooth extraction is also of particular interest: if heavy bleeding has always followed an extraction, there is likely a coagulation problem. A physical exam, as well as blood and urine tests, are also required.

If necessary, the doctor orders further tests (such as a bone marrow sample) and prescribes vitamins.

WHAT IS THE TREATMENT?

Bruising and hematoma

Bruises and hematomas generally heal by themselves and do not require treatment. Certain deep muscle hematomas may require surgery to drain the blood effusion and prevent tissue damage.

However, if the patient has coagulation problems, the doctor will prescribe medication to replace the missing element (plasma or concentrated coagulation factors).

Petechiae

The underlying cause determines the treatment. For example, chemotherapy is indicated for leukemia, vitamin B_{12} injections for persistent anemia, and interferon or blood platelet transfusions for hepatitis B.

Bulging Eyes (Exophthalmos)

Exophthalmos describes the abnormal protrusion of the eyeball from its socket and is often accompanied by diplopia (double vision). Since the lids can no longer entirely close to blink, the eyes become dry, red, sensitive to light (photophobia), sometimes painful and, in a few cases, displaced downwards, upwards or to the sides. Bulging eyes can also create a fixed gaze or staring look.

Exophthalmos can affect both eyes (particularly if congenital or caused by an underlying disease) or only one (in the case of a cyst, tumour, or trauma,).

WHAT ARE THE CAUSES?

- *Thyroid gland disorder.* Thyroid problems can inflame the tissues and muscles behind the eyes, sometimes only affecting one eye.
- *Congenital deformity.* One or both eyes are naturally bigger or the sides of the face are unsymmetrical.
- *Trauma to the eye or face* (eye socket or cheekbone fracture, for example) can cause a hematoma (accumulation of blood) inside the socket, resulting in bulging eyes.
- *Extreme myopia.* Extremely myopic people have larger eyes.
- *Inflammation of the sinus (sinusitis).*
- *Cyst or tumour behind the eye.*

PRACTICAL ADVICE

Do not use "eye whitening" drops as they can have an adverse effect on blood pressure and heart rate. These products can also mask vasodilation.

Do not use plasters or adhesive bandages to keep the eyes closed as they can slip and get into your eye.

Get out the photo album! Find photos of yourself taken recently and over the last few years to help the doctor determine how long you have had the problem and whether or not it is congenital.

Use artificial tears and ointment. Because sufferers cannot close their lids completely, it is hard for them to keep their eyes lubricated. As a palliative solution, ophthalmologists suggest the daytime use of artificial tears or an ointment (used in conjunction with an applicator tube). These products are available over the counter in pharmacies. Using an ointment at bedtime is preferable, since it is absorbed more slowly and lasts longer.

Wear sunglasses to protect the eyes from wind and glare and conceal the protrusion.

Do not walk around like a one-eyed pirate! An eye-patch may hide your condition, but if it is held in place with an elastic band, it can exert uncomfortable pressure. Wear sunglasses instead.

Sleep with an extra pillow. If your lids are swollen, sleep with two pillows or elevate the head of the bed with wood blocks to reduce the accumulation of fluid in the eyelids.

Fixed Stare or Gaze

The impression of a fixed stare or gaze is generally attributable to one eye being open wider or protruding more than the other. It can also result from a thyroid gland disorder or facial paralysis, which prevents complete closure of the lid. Blinking on this side is not possible so the eye remains partially exposed. During the medical examination, the doctor will observe lid movement to determine whether they are retracted or paralyzed.

Cortisone tablets will be prescribed for facial paralysis to reduce inflammation of the facial nerve (often caused by a virus). The paralysis is generally temporary and disappears in 90% of cases after a few months if medical attention is sought promptly. Care must be taken to ensure the eye is properly lubricated during the recovery period.

Adapt your diet. Eliminate salt, sugar, and spicy food, as they can cause water retention and therefore puffy eyelids.

WHEN TO CONSULT?

► Your eyes are red and sore.
► Your vision is diminished or you see double.
► You or those close to you notice your eyes are bulging.
► Your eyes are bulging but you have no other symptoms. (*See an ophthalmologist to determine the cause.*)

WHAT HAPPENS DURING THE EXAM?

The doctor will first try to assess the degree of exophthalmos by examining the protrusion in profile (sideways) and recording the corresponding change in gaze or facial appearance. If only one eye appears to be affected, the doctor will use a special ruler (exophthalomometer) to measure the degree of protrusion. He or she will then look for ocular signs of a thyroid disorder (retracted lids, muscular congestion), check the eyes for dryness, and palpate the area for any cysts. In most cases, he or she will order an X-ray to confirm or rule out sinusitis or any tissue abnormality behind the eye.

WHAT IS THE TREATMENT?

Thyroid gland disorder

The doctor will perform an in-depth assessment of thyroid function. Medication or radioactive iodine treatments are prescribed, depending on the case. During recovery, the patient may also use eye drops or ointments to ease dryness.

Congenital deformity and eye or face trauma.

The patient can simply use make-up techniques to conceal the problem or resort to cosmetic surgery. The latter can significantly reduce bulging and techniques include orbital decompression (involving the removal of part of the bone so the eye can fall back into place in the socket), or lid retraction. If the patient also suffers from double vision, this can be permanently corrected during surgery.

Extreme myopia

Certain types of corrective lenses and make-up techniques can make the bulging less apparent.

Sinus inflammation (sinusitis)

Antibiotics are prescribed for infectious sinusitis and antihistamines and/or nasal spray corticosteroids for allergic sinusitis.

Cyst or tumour behind the eye

Treatment involves surgery to remove the mass. Sometimes, radiation therapy is indicated (lymphoma, for example) and less frequently, cortisone-based oral treatment can be prescribed.

Burning With Urination

Nearly everyone has felt a burning sensation during urination at least once in their lives. The phenomenon is more common in women because the female urethra (the duct emptying the bladder) is much shorter (4 cm) than the male (16 cm). In women, sexual activity or a gynecological examination can move the bacteria normally present at the tip of the urethra to the inside of this duct, possibly leading to infection.

WHAT ARE THE CAUSES?

► *Urinary tract infection.* There are two types: lower and upper urinary tract infections.

An infection of the lower urinary tract can affect the urethra (urethritis) or the bladder (cystitis). Symptoms include a frequent need to urinate and, in some cases, pain above the pubic area caused by the contraction of the bladder muscles as it expels urine. There may be blood in the urine. The burning sensation is directly linked to the swelling of the bladder wall caused by infection. If properly treated, there is no cause for concern.

An upper urinary tract infection, or kidney infection (also known as pyelonephritis), is much more serious. Its symptoms include fever, back pain, cloudy, milky, or bloody urine, nausea and general malaise.

► *Infection of the vagina (vaginitis) or vulva (vulvitis).* In these cases, pain is caused when urine comes in contact with the irritated area. Other symptoms include lesions on the vulva or vagina and unusual vaginal discharge. See the chapter on "Vaginal Ailments."

► *Cystocele,* also known as "fallen bladder," is an exclusively female condition, occurring in older women when the perineum (the muscle and tissue supporting the bladder) loses tone and elasticity. The condition can lead to infection, which in turn causes burning with urination.

► *Sexually transmitted infections.* In men, burning with urination may be accompanied by discharge from the penis. In women, these infections frequently cause urethritis.

► *Prostate infection (prostatitis).* In addition to burning with urination, symptoms include fever, frequent need to urinate, difficulty urinating, blood in the urine, discharge from the penis and pain in the perineum (between the legs).

PRACTICAL ADVICE

Drink plenty of liquids and urinate frequently. Staying well-hydrated cleans out the system, naturally washing away bacteria and reducing the risk of infection. If you increase your intake of liquids, it is important to remember to evacuate more often as well. An empty bladder is better able to defend itself against infection than a full one.

Drink plenty of cranberry juice. This also makes the bladder more resistant to infection.

Urinate to clean the system. Remember to urinate after any activity that may have caused bacteria to move into the urethra and closer to the bladder (sexual intercourse or a gynecological exam, for example). This is especially important for women who suffer from recurring bladder infections.

Avoid consuming irritants. Some foods can irritate the urinary tract. Alcohol, coffee, tea, chocolate, soft drinks, citrus fruit, tomatoes, hot peppers, spicy dishes, vinegar, aspartame and sugar can all aggravate the pain experienced during urination. Eliminate these foods, and once the pain disappears, resume your usual diet one item at a time to determine which substance is responsible.

To ease the pain. Try urinating standing up in the shower or in a lukewarm bath.

Use bathroom tissue properly. For women, the proper way to clean after urinating is to move the bathroom tissue front to back. Wiping in the opposite direction can bring bacteria from the rectum to the urethra.

Do not use irritating products. Many types of soap, body wash, bubble bath and sanitary napkins contain perfume or other additives that can irritate the urethra and the delicate skin around the genital organs. Even products that claim to be gentle can be irritating. In particular, vaginal douches and other internal hygiene products should usually be avoided. Wash with water alone, or use gentle, unscented cleansers like Cetaphil or Spectrojel.

Keep dry. Humidity and chlorine stimulate bacterial infection. Change out of your wet bathing suit after swimming, and keep an extra suit handy.

WHEN TO CONSULT?

- ► You experience a burning sensation during urination lasting for two days or more.
- ► You have a fever and back pain.
- ► Your urine is cloudy, milky or foul-smelling.
- ► There is blood in your urine.
- ► You have or suspect you have a sexually transmitted infection.
- ► For men: the burning sensation is accompanied by discharge from the penis.

WHAT HAPPENS DURING THE EXAM?

The patient answers an assessment questionnaire from the physician. The doctor performs a basic physical examination, checking vital signs and paying particular attention to any sensitivity or pain in the kidney region (in the back, just below the ribs) and just above the pubic area. In most cases, a urine culture is required to confirm the presence of an infection and identify the bacteria. After treatment, the doctor may order another urine culture to be sure the bacteria has been eliminated.

WHAT IS THE TREATMENT?
Urinary tract infection
Lower urinary tract infection (urethritis, cystitis). If mild, the infection will clear up on its own in a day or two. In most cases, however, oral antibiotics are required.

Upper urinary tract infection (pyelonephritis). Antibiotics will be prescribed. The patient must follow instructions carefully to avoid complications.

Infection of the vagina (vaginitis) or vulva (vulvitis)
The doctor will prescribe topical or oral antibiotics.

Cystocele (fallen bladder)
In more serious cases, corrective surgery is required. In milder cases, the doctor may recommend exercises to strengthen the perineum.

Sexually transmitted infections
Antibiotics are prescribed.

Prostate infection (prostatitis)
The doctor will prescribe antibiotics, sometimes on a long-term basis (especially if the infection is chronic).

Cellulite

More of an aesthetic problem than a health concern, cellulite appears after puberty, and affects 80% to 90% of women to varying degrees. A small percentage of men suffering from so-called "monstrous" obesity may develop it on their lower abdomens. Cellulite usually appears on the buttocks, thighs, stomach or backs of the knees. It is not painful, except in extreme cases (people weighing over 110 kilograms).

It should be noted that this chapter does not deal with cellulitis, a subcutaneous infection arising when bacteria infiltrates the body through broken skin, causing fever and hot, swollen, tender, red patches on the skin. This is a medical emergency.

Cellulite, on the other hand, has the following symptoms:

Minor cellulite
► Irregular, orange-peel like surface of the skin when pinched.

Severe cellulite
► Irregular surface of the skin without pinching.

WHAT ARE THE CAUSES?

► *Hormones.* Between puberty and menopause, female hormones (estrogen and progesterone) cause adipose cells and water to build up in vulnerable areas. Pregnancy and oral contraceptives exacerbate the development of cellulite and hormone replacement therapy after menopause prolongs the process. If a woman does not undergo hormone therapy, her cellulite will stop developing.

► *Anatomy.* In women, the strands of fibrous tissue attaching the skin to the subcutaneous tissue have spaces between them, leading to dimpling when fat cells accumulate. (In men, the fibrous strands are crisscrossed, forming a kind of net that keeps the skin surface smooth.) Circulation is poor in the dimpled areas, leading to a lack of oxygen and drainage. The tissues therefore retain water, and the bulges eventually harden and become permanent.

► *Obesity.* Since cellulite is basically fat, every excess kilogram accentuates the problem.

PRACTICAL ADVICE

Be active. Lack of exercise slows the metabolism and circulation.

Avoid stress. It is believed to stimulate tissue congestion.

Avoid salt and alcohol. Salt causes the body to retain water and alcohol leads to tissue congestion.

Do not spend a fortune. Avoid wasting your money on expensive but ineffective appliances that promise to get rid of cellulite. If you cannot resist trying one, your best bet is Cellesse (manufactured by Phillips), a relatively inexpensive machine that stimulates circulation by massaging the skin between rollers. Use daily for effect.

Beware of miracle treatments. Liposuction, a fat-removing surgical treatment, may shrink targeted areas of the body but it does not get rid of cellulite (although it is less apparent). Laser treatments or seaweed wraps subject the skin to intense heat and eliminate only a small amount of water, which is quickly regained.

Maintain a healthy diet. Follow the Canada Food Guide. Eat lean, protein-rich food (fish, chicken, seafood) and slowly-assimilated sugars (pasta, rice) over quickly-assimilated sugars (pastries, etc.). Eat plenty of fruit and vegetables.

Eat plenty of fiber. Raw vegetables and bran or whole wheat cereals help the body eliminate waste.

Drink two to three litres of water a day. The more water you drink, the more you will eliminate and the better the tissues will be drained. Always have a glass within reach.

Control your weight. Almost all women have some cellulite. However, the slimmer the woman, the less likely she is to have a problem.

Exercise. There are no specific exercises that target cellulite, although using all your muscles in regular physical activity (in-line skating, swimming, or cross-country skiing, for example) will encourage healthy circulation and oxygenation of the tissues. Choose a sport you enjoy—you will be more likely to keep it up.

Give yourself a massage. Using your bare hands or a massage glove, massage the affected areas to promote circulation.

Are anti-cellulite creams any good? Various cosmetics companies market slimming creams, but only those with a base of theophylline or caffeine have any real decongestive effect. The cream must be applied daily and its beneficial effects will disappear as soon as use is discontinued.

WHEN TO CONSULT?
► You suffer from obesity.
► Your weight is normal, but you are bothered by cellulite. Do not wait too long before consulting; once the fat dimples have hardened, they are difficult to remove.

WHAT HAPPENS DURING THE EXAM?
The doctor will evaluate the extent of the problem and its stage of evolution to determine which treatment is appropriate.

WHAT IS THE TREATMENT?
Obesity
The patient will be put on a medically-supervised diet.

Minor Cellulite
This responds relatively well to diet, massage (manual or using Cellesse), exercise, and xanthine-based (caffeine, theophylline) slimming creams.

Severe Cellulite

Caffeine, lactic acid or retinol (Prodermafiline) creams bring about lipolysis by releasing the content of fat cells. They are very effective, although successful treatment is proportional to the amount and progression of cellulite. The creams must be used over the long term, as they cannot get rid of cellulite for good. Lymphatic drainage, performed by an experienced technician, is another method to help the body purify waste.

Changes to Urine

Every person's urine is a different colour (pale or golden yellow, for example). It generally carries a light odour of ammonia, which is more pronounced in the morning because the urine is more concentrated.

The colour and the odour of a person's urine can change. It can become paler or darker, or emit a strong and unpleasant smell. In most cases, there is no need to worry.

The following changes may occur:

- ► Orange urine.
- ► Reddish urine (not due to blood).
- ► Brownish-black urine.
- ► Strong, unpleasant odour.
- ► Sweetish odour.

WHAT ARE THE CAUSES?

- ► *Mild dehydration.* Insufficient hydration means that the urine produced by the kidneys is less diluted. Because the urine is more concentrated, it is darker and stronger-smelling. This is absolutely harmless.
- ► *Destruction of red blood cells.* The male hormone testosterone produces a large number of red blood cells. Every 120 days or so, the cells die off and are eliminated through the urine. When this occurs, men's urine (golden in colour to begin with) takes on a more orange tint. This may also occur in pregnant women during the third trimester, when the foetus (either male or female) begins producing a large number of red blood cells. This is a normal phenomenon.
- ► *Food.* After eating beets, urine will remain very dark (almost red) for three or four eliminations. Asparagus and vegetables from the cabbage family give urine an unpleasant smell. This effect is temporary, lasting as long as the digestion process.
- ► *Drugs.* Most medications and some vitamins give urine an orange colour and a stronger odour. This is particularly noticeable with penicillin and phenazopyridine (or Pyridium, prescribed for pain due to urinary infections).

► **Urinary tract problems.** Symptoms of urinary infections include cloudy, bad-smelling urine and pain with urination. A bladder obstruction (due to prostate hypertrophy, constipation, or a neurological disease, for example) prevents the bladder from emptying completely. Urine therefore remains in the bladder for a longer period of time, becoming orange and stronger-smelling. A bloated stomach and difficulty urinating are other symptoms of a bladder obstruction.

► **Liver problems.** Gallstones and pancreatic cancer can obstruct the bile duct, preventing the movement of gallbladder secretions (bile) to the intestines. Absorbed by the blood, these secretions are filtered by the kidneys and eliminated with the urine, giving it a brownish-black colour. Stomach pain and whitish stool are also symptoms of gallstones. Yellowish complexion and generalized itchiness frequently accompany pancreatic cancer (bile acids in the blood release histamines, causing itchiness).

► **Diabetes.** This disease is characterized by the body's inability to properly process sugar and other fuels. Unused sugar is absorbed by the blood and the urine, which emits a sweetish odour (a little like maple sap).

► **Metabolic disorders.** In extremely rare cases, a deficiency of certain liver enzymes changes the urine to a brownish-black colour. There is no change in odour.

PRACTICAL ADVICE

Review your diet. Diet is the most common reason for changes in colour or odour. Check to see if you have eaten a new type of food.

Get information about side effects. Ask your doctor or pharmacist if your medication may be responsible for changes in your urine.

Drink plenty of liquids. Drink at least six glasses of water a day. A well-hydrated body produces lighter and milder-smelling urine.

For diabetics. Both type 1 and type 2 diabetics must follow a balanced diet, do regular exercise and maintain a healthy weight.

WHEN TO CONSULT?

► You notice blood in your urine.
► The unusual colour or odour persists.
► The change to your urine worries you.

WHAT HAPPENS DURING THE EXAM?

The doctor will ask pertinent questions and perform a complete physical examination, including blood and urine tests. If necessary, more in-depth liver or kidney tests will be ordered.

WHAT IS THE TREATMENT?

Change in the colour or odour of urine is usually the result of a benign condition such as mild dehydration, the destruction of red blood cells, food, medication, or vitamins. In such cases, no treatment is necessary.

Urinary tract problems

A bladder infection is treated with antibiotics. Treatment for an obstructed bladder varies, depending on the cause: the doctor may prescribe medication, a catheter (to empty the bladder), or surgery (to remove the hypertrophied section of the prostate gland).

Liver problems

Gallstones are usually removed in a day-surgery procedure (no hospitalization required) and the patient recovers quickly. In cases of pancreatic cancer, the tumour is removed surgically, and chemotherapy and radiation therapy may also be necessary.

Diabetes

Type 1 diabetics are prescribed insulin to replace what the pancreas cannot produce. Type 2 diabetics may require orally-administered hypoglycemic agents to lower their blood sugar levels if lifestyle changes alone are not effective. Insulin may be required.

Metabolic disorders

There is no treatment.

Changes to the Hair

Like skin and nails, the hair is a living part of the body, subject to possibly unattractive or bothersome changes in appearance. While colour and texture are hereditary characteristics, other aspects react to internal or external factors. The scalp may also be affected.

The following problems frequently affect the texture of the hair, its colour, and the scalp:

Texture
- Hair is thin, limp and flat.
- Hair is dry and brittle with split ends.
- Hair is greasy.

Colour
- Progressive greying of the hair, beginning between the ages of 30 and 40.
- Rapid greying of the hair (changes colour "overnight").
- Hair has a greenish tint in the light.
- Hair has a reddish tint in the light.

Scalp
- Dandruff
  - Excessive flakiness of the scalp.
  - May be accompanied by itching.
  - Affects 20% of the population.
- Extreme itchiness.

WHAT ARE THE CAUSES?
Texture
Thin, limp hair
- **Heredity**
- **Lack of nutrition.** A diet poor in protein may make the hair thinner.

Dry and brittle hair

- ► *Overuse of styling instruments* or products, such as hairdryers, curling irons, or hair dye.
- ► *Excessive exposure* to sun and wind.

Greasy hair

- ► *Hormones,* especially during adolescence or pregnancy.
- ► *Regular intense physical activity* stimulates the sebaceous glands.
- ► *Heat, humidity and perspiration* also stimulate the sebaceous glands.
- ► *Residue from hair products* (shampoo, conditioner, hairspray, mousse, gel, etc.).

Colour

- ► *Aging.* Hair usually begins to go grey between the ages of 30 and 40, becoming completely white at a genetically determined age.
- ► *Extreme stress.* While stress does not make the hair turn white, it may cause large amounts of coloured hairs (more easily dislodged than the grey) to fall out, leaving the impression that the hair has changed colour "overnight".
- ► *Chlorine in swimming pools* can give a greenish tint to blonde hair.
- ► *Iron in the water* (from a well, for example) can give the hair a reddish tint.

Scalp

Dandruff

- ► *Yeast infections* may cause inflammation and increase the speed of cell reproduction and turnover.
- ► *Stress* can also accelerate this process.
- ► *Psoriasis.*
- ► *Residue from hair products* may be the real problem, and not dandruff at all.

Itchiness

- ► *Inflammation* due to inadequate care or overuse of chemical products on the hair.

▶ *Dandruff*

▶ *Eczema* is a hereditary disease characterized by red plaque on the scalp and other places on the body. Stress is a trigger or aggravating factor

▶ *Psoriasis* is a hereditary auto-immune disease (inability of the body's immune system to distinguish its own cells from foreign cells). It is characterized by flaking lesions on the scalp and other places on the body. Stress is a trigger or aggravating factor.

PRACTICAL ADVICE

Colour or perm fine hair. These treatments give the hair more body.

Do a spot test before dying your hair. This will guard against allergic reactions causing persistent itchiness.

Avoid acid-based permanent formulas. The chemicals are especially irritating to skin affected by eczema. Choose products with natural ingredients.

Choise your shampoo carefully. The pH balance should be between 4.5 and 5.5. Use a special litmus test available at the drugstore to check.

Rinse with beer. Beer is an excellent (and odourless) leave-in conditioner that adds curl, shine, and body.

Do not over-condition your hair. Commercial conditioners weigh down and flatten the hair. Avoid excessively rich products, and use light conditioners sparingly.

Add volume. Set your hair-dryer at medium heat, and hold it at least 10 cm away from your hair. Lift the hair upwards from the roots with a round brush.

Avoid overheating. Applying too much heat to the hair makes it dry and brittle. Never use curling irons or hot rollers, and set your hairdryer at medium heat.

Treat dry and brittle hair with mayonnaise. Mayonnaise is an excellent conditioner. Massage one tablespoon into your hair and leave on anywhere between five minutes to an hour, then shampoo. You can also use raw eggs alone as a nourishing treatment.

Trim or cut your hair every six weeks. It will avoid split ends.

Protect your hair. Wear a hat to protect your hair from the drying effects of the wind or the hot sun.

Wash greasy hair every day. Clear or transparent shampoos (such as Neutrogena) are effective and leave the least residue. Lather twice, leaving the shampoo on the hair for a few minutes before rinsing. Rinse your hair with a solution of one teaspoon of cider vinegar to a half litre of water, or the juice of two lemons to every half litre of water.

Get rid of styling product residue. Leftover hair spray, mousse and conditioners can change the colour of your hair and accumulate on the scalp. Once a week, use a specially-formulated clarifying shampoo to wash the residue away.

Colour grey hair. If having grey hair bothers you, a number of dyes offer gentle and easy-to-use alternatives. Obvious signs of re-growth can be avoided if the colour is re-applied every six weeks.

Wait for your hair to grow back. Most people whose hair has rapidly turned grey due to extreme shock and stress experience a partial re-growth of coloured hair.

Coat your hair with conditioner before swimming in a chlorinated pool. This creates a barrier between your hair and the chlorine, and protects blonde hair from developing a greenish tint.

Shampoo daily to treat dandruff. This may be sufficient in mild cases. If the problem continues, a selenium sulfide-based shampoo will directly attack the yeast on the scalp. Use for three weeks, alternating anti-dandruff shampoos containing agents such as zinc pyrithione, tar, and salicylic acid. Leave medicated shampoos on for five minutes before rinsing. Exposing the hair to sunlight is also beneficial in cases of severe dandruff (the heat and light have an antifungal effect).

Harness the medicinal properties of thyme. Boil 4 teaspoons of dried thyme in 2 cups of water for 10 minutes. Filter through a strainer and let cool while you shampoo. Massage the thyme water into a damp scalp. Do not rinse.

Relieve itchiness. Massage the scalp with lukewarm olive oil and leave on for 20 minutes. Shampoo.

Reduce flakiness. Tar oil shampoo reduces flakiness caused by psoriasis.

Avoid stress. Exercise, engage in your favourite pastimes, take a vacation.

WHEN TO CONSULT?
► You have persistent dandruff.
► Your scalp is persistently itchy.
► You have lesions (red blotches or patches of flakiness) on your scalp.

WHAT HAPPENS DURING THE EXAM?
The doctor examines the scalp to determine whether the problem is dandruff, eczema, or psoriasis.

WHAT IS THE TREATMENT?
Persistent dandruff is treated with Nizoral shampoo. In cases of extreme inflammation, the doctor will prescribe 1% cortisone cream.
    Itchiness may require antihistamine treatment.

Eczema and psoriasis of the scalp are experienced in recurring and progressive episodes. There is no definitive treatment, although the lesions can be subdued or controlled using cortisone-based lotions and creams.

Chapped Lips

The lips are covered by a natural, protective layer of oil. Dehydration can lead to the loss of this protective layer and cause dryness and chapping.

The lips become covered with flakes of dead skin which cause cracks or fissures when they detach. Redness, irritation and scabs may follow, sometimes beyond the lip line. Irritated, chapped lips can last several weeks or months.

WHAT ARE THE CAUSES?

- *Hereditary factors,* such as a predisposition towards eczema or sensitive and fragile skin.
- *Licking the lips.* Saliva contains irritating substances that prepare food for the digestive process. Frequently licking your lips dries out the mucous membranes.
- *Cold temperatures and overheating in winter.*
- *Upper respiratory tract problems* such as sinusitis or allergic rhinitis require sufferers to breathe through their mouths. The constant passage of air dries out the mucous membranes.
- *Trigger factors* such as children's winter sports. Children often forget to use balm on their lips during outdoor activities, licking their lips instead to keep them moist.
- *Allergies to toothpaste, mouthwash or lipstick* affect the lips, chin, and corners of the mouth. The inside of the mouth is generally spared. Some lipsticks cause photodermatitis after exposure to the sun.
- *Fruit and vegetables,* such as mango, celery and limes.
- *Certain medications,* such as Accutane (used in the treatment of acne), antihistamines, antidepressants, and cholesterol-lowering medications.
- *Vitamin B deficiency.* This is rare in developed countries.

PRACTICAL ADVICE

Avoid licking your lips. The more you lick them, the more they dry out.

Avoid scratching, touching, or pulling at chapped lips. Pulling off the dead skin will impede the healing process and increase the risk of infection.

Use a humidifier. It will preserve the natural hydration of the lips.

Use lip balm as needed. Your lips will be protected from dehydration.

Avoid stretching the lips and reopening the fissures. Apply lip balm first.

Avoid hot drinks and acidic foods. That can cause burning or irritation.

WHEN TO CONSULT?

► You have followed the advice in this chapter and your lips are still chapped.
► Your lips become chapped after developing a skin disease or taking medication.

What is perleche?

Perleche is caused by a bacterial (streptococcus, staphylococcus) or yeast infection (Candida albicans) and causes chapping at the corners of the mouth, as well as the formation of cracks and wet scabs. It is sometimes confused with a cold sore (herpes), which is a viral infection characterized by small transparent vesicles on a red base that can also appear on the lips or corners of the mouth.

The shape of the mouth plays a role in the development of perleche. Poorly-fitting dental prostheses can lead to the progressive atrophying of the gums and underlying bone structure, causing the skin at the corners of the mouth to fold in. This part of the lips then comes into constant contact with saliva, resulting in irritation (*see What is the Treatment?*).

WHAT HAPPENS DURING THE EXAM?

The doctor interviews the patient about his or her oral hygiene products/habits, and assesses whether the problem is due to heredity, vitamin deficiency or an underlying disease. If the lips are itchy, tests are used to determine the presence of a disease or allergy. The doctor discusses products used by the patient that are causing the chapping, if appropriate.

WHAT IS THE TREATMENT?

In general, lip balm (with or without cortisone) or vaseline must be applied regularly.

Hereditary eczema

The doctor will prescribe a protective and moisturizing cortisone ointment and anti-inflammatories.

Perleche

Both the infection and the chapping must be treated. Antibiotics are used to clear up bacteria and topical antifungals for yeast infections. If a dental prosthesis is causing the problem, the fit is adjusted. If the lips are severely cracked, the doctor may apply a bandage to immobilize the area and speed the healing process. Perleche is also common among people with Down's syndrome.

Beware of the sun!

Those who are particularly sensitive to the sun, such as the elderly, the fair-skinned, or people who work outdoors (construction workers, for example), may notice changes in their lips. Sometimes indicating nothing more than dryness, these changes can also signal a pre-cancerous condition. Applying a lip balm with sunscreen will help prevent the condition from getting worse, but it is important to monitor the appearance of your lips carefully and consult immediately if you notice any change.

Pre-cancerous condition

Pre-cancerous changes are detected using a topical application of 5-fluorouracil, which reacts only to cancerous cells. If necessary, a biopsy confirms the diagnosis.

Chest Pain (Not Related to Heart Trouble)

Chest pain that is not caused by heart trouble usually occurs during rest. Palpating (touching the painful area with your hand), breathing, changing positions, or eating may either increase or decrease the pain. Any part of the thorax (the upper section of the trunk, from just under the ribs to the shoulders, including the upper spine) can be affected, and the pain may be diffused or concentrated in one area.

Chest pain occurs in many forms, including cramps, a burning sensation, and stabbing pain. Because it is sometimes accompanied by a feeling of heaviness or tightness, it can be confused with heart trouble. A useful tip: remember that eating or changing position will not change the intensity of the pain if a person is suffering from heart disease.

Chest pain is caused by any one of a number of problems. The most common are listed below.

Musculoskeletal pain
- The pain begins in the bone, cartilage, or muscles.
- It is generally felt in the ribs or at the point where two vertebrae or bones meet (for example, the clavicle and the sternum).
- The pain is concentrated in one area of the thorax.
- It can be aggravated by touching or change of position.

Pain in the lungs
- Usually accompanied by coughing, expectoration (coughing up sputum), breathlessness, and sometimes fever and chills, if there is an infection.
- In cases of pneumothorax, the pain is very intense, sudden and acute, and the sufferer becomes breathless at the slightest effort.

Digestive pain
- Pain originates in the esophagus or the stomach and is generally accompanied by belching, nausea, vomiting, and a sensation of burning in the pit of the stomach.

► In cases of stomach spasms, the feeling of heaviness or tightness in the thorax can be confused with heart trouble.

Vascular pain
► Usually accompanied by breathlessness, coughing, bloody expectoration, and pain when breathing in deeply.

Pain on the skin (shingles)
► Generally accompanied by redness, lesions or blisters in the affected area. The pain appears a few days before the rash.

WHAT ARE THE CAUSES?
Musculoskeletal pain
► *Fracture.*
► *Arthritis* (joint inflammation).
► *Osteoarthritis* in the spinal column (bone degeneration).

Pain in the lungs
► *Lung infections* are caused by viruses or bacteria, such as pneumonia or tracheobronchitis.
► *Pneumothorax* occurs when air enters between the membrane surrounding the lungs (the pleura) and the lung itself. It can be caused by a trauma, emphysema, asthma, or it may occur spontaneously.

Digestive pain
► *Gastric hyperacidity.* Smoking and drinking coffee increases the amount of acid in the stomach.
► *Acid reflux.* The reflux of gastric acid into the esophagus is usually linked to obesity or a hiatus hernia (a stomach hernia where part of this organ protrudes from the abdominal cavity into the thorax).
► *Ingestion of very hot or very cold food.*
► *Anxiety, strong emotions.*
► *Spasms in the esophagus.* The strong and sustained contraction of the muscles in the esophagus causes a feeling of heaviness and tightness that most closely resembles the pain caused by heart trouble.

► *Ulcer.* Ulcers, frequently caused by the *Helicobacter pylori* bacteria, are characterized by a loss of the mucous lining of the stomach or duodenum (the first section of the intestine), making healing difficult. Stress can aggravate the problem by increasing the level of acidity, irritating the stomach.

Vascular pain
► *Pulmonary embolism.* This is generally caused by blood clots obstructing one or more branches of the pulmonary artery.
► *Extended bed rest* or any other event or activity that interferes with proper blood circulation (surgery, for example).

Pain on the skin surface
► *Shingles.* This infectious disease is caused by a reactivation of the varicella (chicken pox) virus due to an immune system deficiency. Only people who have had chicken pox as children can develop shingles later in life.

PRACTICAL ADVICE
Perform a self-exam. Check your temperature. A fever is generally a sign of some kind of infection. Check to see if the pain increases when you cough, expectorate, or palpate the painful area with your hand. Look for redness, lesions or blisters in the sensitive area. If present, this could indicate shingles. Note which variables (foods, spices or alcohol, for example), aggravate or ease the pain and try changing positions to see which are best. Eat lightly to check whether the pain is digestive. Finally, remember that there is not always a correlation between the intensity of the pain and the severity of the problem. Do not dismiss consulting a doctor just because the pain is not excruciating.

Rest. Physical activity requires effort and can aggravate the pain.

Ease the pain. If you are certain that your pain is not due to heart disease, take acetaminophen. One or two acetaminophen tablets

(325 mg to 500 mg), four times a day, should soothe the pain. Never exceed 4 grams daily. If the pain is digestive in origin, aspirin, codeine, and non-steroidal anti-inflammatories like ibuprofen are contra-indicated. Instead, drink milk for its short-term analgesic effects. Musculoskeletal pain may require cold or hot compresses, depending on the specific cause. If the pain is shooting and diffuse (as in arthritis), use a heating pad. If the pain is sharp, concentrated in one area, and accompanied by redness and swelling (as in the case of a fracture), apply ice.

WHEN TO CONSULT?

► You suspect that the pain may be due to heart trouble. Piercing pain moves from the front to the back, possibly radiating to the arms (especially the left) or the neck, and is accompanied by a feeling of heaviness or tightness. Go to the hospital immediately.
► Your temperature remains higher than 38.3 °C for more than 48 hours.
► Your high temperature is associated with coughing and sputum production.
► You are coughing up blood.
► You are out of breath, even after minor effort or at rest.
► You feel a piercing pain in your back.
► The pain does not go away after three days, no matter what type it is.

WHAT HAPPENS DURING THE EXAM?

The doctor interviews the patient to understand the kind of pain, its location, and the factors that trigger, ease or aggravate it. He or she also performs a complete physical exam. Depending on the cause suspected, the doctor will order blood tests, X-rays, an electrocardiogram, or other, more specialized exams.

WHAT IS THE TREATMENT?
Musculoskeletal pain
The doctor will prescribe rest, hot or cold compresses (depending on the cause of the pain), and painkillers (acetaminophen and sometimes anti-inflammatories.

Pain in the lungs

The doctor may prescribe plenty of liquids, rest, cough medicine and, if needed, antibiotics.

Digestive pain

Small amounts of food at a time are recommended and irritants (coffee, tea, tobacco, alcohol) are contra-indicated. If necessary, the doctor will prescribe anti-ulcer medication to neutralize or stop the production of acids.

Vascular pain

A pulmonary embolism requires immediate hospitalization.

Pain on the skin

If shingles is caught within 72 hours of the first eruption, antiviral medication can prevent the further development of lesions. The doctor may also prescribe an ointment to relieve the pain.

Chronic Lower Abdominal Pain (Women)

A number of women experience more or less regular pain in the lower abdominal (pelvic) area, negatively affecting their quality of life. This type of pain can vary in intensity.

WHAT ARE THE CAUSES?

- ► *Adhesions* are abnormal web-like growths of inflammatory tissue over the ovaries, fallopian tubes and pelvic wall. They impede organ mobility and are caused by poorly-treated infections or abdominal surgery.
- ► *Varicose veins around the uterus.* This phenomenon is most common in women who have given birth to several children. The pain occurs during certain phases of the menstrual cycle, such as after ovulation when estrogen and progesterone cause the veins to swell. Sexual arousal can also lead to vascular swelling, though the veins drain fairly quickly after orgasm. If the woman does not climax, however, she may experience abdominal pain.
- ► *Endometriosis.* This condition, apparently hereditary, is characterized by the abnormal growth of endometrial cells outside the uterus. Although the exact cause is still unknown, the problem has been linked to various factors such as genetics, a reflux of menstrual blood in the fallopian tubes, and abnormal uterine cell deposits in the abdominal cavity due to surgery. Another hypothesis is that abdominal cells take on the characteristics of uterine cells and begin to build up outside the uterus in response to a hormonal stimulus, much like the cells of the uterine lining. Whatever the cause, the stimulation of these cells leads to painful inflammation. The pain varies according to the phases of the menstrual cycle.
- ► *Intrauterine devices (IUDs).* An IUD may cause chronic lower abdominal pain because the body perceives it as a foreign object, triggering uterine contractions. IUDs can aggravate the pain of endometriosis and are therefore contra-indicated.

► *Menstruation.* Menstrual pain, also known as dysmenorrhea, is caused by inflammation resulting from cell death.

► *Sexual assault.* Sexual assault can leave permanent psychological scars which may result in chronic lower abdominal pain.

► *Infection.* Interstitial cystitis is a chronic bladder infection causing pain in the pelvic area. Certain sexually transmitted infections also cause lower abdominal pain; in some cases, this is the only symptom. Note that in this case, the pain does not vary with the phases of the menstrual cycle.

► *Irritable bowel syndrome* is a disease affecting the large intestine that manifests in cramps, diarrhea, and mucus in the stool. It causes chronic lower abdominal pain and can be aggravated by certain foods or stress.

► *Other diseases.* Chronic pain may also be caused by appendicitis operations (leaving abdominal scars), diverticulitis, and colon cancer.

PRACTICAL ADVICE

Protect yourself against sexually transmitted infections. These infections can cause chronic or acute lower abdominal pain and carry a long-term risk of adhesions. Protect yourself any way you can.

Pelvic infections: follow prescribed treatment to the letter. Be sure to complete your treatment to avoid long-term negative effects.

Avoid vaginal douches. The flora of the vagina is a natural defense against micro-organisms. Vaginal douches can disturb this balance or transport bacteria up the uterus.

Consult a psychotherapist. This may be necessary in cases of sexual assault.

WHEN TO CONSULT?

► You have been experiencing lower abdominal pain for some time. It is accompanied by other symptoms (fever or somewhat foul-smelling vaginal discharge), or has appeared with the arrival of a new lover.

► Your menstrual cramps are very bothersome.
► You frequently experience pain during sexual intercourse, bowel movements or simple activities such as walking.

WHAT HAPPENS DURING THE EXAM?

The doctor takes a history to determine when the pain first began, also performing a gynecological exam to check the cervix, palpate the organs for adhesions, and observe the size and location of the organs. This is generally enough for a precise diagnosis, although the doctor may try to verify whether the patient was sexually assaulted as a child or adolescent. If endometriosis is suspected, a laparoscopy (internal exam using fibre optics) is recommended.

WHAT IS THE TREATMENT?

A number of studies have shown that medroxyprogesterone acetate is an effective long-term treatment in many cases of chronic lower abdominal pain.

Adhesions

Surgery is the only option, although success rates are rather low: in more than half the cases, the adhesions reappear. It is best to prevent their development in the first place by protecting yourself against sexually transmitted infections and carefully treating any gynecological infection.

Varicose veins around the uterus

This painful condition is not easily treated. Unlike varicose veins in the legs, dilated veins around the uterus cannot be removed, since there are no other blood vessels in this area to take their place. If the pain is intolerable, removal of the uterus is the only option, resulting, of course, in permanent infertility.

Endometriosis

The two treatment options are surgery and medication.

If infertility is a serious concern, surgery is recommended to remove endometrial cells from the abdominal cavity, followed by three to six months of drug therapy with an LH-RH (luteinizing hormone-releasing hormone) agonist. This medication heightens the effects of the hormone that impedes oestrogen production, thereby destroying any endometrial cells remaining in the abdominal cavity.

If pain management is the primary goal, the doctor will prescribe androgen-based (danazol) medication or an LH-RH agonist. In young women, oral contraceptives containing progestin and low doses of estrogen can help ease the pain and stop the progression of the disease. The most radical treatment involves removing the uterus and ovaries altogether, provided, of course, the woman does not wish to have children in the future. This surgery will bring about premature menopause and the woman will be required to undergo hormone replacement therapy to control the risk of osteoporosis. The patient should discuss her various options for treatment with her physician to become fully aware of the consequences of each.

IUD

If an IUD is responsible for the pain, the doctor will remove the device and recommend another contraceptive method.

Menstruation

Nonsteroidal anti-inflammatory drugs (NSAIDs) ease menstrual pain by inhibiting the production of prostaglandin, a substance associated with inflammation and pain.

Sexual assault

In many cases, particularly those involving abuse at a young age, long-term psychological treatment is advised. With time, the abdominal pain may subside.

Infections

The pain caused by chronic insterstitial cystitis is controlled with cortisone drugs and antidepressants (prescribed for their analgesic effects). In the rare cases that do not respond to treatment, an operation to remove a section of the bladder is required. Sexually transmitted infections are treated with antibiotics.

Irritable bowel syndrome

Antispasmodic drugs can prevent intestinal contractions and irritability.

Other diseases

Medications may be prescribed to control pain caused by appendicitis surgery. Diverticulitis is treated with antibiotics. In cases of colon cancer, the appropriate treatment (chemotherapy, radiation therapy, or surgery) is undertaken immediately.

Clicking Joints

Frequent clicking (or cracking) of joints is usually a completely harmless symptom. However, in some cases, pain or other symptoms are experienced at the same time, possibly indicating a more serious problem.

There are two forms of clicking:
- Movement of the joint (knee, shoulder, neck, hand, hip, elbow) causes a cracking noise or feeling.
- Clicking that is accompanied by pain, stiffness, locking of the joint, edema, or sometimes loss of muscle tone.

WHAT ARE THE CAUSES?
Direct causes
- *Growth or aging.* In adolescence, clicking joints may occur because the tendons, ligaments and bones all grow at different rates. In the elderly, it is usually caused by the thinning, cracking and deformation of the cartilage.
- *Osteoarthritis.* Wear and tear on the cartilage is associated with hampered movement.
- *Arthritis.* The various forms of arthritic diseases (rheumatoid, gouty, or psoriatic arthritis, for example) damage the joints.
- *Joint mice* is the term currently used to refer to calcium deposits in the joints, occurring either spontaneously or as a result of trauma. These deposits disturb the function of the affected joint.
- *Dislocation* occurs when the bone completely detaches from the joint. This is usually caused by trauma.
- *Subluxation (partial dislocation)* occurs when the bone partially detaches from the joint and then returns to its place. A frequent example is jaw subluxation, usually due to faulty occlusion.
- *Ligamentous laxity (loose ligaments).* Some people have longer and more flexible tendons than average. As a result, joints become displaced more easily and click more frequently. This is also known as Paganini's syndrome, named after the famous 19th century violinist whose phenomenal virtuosity has been attributed to extremely loose ligaments.

► *Hereditary morphology.* In certain families, there is a tendency towards deformed joints, even in young people.

Indirect causes
► *Obesity.* Excess weight on the joints makes the development of arthritis more likely and aggravates existing arthritic conditions.
► *Jarring physical activity.* Sports that require players to jump and move around swiftly often lead to arthritis.

PRACTICAL ADVICE
Do not ignore clicking if accompanied by other symptoms. You may be suffering from a health problem requiring medical attention.

Watch your weight. This will help control the progression of arthritis, particularly in the hips and knees.

Play low-impact sports. Be gentle with your joints and minimize the risk of trauma.

Stretch and do muscle-building exercises. Ligaments and muscles stabilize the bones. If they are tight or weak, the joints are subject to more stress.

Stay in shape. The fitter you are, the more capable of activity you are likely to be.

Continue your regular activities. If your only symptom is clicking, there is no reason to stop any of your activities. In fact, inactivity will only lead to more serious symptoms.

WHEN TO CONSULT?
► You have been experiencing clicks in one or several joints for a long time. It is beginning to annoy you.
► The clicking is accompanied by pain, stiffness, locking of the joint, edema, or a feeling of joint dislocation.
► The clicking began after trauma.

WHAT HAPPENS DURING THE EXAM?

The doctor interviews the patient, focussing on personal and family history, and then performs a physical exam of the joints. Depending on the results, the physician orders an X-ray, an arthrographic test (involving the injection of coloured liquid into the joints), or arthroscopy (which uses a miniature camera to examine the inside of the joints). A scanner or magnetic resonance imaging (MRI) test may also be necessary.

WHAT IS THE TREATMENT?

Direct causes

If clicking is the only symptom, there is no danger and treatment is not necessary. Arthritis is treated directly. A joint mouse, dislocation or subluxation may require surgery. In the case of a subluxation of the jaw due to faulty occlusion or loose ligaments, a visit to the dentist is in order, where a dental plate may be inserted. Loose ligaments usually spontaneously tighten when the subject reaches his or her late twenties.

Indirect causes

The patient is usually advised to lose weight and engage in low impact physical activity.

Colic

Colic, a general term referring to intense abdominal pain, accounts for approximately 20% of all medical consultations. Colic is usually the result of strong intestinal contractions due to abdominal problems.

The pain, either diffused or localized, is most commonly experienced in the form of cramps and may be accompanied by constipation or diarrhea. The face frequently becomes quite pale, there may be excessive sweating and in rare cases, nausea, vomiting and headache. People suffering from irritable bowel syndrome (alternating diarrhea and constipation throughout the day) are particularly subject to colic.

There are two forms:

Acute colic:
► Intense and sudden abdominal pain.

Chronic colic:
► Constant or intermittent pain lasting over a week, and possibly as long as several months or years.

WHAT ARE THE CAUSES?
► *Lifestyle,* including overeating or over-consumption of alcohol. It may also be caused by bad dietary habits, such as eating only one large meal in the evening.
► *Excessive consumption* of certain foods, vitamins, dietary supplements or over-the-counter medications.
► *Medications such as laxatives, high doses of painkillers, and antiulcerative drugs.*
► *Illicit drugs* such as amphetamines (speed), barbiturates (goofballs), benzodiazepine (tranquilizers), cocaine, or solvents.
► *Migraine headaches* linked to irritable bowel syndrome.
► *Gastroenteritis or chronic constipation.*
► *Certain health problems* such as appendicitis, cholecystitis (inflammation of the gall bladder), gallstones, pancreatitis,

diverticulitis, gastroduodenal ulcer, or intestinal obstruction, among others.

▶ *Stress or psychosocial problems,* including divorce, the illness of a child, or the death of a loved one may lead to a somatic disorder (physical manifestation of emotional difficulty).

PRACTICAL ADVICE

Watch what you eat and drink. Alcohol, tea, coffee, soft drinks, excessive amounts of fibre, dairy products and berries all stimulate intestinal peristalsis (the activity of the intestines).

Avoid large quantities of fruit juice. Drink small amounts of juice at room temperature.

Avoid oral laxatives. Oral laxatives will only aggravate the problem, intensifying cramps and abdominal pain. Even mild laxatives should be avoided, especially if the origin of the colic is unknown. An enema is a safer option to deal with constipation. Kits are available in drugstores or can be easily prepared at home with a bulb syringe and warm, soapy water (soap, an irritant, will help provoke the evacuation of stool).

Avoid emetics. Self-induced vomiting can lead to regurgitation into the bronchi; avoid stimulating this reflex.

Avoid cold compresses on the abdomen. Cold constricts the blood vessels, making the cramps more intense. Apply heat to dilate the blood vessels, relax the muscles, and ease intestinal contractions. Use a hot water bottle, reusable compress, or heating pad.

Try to relax. Stress increases cramping. Although the pain may be significant, remember that the problem is probably not serious. You will feel a little better if you relax.

Get comfortable. Lying in a foetal position (on your side with your knees curled into your chest) relieves pressure on the muscle walls and can ease the pain a little.

Drink plenty of liquid. Diarrhea leads to dehydration; it is therefore important to drink plenty of water. Rice water helps form solid stool, and bouillon and flat 7-Up or ginger ale can be soothing. Mineral water replaces lost sodium and potassium, necessary for proper hydration and maintaining energy levels.

Liquid diets for young children with diarrhea or abdominal cramps. Replace regular food with Pedialyte or Gastrolyte, available over-the-counter in drugstores. The new, flavoured ice Pedialyte preparations taste better than before, and allow the formula to be absorbed at a slower, more continuous rate. A similar mixture can be prepared at home: mix 360 ml (12 ounces) of unsweetened orange juice with 600 ml (20 ounces) of water and half a level teaspoon of table salt. If there is no vomiting, have the child drink some of the solution every 20 to 30 minutes. If there is vomiting, drop 5 to 20 ml on the

---

Colicky babies

Outward signs of colic in babies include screaming and crying. The causes of infant colic include immature intestines, hunger, air in the intestine, and allergy to the milk proteins in baby formula. Colic attacks are generally most intense between the ages of three weeks and three months, and cease after six months.

Applying heat to the stomach generally soothes the baby. Some physicians recommend using a water bottle filled with warm (not boiling) water wrapped in a towel. The heat and pressure of the compress help ease the pain.

Remember that playing with the child will not distract him or her from the pain. A colicky baby should not be stimulated. Holding the baby against the chest to stop the crying is a tried and, in many cases, true method.

If food is the source of the problem, cow milk proteins should be eliminated for a short period of time. If the child is breast-fed, the mother should adapt her diet.

tongue (using a spoon or syringe) every 2 to 10 minutes. Keep the child on Pedialyte alone for 24 hours. Continue treatment for longer only if advised by a doctor. Never use orange juice substitutes.

Allow your digestive tract to rest. Fast for a few hours, but continue to drink plenty of liquids. Consult a doctor if you see no improvement.

Take acetaminophen. To relieve the pain, take one or two acetaminophen tablets (325 mg to 500 mg) four times a day. Do not exceed 4 grams daily. Anti-inflammatories (such as aspirin or ibuprofen) cause side effects and are not recommended.

See a doctor immediately if your condition gets worse. Use your judgement and intuition. Waiting too long before consulting may make the condition worse.

WHEN TO CONSULT?

► You have followed all the tips listed above but nothing has helped.
► The pain becomes intolerable.
► Lying in a foetal position is the only way you can get any relief from the pain.
► The pain is so intense you cannot remain still. You do not feel comfortable in any position.
► Your urine is very concentrated or red in colour.
► The pain radiates to the back or other parts of the body.

Consult immediately if:
► Your stomach becomes bloated or hard.
► You are unable to swallow food and liquid or to keep anything down.
► Other symptoms develop, such as nausea, vomiting, diarrhea, constipation, or rapid breathing.

WHAT HAPPENS DURING THE EXAM?

The doctor interviews the patient, checks vital signs (pulse, blood pressure, respiratory and heart rhythms, etc.), and performs an abdominal and digital rectal exam. Women may require a digital vaginal examination. Blood tests, abdominal X-rays or ultrasound, and intravenous solutions are routine procedure. Endoscopy and radiology imaging tests may be required, as well as a lung X-ray. In some cases, the doctor performs a second physical exam and orders further blood tests to confirm the diagnosis.

WHAT IS THE TREATMENT?

The doctor may prescribe a liquid diet lasting a few hours or days. The patient will probably be advised to change general eating habits to smaller portions of easily digested foods.

The physician may prescribe acetaminophen or antispasmodics. Medications such as opiates and codeine must be avoided as they cause intestinal paralysis.

In serious cases (such as appendicitis, acute diverticulitis, intestinal obstruction or pancreatitis), hospitalization and surgery are necessary.

If the doctor believes the problem is psychosomatic, he or she will help the patient become aware of the underlying issue and take steps to resolve it.

Conditions Affecting the Anal Region

Pain, bleeding, lumps, and itchiness are the most common symptoms experienced in the anal region. Contrary to popular belief, they are not always caused by hemorrhoids, but may be the result of a fissure, abscess, ulcer, marisca, or condyloma, among other more rare causes.

WHAT ARE THE CAUSES?

Pain with or without bleeding.

► *Thrombosed hemorrhoid.* A clot may form inside an external hemorrhoid and provoke sharp stabbing pain. The clot may rupture under pressure (most commonly during defecation), which will ease the pain but cause bleeding.

► *Anal fissure.* Pain occurring at the moment of defecation or immediately after is a characteristic symptom of anal fissures. The small tear in the mucous membrane is usually caused by the passage of a hard stool. In many cases, traces of blood can be seen on the toilet paper or surface of the stools.

► *Anal abscess.* Small glands of unknown function located around the anus drain through very narrow interior canals. If one of these canals becomes obstructed, the gland becomes infected and an abscess forms. The pain is constant, increases gradually, and is not associated with the evacuation of stools. In most cases, there is no bleeding.

► *Anal ulcer.* This type of ulcer is a small hole that may cause pain but does not lead to bleeding. It may result from herpes, cancer, or anal sex.

Bleeding with no pain

► *Internal hemorrhoids.* Hemorrhoids are veins near the anus and rectum that gradually become dilated with repeated strain (defecation or childbirth, for example). This painless dilation first occurs inside the rectum and is indicated by the presence of bright red blood on the underwear, toilet paper or in the toilet bowl.

► *Benign or malignant rectal or colonic tumours or polyps.* Early detection and treatment of malignant polyps can avoid serious, even fatal, complications. Bleeding may be apparent (blood in the stool) or invisible (indicated by anemia or detected in a screening test). In some cases, there is a change in the shape or size of the stool.

Lumps or swelling

► *External hemorrhoids.* Physical exertion may cause hemorrhoids to protrude out of the anal opening. Detectable to the touch, they may be the size of a pea or even an egg. Although they are usually not painful, they may cause some discomfort and itching. There is usually no bleeding.

► *Marisca.* Most lumps in the anal region are caused by stretched skin tissue and do not cause pain or bleeding. They usually occur after a hemorrhoidal thrombosis clot has been reabsorbed, or if there is a chronic anal fissure.

► *Condylomata.* Almost always transmitted sexually, these are caused by a virus contained in the secretions of the partner. The small bumps can be found in the anal area even if there has been no anal contact, as the moist folds of skin in the area encourage viral growth.

► *Persistent anal lump.* This may be cancer of the anus, an extremely rare condition.

► *Thrombosed hemorrhoid.*

Itching

► *Poor hygiene.*

► *Excessive hygiene.*

► *Too much coffee.* Caffeine increases nerve-ending sensitivity

► *Prolonged use of corticosteroid creams and ointments.* Used to soothe the itching, these products can actually create a vicious circle. Because the cream is applied in a location with little exposure to the air (between the buttocks), it does not evaporate and greater quantities are absorbed into the skin. This can lead to increased itchiness and scratching that damages the tissue and aggravates the lesions, as well as to the appearance of a gluteal granuloma (small nodule). Using more cream to soothe the itching only begins the cycle again.

▸ *Various conditions or diseases,* such as diabetes, yeast infections, parasites (worms), hemorrhoids.

PRACTICAL ADVICE

Pain

Take warm or lukewarm sitzbaths. This will help the clot re-absorb in cases of hemorrhoidal thrombosis and relieve the pain of anal sphincter spasms due to anal fissures.

Take painkillers. Take one or two acetaminophen tablets (325 mg to 500 mg) four times a day, never exceeding 4 grams daily. Anti-inflammatories can also ease the pain; follow the dosage recommended by the manufacturer. Take both medications if the pain is difficult to control.

Treat hemorrhoid pain. Hemorrhoids and thrombosed hemorrhoids can be treated with Anurex suppositories, which anesthetize the area and cause the veins to constrict, reducing inflammation. The product, sold over the counter in pharmacies, should be stored in the refrigerator. Another helpful product is Tucks, which consists of small, round, easily-applied pads that are medicated with calamine and hamamelis for their analgesic properties. These are also sold without prescription in pharmacies.

Apply zinc oxide. While most creams or ointments do not treat the underlying problem, zinc oxide (a cream frequently used to treat diaper rash) effectively protects and moisturizes, soothing pain and preventing various problems from developing. Avoid corticosteroid products, as they will lead to tissue damage and persistent itching.

Soften the stool. Eat foods rich in fibre, such as fruit, vegetables, legumes, whole wheat cereals, and nuts. Drink 6 to 8 glasses of water every day. Add a fibre supplement if necessary.

Don't spend too long on the toilet. If you still haven't passed a stool after a few minutes, get up, do something else, and try again later. Don't just sit and read—remaining in this position for a long time and repeatedly straining leads to congestion of the hemorrhoidal veins and can aggravate your symptoms.

Apply hot compresses to an abscess. If you think you have an abscess, consult a doctor, who will drain it, if necessary. In the meantime, hot compresses can provide partial pain relief.

Itchiness

Avoid scratching. This may be difficult, but remember that scratching will only aggravate the problem.

Clean and dry yourself thoroughly (but don't rub). After passing a stool, sponge the anus with a wet tissue—do not rub—and then pat dry with a tissue or use a blow dryer.

Wear cotton underwear. White underwear is best, since the dyes in coloured underwear can cause or aggravate itchiness. Wash with unscented laundry detergent.

Avoid long-term use of corticosteroid creams and ointments. Although they can provide temporary relief, prolonged use can lead to chronic anal itching. Use zinc oxide instead.

Take warm or lukewarm sitzbaths. This will help the clot re-absorb in cases of hemorrhoidal thrombosis and relieve the pain of anal sphincter spasms due to anal fissures.

Avoid using soap. Excessive use of soap or vigorous rubbing while washing can irritate the skin.

Do not wear tight clothing. Avoid wearing tight jeans or thongs, with a seam or band between the buttocks.

WHEN TO CONSULT?

► You notice blood in your stool. This must be checked by a doctor and should not be treated until the cause has been identified.

► You notice a change in the size or regularity of your stool, or have difficulty evacuating.

► You notice an anal lump or sore that does not heal, or experience persistent anal pain.

► You have an anal abscess or ulcer.

► You continue to experience pain or bleeding upon defecation, even after constipation has resolved.

► You suspect you may have parasites (worms).

WHAT HAPPENS DURING THE EXAM?

The doctor takes a detailed history of your symptoms and intestinal habits. He or she will perform a clinical examination, including a digital rectal examination (using the finger), and in some cases, administer an anuscopy, rectoscopy, colonoscopy and barium enema. Anuscopies, rectoscopies and colonoscopies are performed either with rigid instruments or fibre optics, which are inserted into the intestine via the anus to investigate the area and, if necessary, take small samples. A biopsy is performed if cancer or herpes is suspected.

WHAT IS THE TREATMENT?

Hemorrhoids and thrombosed hemorrhoids

In the vast majority of cases, thrombosed hemorrhoids spontaneously re-absorb, within a few days of which the pain and swelling disappear. In some cases, pain is treated with high doses of ibuprofen or analgesic or cortisone creams; in others, the doctor must pierce the thrombosis with a surgical knife to relieve the pressure, ease the pain and begin the healing process. Bleeding internal hemorrhoids are often ligated, using a specialized instrument to grip the hemorrhoid and wrap a tight rubber band around it. This prevents the blood from circulating, causing the hemorrhoid to atrophy, dry out and fall off. Although this treatment is painless for internal hemorrhoids, it is too painful for external ones. In the latter case, the physician will prescribe creams and if they are very large, surgery will be required.

Anal fissure

In most cases, a diet rich in fibre and water will clear up anal fissures after a few days, although they can become chronic for unknown reasons. If persistent or recurrent, surgery or drugs may be necessary.

Anal abscess

To stop the pain, anal abscesses must be drained. Although this may occur spontaneously, minor surgery under local anesthesia is usually necessary.

Anal ulcer

The underlying cause determines the appropriate treatment. If caused by anal sex, the ulcer will heal on its own. The doctor may recommend the patient use a lubricating cream.

Benign or malignant tumours or polyps

Anal polyps that cause symptoms are removed in a minor surgical procedure. Rectal polyps can also be removed, in most cases. If the tumour is benign, the appropriate treatment will be immediately undertaken.

Marisca

No treatment is necessary. If the symptoms are severe, they may be surgically removed.

Condyloma

The infected cells containing the virus must be destroyed using chemicals, electrocauterization, cryotherapy, or laser. Complete treatment requires several sessions and the follow up should last several months. The patient must practice safe sex until the condylomata are completely gone, as they are sexually transmitted.

Various diseases causing itching

The itching can be relieved by treating the underlying ailment, whether it is diabetes, yeast infection, or parasites (worms). In many cases, the precise cause cannot be determined, and treatment will take the form of the practical advice listed above.

Conditions Affecting the Penis

Problems affecting the penis can manifest in three ways: pain, abnormal discharge, or prolonged erection without sexual desire, known as priapism. Contrary to popular belief, priapism is not a sign of sexual virility, but rather a potentially serious erectile problem.

Symptoms related to Peyronie's disease

- Pain at the time of erection. In rare cases, there is pain even when not erect.
- Development of a plaque of fibrous scar tissue detectable to the touch, causing the penis to curve; after this stage, the pain diminishes.
- In some cases, the curvature prevents penetration.

Symptoms related to trauma

- Intense pain.
- May be accompanied by a cracking sound at the moment of trauma, swelling of the penis at the site, bluish discoloration, or internal or external tears.
- In the case of a ruptured urethra, intermittent discharge of blood (depending on the fullness of the bladder). If the urethra is only partially ruptured, the man can continue to urinate normally, although it is more difficult to control the direction of the flow. If the rupture is complete, he is unable to urinate and will experience abdominal pain.

Abnormal discharge

- Discharge may be transparent, yellowish, bloody, greenish, very thick (in the case of gonorrhea), or sticky and clear (Chlamydia).
- It may be accompanied by pain in the urethra upon urination.

Priapism

▶ Prolonged erection (longer than four hours), not provoked by sexual desire; failure of blood to drain from the penis back into the circulatory system.

▶ Persistent pain, even when not engaging in sexual activity.

▶ Sudden onset of pain, possibly following sexual intercourse.

WHAT ARE THE CAUSES?

Peyronie's disease

▶ *Repeated light trauma* during sexual relations is a possible explanation for the development of fibrous scar tissue in the penis, which prevents penile expansion during erection and causes the penis to bend. This is the most common cause of pain felt in the penis.

Trauma

▶ *"Fractured penis."* This term is used to describe a rupture of the rigid tunica (membrane) under the skin of the penis that plays a role in erection. This injury can occur due to an improperly positioned penis during sexual intercourse or excessively vigorous sexual relations.

▶ *Ruptured or lacerated urethra.*

Abnormal discharge

▶ *Sexually transmitted infections* are the most common causes of abnormal discharge from the penis, with Chlamydia infection ranking as number one. With some infections, the source is located in the throat or anus, and can therefore be transmitted orally or through anal–genital contact. The Chlamydia virus has an incubation period of two to four weeks (sometimes more) after contact, during which the carrier remains asymptomatic. The symptoms of gonorrhea appear two to five days after contact.

▶ *Persistent prostate fluid discharge.* This is very rare and is not usually associated with a disease.

Priapism

► *Self-administered medications* injected directly into the penis to treat erectile dysfunction (such as papaverine or prostaglandin E_1).

► *Internal or external trauma* of the penis rupturing an artery. This increases blood flow to the penis and the organ does not have the capacity to absorb it all.

► *Oral medications,* including certain psychotropic, neuroleptic and anticoagulant drugs.

► *Predisposing factors,* such as diabetes or African or Mediterranean ancestry.

PRACTICAL ADVICE

Peyronie's disease
Do not go into hiding. Discuss your worries with your doctor before giving up sex altogether. He or she should be able to reassure you about resuming a normal sex life.

Trauma
See your doctor immediately. If the trauma is minor, wrap ice in a towel and apply it directly to the site. Avoid sexual relations and take your usual painkillers.

Remember: sex is not an Olympic event. Be gentle with yourself.

Abnormal discharge
Abstain from sexual intercourse of any kind. Remember that condoms can break, and you could still infect your partner.

Complete the treatment prescribed. Do not attempt to treat yourself. Take the full course of medications even if the symptoms disappear. Stopping treatment increases the risk of recurrence.

Maintain good hygiene. Wash with soap and water frequently (four times a day until discharge ceases). To prevent recurrence, always wear a condom when you have sexual intercourse.

Priapism
Try to drain the penis of blood. Apply ice wrapped in a towel. Ejaculation might provide some relief, if it is possible. If no change occurs within an hour, go to the hospital. This condition can cause damage to the erectile tissues.

WHEN TO CONSULT?
► You have suffered trauma to the penis.
► You feel pain at the time of erection.
► Your penis bends when erect.
► You have trouble urinating, or are unable to urinate.
► There is abnormal discharge from the penis.

WHAT HAPPENS DURING THE EXAM?
The doctor will thoroughly assess any trauma, even if minor. If Peyronie's disease is suspected, the patient will undergo a physical examination and detailed interview.

Testing for sexually transmitted infections requires a culture from the secretions. Samples are taken by inserting a swab into the urethra, a process that generally causes discomfort in the patient. A Chlamydia test requires a morning urine sample. The patient must inform all his partners and they too must be tested. In cases of prostate fluid discharge, a urine analysis will be ordered, even though this condition is rarely associated with infections.

WHAT IS THE TREATMENT?
Peyronie's disease
If the curvature in the penis is not pronounced and sexual inter-course is possible, no treatment is necessary. The problem should resolve on its own within a year, the scarred tissue regaining its elasticity. If the condition worsens, high doses of vitamin E (an antioxidant) and ultrasound treatment may help. If the curvature is significant, the fibrous tissues can be surgically removed and the penis straightened. The condition is almost always benign.

Trauma

Serious trauma (such as a ruptured artery, a large tear of the inner tunica, or a "fractured penis") requires immediate attention. Delay may allow scarring to take place, definitively robbing the penis of elasticity and rendering surgery ineffective. Unsightly scars, a deviated penis (making penetration impossible), or, in rare cases, erectile dysfunction are possible consequences.

Abnormal discharge

Sexually transmitted infections are always treated with antibiotics. Urethritis and prostate fluid discharge are benign and do not usually require treatment.

Priapism

If treated within four hours, there is no risk of damage to erectile function. Without treatment, there is a 25% to 75% risk of tissue necrosis, depending on the time elapsed before consultation. The doctor may choose to aspirate the blood from the penis and inject medication. If this treatment fails, he or she may resort to surgery to encourage blood circulation. Relapses are possible. Of course, if the condition was caused by a specific drug, the patient should stop taking the medication.

Conditions Affecting the Skin of the Feet

Skin conditions on the feet are rarely serious, but they certainly can be annoying!

The most common symptoms are the following:
- Strong, persistent odour.
- Skin between the toes is cracked, red and itchy. It may also be macerated (white and slightly puffy, as though the feet have been soaking in water).
- Irritation and red blotches.
- Blisters, corns and calluses.

WHAT ARE THE CAUSES?

Strong, persistent odour
- *Poor hygiene.*
- *Intense physical activity.*
- *Bacteria* (Corynebacterium minutissimum) causing a change in sweat molecules leading to strong and persistent odour.
- *Skin reactions* to certain shoes or socks.

Cracked skin between the toes, itchiness, macerated skin, redness
- *Athlete's foot* is caused by a contagious yeast infection. Damp environments and perspiration create a breeding ground for yeast.

Itchiness, irritation and red blotches
- *Allergies* to products used in the manufacture of shoes, coloured socks, nylon stockings, scented moisturizing creams, etc.
- *Yeast infection, eczema, hives, and other forms of dermatitis.* If the symptoms appear on the top of the foot, the problem is probably dermatitis, since this area has very few sweat glands. However, if the symptoms develop on the sole of the foot, it is very likely a yeast infection.

Blisters, corns and calluses

- **Obesity.** Excess weight compresses the tissues on the sole of the foot.
- **Shoes.** Narrow or high-heeled footwear puts excessive pressure on the feet. Repeated rubbing leads to a thickening of the skin under the toes (corns), under the foot, or in between the toes (calluses). The lesions sometimes resemble warts.

PRACTICAL ADVICE

Strong, persistent odour and athlete's foot

Maintain good hygiene. Humidity creates a breeding ground for bacteria and yeast. After washing your feet and toes thoroughly with antibacterial soap, be sure to dry them well. Trim your toenails every two or three days, but be careful not to cut them too short as this can lead to ingrown toenails.

Avoid spreading the infection. Athlete's foot is contagious. Clean your bathtub well after using it and never share your towels, socks or shoes with others. Do not walk around barefoot, and always wear bath sandals in public showers and locker rooms.

After the infection is cured. After medical treatment clears up the infection, care is needed to avoid re-infection. Use tinctures, such as 1% mercurochrome or tincture of iodine between the toes once or twice a day to help the drying process. Continue until the skin between the toes is completely dry. Dry skin scales still harbour yeast, and must be removed. Use a brush to scrub your toes and feet.

Take care of your feet. Before putting on socks, sprinkle your feet and toes with corn starch or an unscented antifungal powder. An aluminum chlorohydrate-based antiperspirant can also be used, though it should be avoided in cases of athlete's foot, as it can cause a burning sensation.

Socks. 100% cotton socks are the most absorbent. Sprinkle the inside with corn starch or antifungal powder. If possible, change your socks two or three times a day.

Shoes. Wear open-toed leather shoes or sandals as much as possible. Boots and running shoes do not allow air to circulate very well, creating a hot and sweaty environment for the feet. Avoid wearing them all day long and never wear them without socks. To fight odour, use activated-charcoal insoles (buy them at a drugstore or from your shoemaker), and to ensure your shoes are well-ventilated, remove the laces and pull out the tongue after you take them off. Avoid wearing the same shoes two days in a row. Sprinkle the inside of your shoes before putting them on, or try spraying them with a disinfectant to kill yeast spores. Ask your pharmacist for advice about the products.

Relax. Many people sweat profusely when they are stressed. Plan leisure time and take care of yourself.

Eat less spicy food. People who eat a lot of strong-smelling food (spicy dishes or onions, for example) may find the same strong odours emanating from the sweat glands in their feet.

Itchiness, irritation and red blotches
Is it an allergy? Although extremely uncommon, some people are allergic to products used in the manufacturing of shoes, socks, nylon stockings, or moisturizing cream. Avoid using the item that may be causing the reaction for a few days and if the blotches and itchiness disappear, stop using it altogether.

Apply cream. Cortisone-based cream, available over-the-counter in drugstores, can be very soothing. But be careful: this product is to be avoided if you are suffering from a yeast infection, as cortisone effects the immune system and encourages the propagation of yeast. If you are not absolutely sure, consult your doctor.

Avoid scented products. Scented powders and antiperspirants can irritate the skin between the toes and cause eczema.

Blisters, corns and calluses

React quickly. As soon as you notice the skin thickening, massage your feet with lanolin. This will soften the skin and make it less sensitive to pressure.

Protect your feet and toes from pressure. A small adhesive bandage (Band-Aid) or dressing can stop the rubbing in one area. Cotton or gauze can be used to separate the toes.

Have your shoes widened. This will help reduce pressure and friction between the toes. See your shoemaker.

Always wear socks with shoes. Going barefoot in shoes increases friction on the skin of your feet.

Remove corns and calluses. Special bandages medicated with salicylic acid will soften the corn or callus. Follow the instructions (note that diabetics should not use this product). Soaking your feet in hot water is also an effective way to soften the skin. Use a nail file or pumice stone to rub the corn or callus lightly, removing the outer layers. Note that rubbing too hard or frequently will thicken the skin even more. Do this no more than once a week. Apply a cream containing 20% urea (Uremol 20%) to soften the skin. Corns can also be trimmed using a razor blade, but this must be done very carefully to avoid cutting yourself and possibly causing infection. Your podiatrist or doctor will show you the correct technique.

Do not burst blisters. Wait until the lymphatic fluid is absorbed by the body. Blisters are the skin's way of protecting itself. The inside is a naturally sterile environment, and as long as it is not broken, there can be no infection. Blisters also encourage the scarring process, making the skin less sensitive. If one bursts accidentally, apply an antibiotic ointment and a bandage.

WHEN TO CONSULT?

► Strong foot odour persists, despite your best efforts.

► Athlete's foot recurs, accompanied by other symptoms, such as swollen feet, fever, and infected fissures.
► You suspect a yeast infection.
► Your dermatitis does not go away.
► Corns and calluses do not disappear.

WHAT HAPPENS DURING THE EXAM?

The doctor will perform a complete dermatological exam of your feet.

WHAT IS THE TREATMENT?

Strong, persistent odour

The doctor will prescribe an antibiotic lotion containing erythromycin to eliminate the bacteria responsible for odours.

Athlete's foot

Antifungal pills or cream treatments are effective.

Yeast infections and dermatitis

Antifungal treatments are used for yeast infections. Creams with high cortisone content are prescribed for dermatitis.

Corns and calluses

The doctor can trim corns or calluses with a razor blade or a scalpel. Orthotics are used in tough cases.

Constipation

Constipation occurs when stools are blocked in the rectum or the sigmoid colon (positioned just ahead of the rectum). It frequently leads to an accumulation of gas above the fecal block, which may cause pain or discomfort.

Some people say they are suffering from constipation if they have hard stool that is difficult to evacuate, whether or not the actual evacuation is painful. Others say they are constipated if they do not have bowel movements at least twice a week. In fact, constipation is defined more in terms of the discomfort experienced. It is not a hereditary condition, although a familial tendency has been observed. It is more common in women than in men.

Constipation manifests in the following ways:
- Abdominal discomfort (gas, cramps or bloating).
- In some cases, hemorrhoids or blood in the stool (caused by hemorrhoids) or, very rarely, colon cancer.

WHAT ARE THE CAUSES?
- *Insufficient Dietary Fibre.*
- *Lack Of Physical Activity.*
- *Stress* is a rare cause, but can change the natural contractions of the intestines.
- *Change of environment.*
- *Bad habits or excessive modesty* causing people to restrain themselves from having bowel movements.
- *Surplus iron in diet.*
- *Certain medications,* especially drugs for psychiatric conditions, high blood pressure, and those containing codeine.
- *Certain diseases* such as irritable bowel syndrome, lazy colon (an intestinal motility disorder), colon cancer, hypothyroidism and diabetes.

PRACTICAL ADVICE

Do not ignore the call of nature. Stool evacuation is a conditioned reflex that is usually triggered in the morning, often by the first sip or even smell of coffee. Many people, however, feel too rushed, do not answer the call, and lose their reflex as a result. Fortunately, it can be recovered. Bring your coffee into the bathroom along with some reading material, and relax. After a few days, everything should return to normal. If, however, you are suffering from hemorrhoids, do not stay on the toilet too long. This can put pressure on the hemorrhoid and cause it to emerge, leading to pain and possibly bleeding. In children, constipation is usually caused by bad eating habits and the tendency to ignore the call of nature in preference for more enjoyable activities.

Get moving. All you need is minimal physical activity to keep the digestive system healthy.

Consume more fibre and liquid. Fibre can be taken in natural form or supplements, such as Metamucil or Prodiem. Increase the amount of liquids consumed along with fibre to avoid aggravating the constipation.

Eat rhubarb. Fresh rhubarb stalks are an effective cure for constipation.

Watch what your children eat. Be sure they have enough fibre in their diets.

Check your medications. Certain medications (particularly antidepressants) cause constipation. Talk to your doctor.

WHEN TO CONSULT?

► There are unexplained changes in the consistency of your stools and the frequency of your bowel movements, possibly accompanied by abdominal pain.

► You are over 50 years old and you notice changes in the consistency of your stools and frequency of your bowel movements, possibly accompanied by blood in the stool.

WHAT HAPPENS DURING THE EXAM?

The doctor may order a barium enema or a colonoscopy to screen for a colon disorder or blockage caused by a cancerous tumour or pre-cancerous polyp. In patients over the age of 50, these exams are almost always required because of the increased risk of cancer. The doctor will also perform a complete health assessment to check for organic causes such as hypothyroidism or diabetes. In the rare cases where lazy colon is suspected, more in-depth tests will be ordered.

WHAT IS THE TREATMENT?

Insufficient dietary fibre

If the colon is anatomically normal, the first stage of treatment involves modifying eating habits. Most North Americans do not eat enough fibre. The amount required for healthy digestion is an average of 25 grams a day in the form of fruit, vegetables or whole grains (found in bran cereals or brown bread). Many do not drink enough liquid, either. Four to six large glasses of water are recommended. Because the elderly tend to eat less in general, they are frequently advised to take fibre supplements such as Metamucil or Prodiem.

Lack of physical exercise, surplus iron in diet, certain medications

People with sedentary lifestyles are advised to get more physical exercise. The doctor will also check the levels of iron in the diet and type of medications the patient may be taking, and make the necessary corrections. If these efforts are not successful, the doctor will begin by prescribing mild laxatives (glycerin suppositories or milk of magnesia). Stool softeners will also facilitate evacuation. As a last resort, the doctor will prescribe laxatives, possibly in the form of teas, containing senna (the active ingredient in 90% of marketed laxatives). These products must be administered with care, since senna is addictive.

Irritable bowel syndrome
Healthy digestive habits (good hydration and dietary fibre, in particular) can alleviate the symptoms.

Tonic dystonia
In the rare cases that drug treatment is unsuccessful, surgery may be required.

Colon cancer
Treatment (including surgery, radiation therapy, chemotherapy) is undertaken immediately.

Cough

Coughing is a defence mechanism against an outside assault on the body. The throat, trachea (windpipe) and respiratory airways all have receptors that send a message to the brain when stimulated. The brain responds by issuing a command to the muscles to contract and produce a cough. This is what happens when someone chokes on food, breathes in cold air (directly irritating the trachea), or inhales an irritant.

WHAT ARE THE CAUSES?

Acute cough

- *Viral or bacterial infection.* Cold, flu, bronchitis and pneumonia cause inflammation of the throat and the bronchi that is often accompanied by fever, muscle aches or stiffness, nasal congestion and expectoration (sputum).
- *False croup* primarily occurs during cold weather and describes a benign inflammation of the larynx (voice box) caused by an airborne virus or bacteria. False croup manifests in a barking cough, wheezing with inhalation (stridor), hoarseness, fever, and difficulty breathing. Children five-years-old and younger are primarily affected because their immune systems are less developed and secretions block their smaller larynxes more easily. Because false croup and epiglottiditis, a much more serious condition, have similar symptoms, a doctor should be consulted immediately.
- *Epiglottiditis* is a very serious bacterial infection of the epiglottis and the throat that can lead to asphyxiation if not treated immediately. It affects young children and symptoms include a barking cough, stridor (noisy, high-pitched wheezing), loss of voice, sore throat, and fever. The child may need to sit down to inhale. This is an emergency.
- *Whooping cough* is a contagious infection caused by a specific bacterium, Bordet-Gengou bacilli. The disease is characterized by fits of dry coughing interspersed with long, wheezing gasps upon inhalation that produce a "whooping" sound. While it is a relatively uncommon disease (most children are vaccinated

against it at an early age), in children under six months and the elderly, it is a serious disease and constitutes a medical emergency.

Chronic cough (longer than a month)

► *Posterior rhionorrhea* describes the discharge of nasal secretions from the base of the throat, often caused by sinusitis or chronic rhinitis (inflammation of the mucous membrane lining the nose). Rhinitis can also be caused by allergies (pets, pollen, dust mites).

► *Asthma* is an inflammatory disease of the bronchi, leading to thickened secretions and a contraction of the bronchial tubes. It manifests in the form of a cough (with or without sputum), wheezing, and shortness of breath. The cough is usually triggered by bronchial irritants (cold, smoke, strong odours, laughter) and sometimes causes asthmatics to wake up during the night. Asthma can result from an allergic reaction (to animal hair, for example). In some cases (particularly children), coughing is the only symptom.

► *Chronic bronchitis* is a disease usually caused by smoking. It is characterized by a moist cough and expectorations resulting from an inflammation of the respiratory airways. Secretions are more common in the morning. As the disease progresses, wheezing and shortness of breath can develop. Non-smokers who inhale large amounts of second-hand smoke can also develop chronic bronchitis, but this is rare.

► *Pulmonary emphysema* refers to the most advanced stage of chronic bronchitis and is characterized by a dry cough, difficulty expectorating, and shortness of breath.

► *Gastroesophageal reflux disease (GERD).* In this condition, gastric acid flows back into the esophagus, irritating the windpipe and precipitating a dry cough. GERD can also be accompanied by heartburn and a bitter taste in the mouth.

► *Certain drugs,* such as angiotensin-converting enzyme (ACE) inhibitors used in the management of hypertension, sometimes produce a dry cough. Beta-blockers for the treatment of angina and hypertension have a similar effect and can aggravate asthma. In some cases, the cough persists even after treatment comes to an end.

► *Lung cancer and tumour.* Lung cancer sometimes manifests in a cough with sputum that may contain blood, along with shortness of breath and fatigue. Smokers need to pay special attention to these symptoms. Tumours obstructing the trachea and the respiratory tract (such as those caused by throat cancer) can cause a chronic cough with or without sputum.

► *Heart failure* causes shortness of breath, as well as coughing at night and with exertion.

► *Hypersensitivity pneumonia.* Contact with certain birds, namely parrots and pigeons, moldy hay, or certain chemical products can induce a pulmonary defence mechanism in the form of a cough, shortness of breath, fatigue and weight loss. Fever is also often a symptom.

► *Tics.* Some people develop a habit of coughing in certain circumstances (for example, when they are nervous, self-conscious, anxious, or stressed). This is similar to compulsive throat clearing.

PRACTICAL ADVICE

Acute cough

Drink plenty of fluids. Water, juice and hot drinks help loosen secretions and promote expectoration. Four to six glasses of liquids a day will help ease congestion if you have an infection.

Use a cough suppressant. Cough suppressants are occasionally recommended for acute, dry coughs. The best formulations contain codeine or a codeine derivative. Dextromethorphan is also effective.

Cough to remove secretions. It is best to expectorate secretions and eliminate them from the body. Note that expectorant syrups generally have little effect.

Chronic cough

Stop smoking. Smoking is the major cause of chronic coughing. A smoking-related cough decreases significantly one to two weeks after quitting and, in more than 50% of cases, entirely disappears. Do not worry if the cough worsens in the first few days. Smoking thickens bronchial secretions, thereby paralyzing the vibrating cilia that move secretions up. When the smoker quits, the sputum becomes more liquid, allowing the cilia to do their job more effectively again. Coughing and expectorating calm down as the body gets rid of the secretions.

Do not tolerate second-hand smoke. Non-smokers need not abide someone smoking in their presence.

WHEN TO CONSULT?

- ► Your cough lasts longer than a week or grows worse from day to day.
- ► Your cough wakes you up at night.
- ► Your cough is accompanied by chest wheezing or shortness of breath.
- ► Your fever lasts more than three or four days.
- ► You are spitting up blood.
- ► You think you have an allergy.
- ► You suspect your medications are making you cough.
- ► Your general condition deteriorates.
- ► You suspect your child has whooping cough or epiglottiditis.

WHAT HAPPENS DURING THE EXAM?

The doctor will take a thorough history and conduct a complete physical examination. He or she may order some additional tests, including a chest X-ray, skin allergy tests, respiratory tests, blood work and, less frequently, a bronchoscopy. A bronchoscopy examines the bronchi by means of a slender tubular instrument with a small light on the end.

WHAT IS THE TREATMENT?

Acute cough
Infection
For viral infections, like a cold or flu, the sufferer should treat the symptoms and be patient. Drugs are only prescribed in very rare cases. A bacterial infection, like acute bronchitis or pneumonia,

is treated with antibiotics. Codeine or one of its derivatives may occasionally be used temporarily to relieve your cough.

False croup
In some cases, vasoconstrictors will be prescribed to make breathing easier as well as anti-inflammatories to reduce the swelling of the larynx.

Epiglottiditis
The patient is hospitalized and receives antibiotics to clear up the infection. In some cases, the patient must be intubated (have a tube inserted into the larynx) to facilitate breathing.

Whooping cough
Whooping cough is treated with antibiotics, notably to keep the contagion in check.

Chronic cough
Posterior rhinorrhea
Nasal discharges are treated with antihistamines and, if need be, spray-form corticosteroids (steroids). If an allergy is responsible for the discharge, the allergen will be identified and eliminated.

Asthma
Asthma is managed first by eliminating the cause (if an allergy is responsible), then with bronchodilators and anti-inflammatories.

Chronic bronchitis and pulmonary emphysema
Quitting smoking will relieve the symptoms. Use bronchodilators and take antibiotics, if necessary.

Gastroesophageal reflux disease (GERD)
GERD, usually caused by poor eating habits and obesity, can be managed by a change in lifestyle. Antacids can be prescribed for serious cases.

Certain drugs
You may require a change of prescription, but do not discontinue treatment without consulting a doctor first.

Lung cancer and tumour
The appropriate treatment (chemotherapy, radiation therapy, or surgery) is immediately undertaken.

Heart failure
Heart failure is managed by limiting fluid intake, controlling blood pressure, and administering the appropriate treatment.

Hypersensitivity pneumonia
The cause determines the treatment. Cortisone may be prescribed.

Tics
There is no physical treatment for this behaviour. It is up to the patient to control it.

Diarrhea/Gastroenteritis

Some people have bowel movements three times a day; others, three times a week. The frequency depends on each person's rate of intestinal activity. Diarrhea—also known as gastroenteritis—is characterized by an increase in the frequency and fluidity of stools. It is not a disease, but rather a sign that the intestine is flushing out bacteria, a virus or parasites.

There are different forms of diarrhea:

Acute gastroenteritis
► Usually accompanied by abdominal cramps and an urgent need to defecate.
► Sometimes accompanied by vomiting.
► Lasts three to four days. Usually does not cause dehydration.
► There is a higher risk of dehydration if the diarrhea lasts longer than a week, particularly in children under three years of age and adults over the age of 60.
► Symptoms of dehydration include dry mouth and diminished urination (even if the sufferer maintains or increases consumption of liquids).

Chronic diarrhea
► Lasts longer than three weeks.
► Sometimes leads to weight loss and anemia (causing very pale skin).

Paradoxical (false) diarrhea
► Increased frequency of stools (normal consistency).
► May be accompanied by abdominal cramps.

Travelers' diarrhea ("turista")
► Lasts four or five days. May occur after returning from a trip.
► May be accompanied by abdominal cramps, fever, and vomiting.

► Travelers in developing countries, campers, children under the age of five, and young adults are particularly at risk.

WHAT ARE THE CAUSES?

Acute gastroenteritis

► *Viruses and bacteria* in water and food (especially meat, seafood, eggs, cheese, and mayonnaise). Buffet and food sold at public events, as well as fast-food may be contaminated by frequent handling. Re-heating does not destroy bacteria.

► *Viruses and bacteria* transmitted through contact with animals and humans. Daycare centres and hospitals for the chronically ill present the highest risk. Anal sex, sexual contact with prostitutes, and sharing syringes are also risky.

► *Gastric surgery* decreases gastric acid, lowering the body's defenses against bacteria.

► *Lactose intolerance.* Lactose is found in dairy products.

► *Antibiotics and antacids* containing magnesium (Maalox, for example) may cause acute gastroenteritis, along with laxatives, diuretics, and certain other medications.

Chronic diarrhea

► *Chronic inflammation* of the intestine due to food intolerance or parasites.

► *Gallbladder surgery* may cause a bile leakage in the intestines leading to diarrhea.

► *Psychological origin.* For example, certain psychological conditions may lead to laxative abuse.

Paradoxical (false) diarrhea

► *Irritated colon* caused by medication.

► *Anal incontinence.*

► *Over-consumption of certain foods* with laxative properties, such as prunes, strawberries, and hot peppers.

► *Nervousness.*

Travelers' diarrhea ("turista")

▶ *Bacteria, viruses or parasites* in the water or food.
▶ *Change in eating habits.*
▶ *Jet lag.*
▶ *Fatigue.*

PRACTICAL ADVICE

Drink plenty of liquids. This will not aggravate the condition. Even if you do not feel thirsty, it is important to avoid dehydration, especially in young children. Drink water, beef stock, juice, flat 7-Up (it is often all children will drink) or commercial electrolyte (mineral salts) preparations like Pedialyte. Pedialyte is now available in flavoured frozen ice form, which not only tastes better, but also enables a slower and more continuous absorption of the liquid. Sweetened sports

---

How to avoid travelers' diarrhea ("turista")

▶ Drink bottled water. Filters that sterilize water do not get rid of viruses.

▶ It is okay to drink small quantities of alcohol, but avoid ice cubes. The water used to make the ice contains bacteria and alcohol will not kill them.

▶ If possible, prepare your meals yourself or go to well-known restaurants. Eat hot meals if you like, but not re-heated ones. Bacteria cannot survive over 65 °C, but re-heated meals never reach that temperature.

▶ Beware of unpeeled fruit, vegetables, raw meat, milk and cheese. Oranges and grapefruit are generally safe, since their high acidity protects them from bacteria.

▶ Avoid cream-based desserts, strawberries, grapes, and watermelon.

▶ A general rule for travellers: eat only cooked food and drink only boiled water.

▶ Before leaving on your trip, consult your family physician or go to a travel clinic for information on how to avoid tropical diseases.

drinks also effectively replace electrolytes and sugar (which help the intestines absorb liquids). Or try the following home remedy, and drink as much as you want:

> 1 litre boiled water
> 5 ml salt
> 5 ml baking soda
> 2 tablespoons sugar
> 120 ml apple juice

Eat. Maintain a light and varied diet, avoiding dairy products and fibre. Stop eating altogether if you are suffering from strong abdominal cramps or vomiting. Once you feel a little better, begin with easily digestible foods, such as clear soups, ripe bananas, and toast. Have six small meals a day instead of three large ones.

Avoid milk, coffee, tea, alcohol, cola and tap water. They stimulate the intestines. Clear soft drinks are not helpful because they do not contain electrolytes.

Avoid dairy products and fibre. It is also a good idea to limit the amount of carbohydrates you consume. Do not eat bread, bran, pasta, cabbage or legumes.

You were very careful, but somehow you still got *turista*

In most major cities of the world, it is easy to find Pepto-Bismol. Take eight tablets a day. Do not be alarmed when your mouth and stools turn black. This is a harmless side effect. Be careful: do not take Pepto-Bismol if you have a fever.

Small packets of mineral salts should also be available. Dissolve them in boiled water and drink. This will help you rehydrate your body.

Yogurt. The active bacterial cultures in yogurt can replace intestinal flora. However, some doctors say that the sterilization process in commercially marketed dairy products kills all living bacteria, rendering it ineffective.

Beware of antidiarrheal medications. Drugs like Imodium can impede the elimination of bacteria and increase the amount of toxins absorbed by the body. If you also have a fever and believe your diarrhea was caused by your diet, avoid these medications, unless recommended by a doctor.

Change your antacid medication. Antacids containing aluminum hydroxide can help you avoid diarrhea related to heartburn. Although less effective than those containing magnesium, they are ultimately preferable.

Avoid contagion. Parasites can also be spread by the hands. Wash your hands carefully when preparing food and use your own soap and towels.

WHEN TO CONSULT?

► Your diarrhea has lasted over a week.
► Your diarrhea is accompanied by a fever, blood in the stool, or strong abdominal cramps.
► There is mucus (transparent liquid) or pus (thick, foul-smelling yellowish or greenish liquid) in your stool.
► Your mouth, lips and tongue are abnormally dry.
► Urination has diminished. You have lost weight.
► You are pregnant and have a number of these symptoms. Consult immediately.

WHAT HAPPENS DURING THE EXAM?

The doctor performs a complete abdominal (and sometimes rectal) examination and may order stool cultures and parasite screenings. Depending on the severity of the condition, he or she may order additional tests (blood tests, for example). Proctoscopy, X-rays, or even an intestinal biopsy may be necessary in cases of chronic diarrhea.

WHAT IS THE TREATMENT?

Usual treatment

Antibiotics, antidiarrheal medications or simply rehydration is often enough to deal with the problem. Patients with severe dehydration, fever, and blood in the stool are hospitalized and rehydrated intravenously.

Lactose intolerance

If lactose intolerance is causing chronic diarrhea, eliminate dairy products from your diet or take Lactaid. Re-introduce milk into your diet slowly. For children, replace milk with soya based drinks.

Travelers' diarrhea ("turista")

Many ask for a prescription to avoid diarrhea before they leave on a trip. Because of the risk of side effects and bacterial resistance, doctors prescribe them only to people at high risk: diabetics taking insulin, AIDS patients, high blood pressure patients taking diuretics, and people with chronic inflammatory diseases like Crohn's disease or ulcerative colitis.

Difficulty Breathing

The lungs perform a double function, simultaneously nourishing the blood with oxygen and eliminating carbon dioxide from the circulatory system. During respiratory failure, carbon dioxide levels in the blood increase while blood oxygen levels diminish, causing the patient to have difficulty breathing (dyspnea). The sufferer becomes short of breath, feels tightness in the chest, a sensation of smothering, and is required to make extra efforts to take in sufficient oxygen. Breathing may also be shallow and rapid. There are a number of possible causes, including intense physical activity and heart or lung disease. This chapter deals specifically with respiratory problems caused by lung disease, since those due to heart disease are examined in another section.

WHAT ARE THE CAUSES?

- ► *Pneumonia* is a bacterial or viral lung infection that can cause shortness of breath, coughing, possibly bloody expectoration (sputum), shivering, and fever.
- ► *Chronic bronchitis* describes inflammation of the bronchial tubes caused by smoking or regular exposure to toxic irritants such as chlorine. It is characterized by a chronic cough, expectoration, and, in severe cases, shortness of breath.
- ► *Emphysema* causes the gradual destruction of the alveoli (tiny sacs at the end of the bronchial tubes) and is particularly common in smokers. The symptoms of this chronic disease are shortness of breath, wheezing, and possibly coughing and expectoration.
- ► *Asthma.* An asthma attack may result from an allergic reaction and is characterized by sudden shortness of breath, tightness in the chest, a smothering sensation, and a dry (no sputum) or wet (sputum) cough.
- ► *Severe respiratory allergies* cause swelling of the face, tongue, larynx, soft tissues of the throat, and vocal cords and are accompanied by a harsh wheeze (known as stridor). This reaction constitutes a medical emergency and is most common in those with allergies to penicillin, nuts and insect bites.
- ► *Pulmonary embolism.* This occurs when a clot forms in a blood vessel (usually in one of the legs), breaks free, and is carried to a

pulmonary artery where it causes an obstruction. Long periods of immobility (during long car trips or bed rest, for example), or leg injuries can lead to the formation of blood clots, with the risk increasing if you have an immediate family history of the problem. Embolisms cause sudden shortness of breath and, depending on the size and location of the clot, chest pain, fever, and bloody expectoration.

► *Pneumothorax* occurs when gas bubbles in the cell tissue at the surface of the lung burst and air becomes trapped in the pleura (the two-layered membrane surrounding the lungs). This causes the lung to collapse and, of course, difficulty breathing. For unknown reasons, tall and thin young adults are particularly susceptible. Because height is hereditary, therefore, several cases of

Choking on a foreign object

If a person becomes suddenly unable to breathe, places a hand on the throat, is unable to speak, and begins to turn blue, it is very likely that he or she is choking on a piece of food or some other foreign object.

Ask the person if he or she is able to cough. If it is possible, encourage the person to do so and stand by to observe. If this does not dislodge the object, perform the Heimlich manoeuvre: stand behind the person, wrap your arms around his or her stomach, hold your hands together, and pull the sufferer firmly and quickly upward and back. The object should be propelled up the windpipe and out the mouth.

If this does not work, lay the person on his or her back, turning the head to one side. Place one knee on the floor on each side of the person's body, place your hands one on top of the other on the person's upper abdomen (between the navel and rib cage), and push upwards firmly and quickly.

Be careful: this should not be done with young children or babies. Lay the child on the stomach sideways over your lap with the head hanging down, and tap him or her on the back. Play it safe, and bring the child to the hospital.

pneumothorax may occur in the same family. Emphysema and chest injuries are other possible causes. Symptoms develop suddenly in this case, with the sufferer becoming short of breath and experiencing intense pain in the area of the ribs.

▶ *Epiglottiditis* is a bacterial infection of the larynx, pharynx and epiglottis (the small flap at the back of the throat covering the vocal cords during swallowing). Symptoms include a whistling sound while breathing (particularly during inhalation), sore throat, and fever. Because there is a danger of asphyxiation, this is a medical emergency. This acute infection is most common in children.

▶ *Hyperventilation syndrome* is a benign phenomenon that generally occurs in people who are extremely anxious. Women tend to be more susceptible than men. Rapid breathing leads to a sharp decrease in carbon dioxide levels in the blood, causing a sensation of smothering, dizziness, weakness, fatigue, heart palpitations, tingling in the arms and hands, chest or abdominal cramps, hot flashes, and occasionally loss of consciousness.

▶ *Pulmonary fibrosis* is a serious chronic disease characterized by the gradual build-up of scar tissue on the lungs. In most cases, the cause is unknown, although it can develop in people with asbestosis (a respiratory disease caused by inhaling asbestos fibres), silicosis (caused by prolonged exposure to silica, found in stone quarries, mines, foundaries and places where masonry is practiced), or allergic alveolitis (triggered by prolonged contact with mouldy hay, pigeons, or parakeets). Eventually, pulmonary fibrosis causes the lungs to stiffen, impeding their ability to function. Symptoms are shallow rapid breathing and intense fatigue that progresses with the disease.

▶ *Cystic fibrosis* is a congenital and hereditary disease characterized by a malfunctioning of the mucus glands in the lungs and digestive system. This causes thick mucus secretions in the bronchioles, which block the passage of oxygen and create a breeding ground for bacteria. The resulting recurrent infections lead to the gradual breakdown of lung tissue. The patient will experience breathing difficulties, digestive problems (such as chronic diarrhea), and growth disorders.

▶ *Morbid obesity.* A significant amount of excess weight causes the abdomen to push upwards against the diaphragm, crushing the lungs and requiring the person to make extra efforts to breathe adequately. Respiratory problems are constant and further aggravated by physical exertion and reduced cardiac and muscle capacity.

▶ *Scoliosis* is a congenital deformity of the spinal column that causes it to bend into an S-shape, sometimes pinching the lungs and limiting their ability to expand, causing a chronic respiratory disorder.

▶ *Muscular dystrophy* is a progressive muscle disease causing weakness that begins in the face, chest and neck, and eventually (over a period of years) becomes generalized. Respiratory problems result from a weakening of the lung muscles.

▶ *Inflammatory diseases of the pleura (pleurisy).* The pleura describe a membrane composed of two thin layers surrounding the lungs and lining the rib cage. The most common symptoms of pleurisy are chest pain (increasing with inhalation), coughing, and shortness of breath (when liquid accumulates in the membrane). In most cases, it is brought on by an infection (virus, pneumonia, or an infection of the pleura itself). Diseases caused by immune system disorders (such as rheumatoid arthritis or systemic lupus erythematosus) can also be responsible. Lung cancer may also affect the pleura.

▶ *Respiratory failure.* Lung problems in general can worsen and cause breathing problems when the lung cannot properly oxygenate the blood. Depending on the nature of the underlying problem, other symptoms may also appear.

PRACTICAL ADVICE

For serious allergies. People with allergies to nuts, insect bites and penicillin should always have an adrenalin syringe (Epipen, sold over the counter in pharmacies) ready for immediate injection in case they come into contact with an allergen. If possible, a dose of oral or syrup antihistamine (Benadryl) should also be taken and the patient should go to the emergency room as quickly as possible. Don't forget to watch for the Epipen product's expiry date.

Take it easy. If you are out of breath, rest for a few minutes before gently resuming your activities.

Prevent blood clots. Be sure to stop frequently during long car trips to get the circulation back in your legs and prevent the formation of blood clots. Injectable or subcutaneous anticoagulants (low molecular weight heparin) can help prevent clotting during long periods of immobility (five hours or more) for people who have previously had deep vein thrombosis or a pulmonary embolism. Speak to your doctor if you are planning a trip. Elderly people and those with a personal or family history of pulmonary embolism should also wear support stockings (particularly if a long period of bed rest is expected). Sold without prescription in pharmacies, these elastic stockings facilitate proper blood circulation and prevent phlebitis (inflammation of the veins associated with blood clotting).

Stay in shape. Good physical condition means greater endurance. If you lead a sedentary life, begin physical activity gradually, doing a minimum of 20 minutes of walking, three times a week. Don't forget to do warm-up stretches beforehand.

Become informed. The provincial branches of the Canadian Lung Association are invaluable sources of information, advice, and support.

Do not smoke. Smoking tobacco obstructs the respiratory tract and shortens life expectancy.

Adapt breathing during hyperventilation. If you are suffering a hyperventilation attack, try to breathe more slowly and less deeply. Breathe through the nose, using the diaphragm and do not sigh. Breathing in and out of a paper bag will lower carbon dioxide levels in the blood, but will not correct the breathing. Speak to your doctor about hyperventilation and diaphragm exercises, and ask if there are respiration clinics in your area.

WHEN TO CONSULT?

▶ Your breathing suddenly becomes rapid and you feel as though you are smothering.

▶ Your shortness of breath lasts for more than 15 minutes.

▶ You make a whistling sound when you breathe.

▶ You are short of breath and have pain in the chest.

▶ Your child has symptoms of epiglottiditis (whistling sound when breathing, sore throat, and fever).

WHAT HAPPENS DURING THE EXAM?

The doctor takes a history and performs a physical examination, requesting lung X-rays, blood analyses and sometimes diagnostic nuclear medicine tests. In emergencies involving a severe allergic reaction, the doctor will take the vital signs and check whether the lungs are receiving adequate air supply.

WHAT IS THE TREATMENT?

Pneumonia

Bacterial pneumonia usually responds well to antibiotic treatments, which are usually prescribed for ten days.

Chronic bronchitis, emphysema, and asthma.

These diseases can be controlled with bronchodilators and anti-inflammatories. In advanced cases of chronic bronchitis and emphysema, oxygen therapy may be necessary, either using a tank or an oxygen concentrator (a machine that sucks the air in from the immediate environment, converting its oxygen levels from 21% to 95%). While some patients require this treatment only during physical exertion, others use the machine or tank while sleeping and some require it permanently.

Severe respiratory allergy

The doctor will inject the patient with adrenaline to dilate the bronchi. Intravenous cortisone treatment or antihistamines will help reduce inflammation of the face, tongue, larynx, soft tissues of the throat, and vocal cords. Spray bronchodilators will also be prescribed.

In severe cases of respiratory failure whereby mechanical breathing assistance is required, the patient is intubated (has a tube inserted through the mouth) or a tracheotomy (surgical opening of the windpipe) is performed to avoid the obstruction in the upper respiratory tract.

Pulmonary embolism
The patient is hospitalized for a few days or treated as an out-patient, depending on the severity of the case. He or she will receive anti-coagulants (intravenous or subcutaneous heparin) to prevent new clots from forming and dissolve those in existence. The doctor will prescribe continued treatments with Coumadin or Sintron (warfarin) for several months to prevent recurrence.

Pneumothorax
In most cases, the air reabsorbs into the body by itself after a few days and the patient will only be kept in hospital for observation over a few hours. In more serious cases, a chest tube is used to release the air and let the lung expand back to its full capacity. Analgesics are usually prescribed, as this is a painful condition.

Epiglottiditis
The patient is hospitalized and treated with antibiotics to clear up the infection. If the upper respiratory tract is severely blocked by a swollen epiglottis, intubation or a tracheotomy may be required.

Hyperventilation syndrome
The doctor will reassure the patient that hyperventilation is benign, advise him or her on breathing control techniques, and provide information on any programs available. Anti-anxiety drugs may be necessary.

Pulmonary fibrosis
Steroid (cortisone) treatment may be beneficial, depending on the underlying cause of the pulmonary fibrosis.

Cystic fibrosis

There is no cure for this disease and life expectancy does not generally exceed the age of 30. Doctors will write lifetime prescriptions for drugs to liquefy secretions. The patient will also require regular "clapping" sessions (a physiotherapy exercise that dislodges thick mucus by clapping the patient firmly on the back or chest).

Morbid obesity

The patient's weight loss is medically supervised and may be supported by weight-loss medication. Stomach reduction surgery or an operation to shorten the intestines (reducing the time food spends in the intestines and therefore the amount absorbed) may also be performed. The doctor may also prescribe oxygen to help the patient breathe.

Scoliosis

In serious cases (when the spine is curved more than 45 degrees), surgery to correct the curvature may be required, particularly in young patients. If breathing is severely impeded, a BiPAP (bi-level positive airway pressure) machine may be useful.

Muscular dystrophy

Physiotherapy will help maintain muscle strength for as long as possible. Once respiratory failure begins, oxygen therapy will be required (using a tank or an oxygen concentrator). In severe cases, a BiPAP machine is used.

Inflammatory diseases of the pleura (pleurisy)

Treatment is immediately undertaken.

Respiratory failure

Depending on the underlying cause, the condition may be temporary (when caused by pneumonia, for example) or chronic (as a symptom of emphysema). The patient must be hospitalized (sometimes in intensive care) for treatment of lung disease.

Walking is a complex process, requiring the coordination of the central nervous system (cortex, sub-cortex, cerebellum, and spinal cord), the peripheral nervous system (nerves), and the musculoskeletal system (muscles, bones, and joints). It also depends, of course, on balance, which is regulated by the inner ear (vestibular system).

Serious problems can be indicated by any one of a number of symptoms, including numbness in the lower limbs, lack of balance or coordination, frequent falls, and stiffness or weakness in one leg causing the limb to drag or move awkwardly.

WHAT ARE THE CAUSES?

Central nervous system problems

- *Aging.* Normal aging alters the neurons that transmit nerve impulses to the extremities and regulate communication between the cerebellum and inner ear. Elderly people are less sure on their feet and walk more slowly. Vision problems such as cataracts often aggravate the situation.
- *Cerebrovascular accident (CVA).* CVAs are caused by a decrease in blood circulation or cerebral hemorrhage that partially disturbs brain function, possibly leading to numbness or paralysis of one or more limbs.
- *Brain tumour.* Tumour growth can cause the compression or death of brain tissue, leading to progressive numbness and loss of sensation or function of the limbs.
- *Multiple sclerosis* affects myelin, the substance that surrounds nerve fibres, disturbing the flow of nerve impulses. Numbness may begin in the feet and move up towards the abdomen, or occur only on one side of the body. The disease can cause weakness, muscle spasms or awkward movements in the lower limbs.
- *Dementia.* Disorders such as Parkinson's disease cause hesitant and jerky movements, eventually rendering walking impossible.
- *Muscular dystrophy* affects the nerves and the brain stem (the base of the brain), causing weakness in the limbs and a shrinking of the

muscles (amyotrophy), as in amyotrophic lateral sclerosis or Lou Gehrig's disease.

▶ *Compression of the spinal cord* caused by a tumour, vertebra, or spinal trauma. Difficulty walking is accompanied by urinary incontinence, persistent constipation, numbness from the feet to the waist, chest or neck, as well as weakness and spasms in the legs (and sometimes arms).

▶ *Labyrinthitis* is a temporary condition caused by a virus that infects the inner ear (labyrinth), causing vertigo (loss of balance). Repeated or chronic bacterial infections may have the same long-term effect.

▶ *Prescription medication, drugs, and alcohol.* Sedatives, psychotropic drugs, and hypotensive medications, for example, can interfere with balance and alertness.

▶ *Conditions affecting the cerebellum* disturb balance and cause difficulty walking.

Peripheral nervous system problems

▶ *Polyneuropathic conditions* are most frequently caused by diabetes, alcoholism, or vitamin B_{12} deficiency (due to a digestive absorption problem or insufficient consumption of the vitamin). As they destroy nerve endings, these conditions cause the sufferer to lose sensation in the feet and become disoriented, which may lead to falls.

Musculoskeletal system problems

▶ *Herniated lumbar disc.* This condition can develop as a result of lumbago or repeated sprains of the lumbar spine. The disc, flattened between two vertebrae, irritates the nerves that run from the spinal column, causing pain and varying degrees of disability in the lower limbs.

▶ *Arthritis.* This disease can attack and incapacitate any joint in the body. Pain and edema in the hips, knees, ankles or toes limit the ability to walk. In advanced stages, the joint can become deformed and eroded by repeated inflammation. Gout is a form of arthritis in which an excess of uric acid (urea) leads to painful calcifications in the joint.

► **Osteoarthritis** causes a progressive hardening of the joint tissue, limiting movement and causing intense pain.

► **Arteriosclerosis in the lower limbs** occurs when the amount of oxygenated blood brought to the legs is reduced. Analogous to angina pectoris, which affects the heart, this phenomenon causes pain that leads to limping (intermittent claudication). Smokers represent 90% of sufferers.

► **Myopathia** causes weakness in certain muscles, making walking difficult.

► **Conditions affecting the feet,** such as sores, bunions, flat feet, and certain foot deformities.

► **Phlebitis** occurs when blood clots form in a vein, causing pain in the calf, possibly accompanied by swelling.

PRACTICAL ADVICE

Exercise regularly, no matter what. Exercise helps maintain bone density, muscle mass and joint flexibility and is one of the best preventive measures available. If you have suffered a CVA or undergone surgery for a tumour, compression or spinal cord injury, all the more reason to get moving! Try to move your legs, even if immediate results are not evident. Remember that you are helping your brain find new ways to deliver its commands. Another person can help you do passive exercises to minimize muscle atrophy. Your number one priority should be your rehabilitation, even if it can only be partial.

Watch your weight. Obesity places extra pressure on the joints and lower extremities.

Get your eyes checked. Maybe you are unsteady on your feet because you cannot see where you are putting them!

Pay attention to arteriosclerosis risk factors. Watch your cholesterol, sugar levels, and blood pressure. Do not smoke and be sure to exercise regularly.

Have your medications checked. Remember that sedatives can interfere with balance. Ask your doctor to prescribe an alternative.

Fight aging. If you have reached your golden years, be sure to wear your glasses and good walking shoes. To avoid falling when moving around, keep your back straight and look ahead of you instead of at the ground. If the walking surface worries you, use a cane to detect problem spots rather than searching for them visually. The best exercises are swimming and stretching, as well as any other activity that combines movement and balance (such as walking, dance, and low-impact aerobics).

Don't let your arthritis tie you down. During attacks, take painkillers or anti-inflammatories. One or two acetaminophen tablets (325 mg to 500 mg) four times a day will help ease the pain. Do not exceed 4 grams daily. It is especially important to follow manufacturer's instructions when taking anti-inflammatories. Take both medications if the symptoms are hard to control. Apply cold compresses and do light exercises to maintain range of movement. After the attack, resume your usual activities like walking, swimming, or cycling to avoid immobilization syndrome.

Take care of lumbar pain, caused by lumbago, sprain, or herniated disc, for example. Take painkillers or anti-inflammatories. Apply cold compresses for twenty minutes every three to four hours during the first two or three days, then hot compresses until the pain disappears. Stay in bed and alternate between two positions: lying on your back with at least two pillows under your thighs and one under your head, and on your side with one or two pillows between your knees and one under your head. Change positions slowly, in stages, avoiding any twisting of your torso. Once the attack has passed, resume your daily activities, and eventually, your exercise programme.

Adopt a healthy lifestyle. Limit your consumption of coffee, as it causes the blood vessels to constrict, reducing blood flow. Also be careful with alcohol and abstain from non-medical drugs altogether.

These substances affect the cerebellum and can significantly disturb your balance.

WHEN TO CONSULT?

► You repeatedly experience osteoarticular pain (pain in the bones of the joints).

► One or both of your legs feel numb or weak.

► You have difficulty walking, turning, or going up stairs.

► You are unsteady on your feet. You frequently bump into objects and fall.

► One of your legs feels stiff or weak. Your muscle seems to be shrinking (amyotrophy).

► Every time you walk, you feel the same pain in your calf. The time it takes for the pain to develop is becoming progressively shorter.

► You experience periods of intense and persistent pain in one joint (usually the big toe) that wakes you up at night.

► You have suffered from lumbago or a lumbar sprain. After three days of rest in bed, you are still unable to resume most of your normal activities.

► One of your joints is hot, swollen, and painful. You have been unable to use it for some time.

WHAT HAPPENS DURING THE EXAM?

The doctor takes your medical history and performs neurological and osteoarticular tests, as well as an examination of the muscles and sense organs. Particular attention is paid to the speed at which the patient walks, the length and height of each step, regularity of movement, postural reflexes, and antalgic limping. The doctor may also order tests to determine the likelihood of falling and the prognosis.

In some cases, the doctor will add complementary tests, such as X-rays, computerized tomography scans, and magnetic resonance imaging (MRI) tests.

WHAT IS THE TREATMENT?

The general objective of treatment is to restore an acceptable walking pattern and the stability to avoid falling, with or without technical aids. Functional re-education aims to help the sufferer maintain his or her autonomy by making it easier to perform everyday domestic and social activities.

Specific treatments vary according to the cause of the problem, from medications to physiotherapy and even surgery in some cases.

Disorders Affecting the Breasts

The breasts are made up of fatty tissue and milk glands, known as alveoli. The glands are clustered around tiny canals that converge into larger ducts called galactophores (15 to 20 of which are found in each breast). The ducts secrete milk through tiny orifices on the surface of the nipple.

Over time, breasts change and the tissue loses its tone. During menopause, the absence of menstrual hormone stimulation causes the glands to atrophy. When the process is over, the breast tissue consists almost exclusively of fat.

Certain problems may affect the breasts at various points in a woman's lifetime:
► Lumps.
► Sensitivity.
► Redness, with or without sensitivity.
► Discharge.

WHAT ARE THE CAUSES?
Lumps
► *Mammary cysts.* Cysts are benign, well defined and movable. Generally about the size of a marble, they may be sensitive to the touch. Caused by the accumulation of colostrum in a gland with a blocked duct, cysts usually develop a few days before menstruation and disappear when it ends. They occur primarily in adolescent and premenopausal women, with some developing cysts every time they menstruate. If the lump does not disappear or persists throughout two menstrual cycles, medical consultation is advised.
► *Fibroadenoma (or adenofibroma).* Well defined, movable, and variable in size, these fleshy lumps are created by the stimulation of the fibroepithelial cells (the fibrous tissue in the breast). They do not disappear over the course of the woman's cycle and may increase

in size or become more sensitive as menstruation approaches. The lumps are almost always benign, although they may become cancerous. Any new lump should be examined by a doctor.

► *Dysplasia.* These benign masses, usually appearing on the upper exterior part of the breast, are poorly defined (difficult to grasp between the fingers) and sensitive to the touch. They frequently increase in size and sensitivity two weeks before menstruation and may disappear when it ends. This condition, caused by changes in the fibrous breast tissue (specifically, the formation of scar tissue), is more common in women over 35.

► *Galactocele.* This unmovable hard mass may be sensitive to the touch. It appears during the breastfeeding period and can persist after weaning. Formed by the accumulation of milk in an obstructed canal, it is completely benign.

► *Cancerous tumour.* Cancerous tumours are hard, poorly defined and more or less movable. The texture of the tumour is different from the rest of the breast tissue. Rarely painful, it can increase in size regardless of the stage of the menstrual cycle. Women between the ages of 50 and 69 are particularly prone: more than 70% of breast cancer cases occur in this age group. Furthermore, after the age of 50, hormone replacement therapy that continues for more than five years increases the risk of breast cancer. Doctors therefore avoid prescribing this therapy to women over 55, unless the patient is experiencing extremely bothersome symptoms, such as hot flashes. In such cases, the patient is followed and the treatment is discontinued as soon as possible. Oral contraceptives do not seem to increase the risk of breast cancer. Any persistent lump must be examined by a doctor.

Sensitivity

► *Hormonal factors.* Many women, particularly those over the age of 35, experience pain and swelling in their breasts during their premenstrual period. There is absolutely no cause for alarm. For unknown reasons, increased sensitivity may also occur at other times during the menstrual cycle. Although bothersome, this phenomenon is not dangerous.

Redness and sensitivity

► *Mammary abscess.* The symptoms of an abscess are redness and sensitivity, possibly accompanied by a fever and/or greenish/yellowish nipple discharge indicating bacterial infection due to an obstructed duct. Consult a doctor.

Redness with no sensitivity

► *Superficial cancer* (near the surface of the skin) causes signs of inflammation. Half of the surface of the breast may become red and take on the texture of an orange peel. Consult a doctor immediately.

Discharge

► *Prolactinoma.* This causes the spontaneous and abundant discharge of a yellowish, serous (watery) and odourless liquid from numerous orifices in both nipples. The condition results from an excessive production of prolactin (the hormone triggering lactation), which is caused by a prolactinoma, or tiny benign tumour in the hypophysis of the brain. This can occur in a woman of any age, whether or not she has had children.

► *Papilloma* refers to a tumour that blocks one of the ducts, bringing about a spontaneous and painless discharge of blood or serous liquid from one nipple. The tumour is generally benign, but the woman should nevertheless consult a doctor as quickly as possible. This is most common in those over 40 years of age.

► *Hormonal stimulation.* Sexual intercourse, showering, or strong emotions can cause a white, odourless liquid (colostrum) to leak from the breasts. Lactating women may continue to excrete milk

---

Mammography

Most provinces have established provincial breast cancer screening programs which provide access to mammography screening. The procedure is easy, quick and, for most women, painless.

in the minutes following a feeding. This is perfectly normal and there is no cause for alarm.

PRACTICAL ADVICE

Do not ignore the problem. In most cases, the disorder causing the problem is minor, but if you are at all worried, consult your doctor.

Lumps
Wait until your next menstrual cycle. In many cases, lumps disappear over the course of the menstrual cycle.

Sensitivity
Use medication. To relieve sensitivity, take one or two acetaminophen tablets (325 mg to 500 mg), four times a day, never exceeding 4 grams daily. Anti-inflammatories are also helpful. Follow the manufacturer's dosage recommendations. Take either of these medications, or both if the sensitivity is difficult to control.

Use alternative methods. Gentle breast massages can help relieve the pain. Also try compresses and cold or lukewarm showers.

Modify your diet. Products containing methylxanthine (wine, cheese, chocolate, tea, coffee) can cause this type of pain in some women. Consume moderately.

Take vitamin supplements. It is important to note, however, that several studies have shown vitamin E to be an ineffective treatment for sensitive breasts.

Wear a good quality bra. Firm support or sports bras can help decrease breast sensitivity. Wearing a bra overnight may also ease breast pain.

Redness
Apply compresses. Lukewarm water compresses applied several times a day for fifteen minutes at a time can be effective.

Discharge

Keep a close watch. Discharge leaking from both breasts is usually not a sign of a serious condition and there is no need to worry. Avoid massaging or manipulating the breasts so as not to further stimulate them. If you feel worried or only one breast is leaking, see a doctor. Note whether the discharge issues from one or many orifices and tell your doctor.

WHEN TO CONSULT?

- The lump does not disappear at the end of your menstrual period.
- The lump appears during the breastfeeding period and persists after weaning.
- There is persistent redness on your breast that may or may not be accompanied by sensitivity.
- There is a discharge of blood from one nipple.
- Breast discharge is worrying you.
- Breast sensitivity has become intolerable.

WHAT HAPPENS DURING THE EXAM?

The doctor will ask some questions and perform a complete physical exam. He or she may order an ultrasound examination of the breasts or a mammography (breast X-ray).

Mammography exams are usually ordered for women over 50 years of age because their breast tissue is less dense and easier to examine using this method.

If there is a lump, the doctor may choose to aspirate the lump with a needle. The procedure is quick, painless, and necessary for the diagnosis of dysplasia, fibroadenoma or breast cancer. Puncture therapy is also used to treat mammary cysts and galactoceles. If the breast has redness without sensitivity, a biopsy is ordered to rule out superficial cancer.

WHAT IS THE TREATMENT?

Lumps

Mammary cysts

This condition is not dangerous and generally does not require surgery or, in many cases, any treatment at all. If treatment does prove necessary, therapeutic puncture is usually sufficient.

Fibroadenoma

Even though this type of lump is benign, the doctor may opt for surgical removal if it grows bigger and causes the patient any pain or worry.

Dysplasia

These masses often disappear on their own over time. Unless there is doubt about the diagnosis, little reason exists to remove them surgically.

Galactocele

The only treatment necessary is therapeutic puncture to drain the accumulated milk. This is a minor and painless procedure that takes place in the doctor's office.

Cancerous tumour

Such cases require a partial mastectomy (also called a lumpectomy), which describes the removal of the lump along with some surrounding tissue and, on occasion, the lymph nodes in the armpit. This surgery, performed under general anesthesia, is generally successful, but complete treatment may require radiation therapy or chemotherapy to minimize the risk of relapse or distant metastases. Nowadays, doctors rarely need to perform total mastectomies (removal of the entire breast).

Sensitivity

The doctor may prescribe drugs like anti-inflammatories, oral contraceptives or Danazol (brand name for a product preventing hormonal fluctuations) to relieve the symptoms.

Redness with sensitivity
Mammary abscess
These are drained surgically and antibiotic treatment may be prescribed.

Redness without sensitivity
Superficial cancer
The appropriate treatment (surgery, chemotherapy or radiation therapy) is immediately undertaken.

Discharge
Prolactinoma
These benign tumours disappear with the appropriate treatment, namely, hormone-based medication. (Note: this is not the same as hormone replacement therapy, used for menopausal women.)

Papilloma
This is a surgical procedure performed under local or general anesthesia that removes the affected duct behind the nipple. It has no impact on the nipple itself.

Disorientation

Disorientation refers to the loss of the sense of time, space, or body schema (recognition and spatial orientation of the body). This symptom may last a few seconds and signal a temporary harmless condition, or it may indicate a much more serious disorder. Disorientation can be acute or chronic.

Acute disorientation
- Sudden onset.
- Usually accompanied by extreme anxiety; sometimes by agitation and rapid speech.

Chronic disorientation
- In many cases, disorientation fluctuates in intensity in the early stages.
- Can progress rapidly. The sufferer may become oblivious to the disorientation after a period of months or years.
- Usually accompanied by apathy and a loss of autonomy brought on by problems with language, memory, balance, and organizational skills.
- Sufferer may require 24-hour care.

WHAT ARE THE CAUSES?
Acute disorientation
- *Reaction to medications.* Certain sedatives, sleeping pills or painkillers (codeine or morphine, for example) frequently cause disorientation, especially in the elderly.
- *Reaction to alcohol or drugs,* particularly cocaine.
- *Epilepsy*. An epileptic seizure is always followed by a period of disorientation that lasts a few minutes. Frequently, the primary symptom of a partial seizure is disorientation, accompanied by automatic hand movements and lip chewing.
- *Cerebrovascular accident.* Disorientation (particularly spatial) lasting a few hours or even days is frequently the only symptom. Difficulty speaking is another important sign of a CVA.

▶ *Transient global amnesia* refers to an acute episode of amnesia that lasts a few hours. It is most common in the elderly. Sufferers ask the same questions repeatedly, unable to recall responses, and have no memory of the episode after the attack. Although the problem seems worrying, the prognosis is good and episodes do not generally recur.

▶ *Moderate hypoglycemia.* Diabetics taking insulin or certain oral medications may experience disorientation.

Chronic disorientation

▶ *Various diseases of the vital organs.* Certain disorders (kidney or heart failure, emphysema, and cirrhosis, for example) prevent the brain from receiving enough oxygen or nutrients to function properly.

▶ *Repeated cerebrovascular accidents.* The degree of disorientation varies from day to day.

▶ *Dementia.* The best-known disorder causing dementia is Alzheimer's disease. In its early stages, temporal, spatial and environmental disorientation fluctuates, occurring more and more frequently with time.

▶ *Cerebral tumour or hematoma.* A cerebral tumour can be benign or malignant. A cerebral hematoma refers to bleeding inside the brain, usually caused by trauma or uncontrolled high blood pressure. Disorientation and problems with language skills can evolve over a few months or even weeks.

PRACTICAL ADVICE
Acute disorientation
Do not panic. If you have mild memory problems, often find yourself looking for your keys, or take a few seconds before you recognize a familiar spot, there is no need to worry. Occasional and fleeting periods of mild disorientation are normal manifestations of fatigue or stress and do not indicate that you are suffering from Alzheimer's disease.

Choose your medications carefully. Even non-prescription medications can cause disorientation. Speak to your pharmacist.

Follow your prescription to the letter. If you suffer from a disease like diabetes or epilepsy, be sure to follow the treatment properly.

Chronic disorientation

Prevent accidents. If someone you know suffers from disorientation, he or she may have a tendency to leave things burning in the kitchen, for example. Unplug the stove, replace it with a microwave, and buy a kettle that shuts off automatically. Because disorientation becomes worse in the dark, leave nightlights on all the time. Be sure familiar objects are within arm's reach.

Avoid moving or changing the décor. Disorientation becomes more intense in unknown environments and during trips or outings.

Never let a sufferer drive a car. Be sure to tell the doctor if a loved one is having trouble behind the wheel. If a person is unable to perform basic tasks (distinguishing a green light from a red light, for example), he or she should not be driving.

Mark your calendar. Circle important dates on the calendar to help them identify the day, season, or year.

Provide stimulation. Speak to sufferers. Make them read the newspaper, listen to the news on the radio, or watch television. This will help them stay in touch with reality.

Ask for help. Day centres offer therapeutic leisure activities for sufferers. This provides them with an opportunity for social contact outside the family and gives their spouses or children a day off.

WHEN TO CONSULT?

► Disorientation comes on suddenly and lasts several minutes, hours or days. Consult as soon as possible.
► Disorientation is associated with a disease like heart failure or emphysema.

► Disorientation has progressed over a few weeks, months, or years, and is accompanied by speech or memory problems.

WHAT HAPPENS DURING THE EXAM?

The doctor will take a detailed history and perform a complete physical examination to reach diagnosis. Lab tests (such as blood sugar and electrolytes, encephalogram or tomography scan) may be ordered. The doctor will also review the patient's medications and ask him or her to perform tests that assess intellectual skill (memory, calculation, language, orientation, attention). A neurological consultation is often recommended for people suffering from epilepsy or acute disorientation.

WHAT IS THE TREATMENT?

Acute disorientation

If medication is the cause, the doctor will modify the prescription. If it results from an epileptic seizure, cerebrovascular accident or transient global amnesia, the doctor will trace the progression of the disease and try to prevent recurrences. Moderate hypoglycemia is treated with an infusion of glucose-based solution or, if the patient is able to eat, oral administration of sweet substances. Alternatively, the doctor may choose to prescribe injectable medication.

Chronic disorientation

The underlying disorder determines the treatment. The physician will prescribe medication to control diseases such as heart failure, diabetes, and emphysema. Surgery is required to remove a tumour, drain a hematoma, or unblock an obstructed or shrunken artery. There are now a number of drugs that can improve quality of life for sufferers of Alzheimer's disease.

Dizziness

It is sometimes difficult to differentiate between loss of balance, vertigo, and dizziness, although these problems and their causes are distinct.

Loss of balance is defined by a difficulty remaining in a stable upright standing position, while vertigo gives a person the feeling that the room is spinning. The latter is often accompanied by nausea and vomiting.

Patients suffering from dizziness complain of the following symptoms:

- Light-headedness.
- Feeling that the head is spinning "on the inside".
- Faintness.
- In some cases, blurred vision and loss of balance.

WHAT ARE THE CAUSES?

- *Certain drugs,* including sedatives, neuroleptics, antihypertensives, and antiepileptics.
- *Rapid changes (increase or decrease) in blood pressure.*
- *Hyperventilation syndrome.*
- *Anemia.*
- *Hypoglycemia.*
- *Dehydration.*
- *Heart disease.*

PRACTICAL ADVICE

Take measures to avoid falling. Dizziness and vertigo can lead to falling. Because of their susceptibility to bone fracture, the elderly in particular should take certain precautions. Possible safety measures include installing a handrail in the hallway, using a cane or a walker, and putting down a non-slip rug in the bathtub. Ask your doctor or local clinic for advice.

Rapid changes in blood pressure. Lie down for a few minutes with your head lower than the rest of your body to facilitate the flow of oxygen to the brain. Sit up slowly and pause before standing (stay on the edge of the bed and count to three). If you have been sitting down for a long time, be sure to stand up slowly—don't jump up and run to the telephone, for example.

Control hyperventilation. As soon as you feel the first symptoms, inhale and exhale normally with your nose and mouth in a paper bag. Continue for five to ten minutes.

Are you suffering from anemia? A balanced diet is the best treatment. Your meals and snacks should contain the four food groups (fruit and vegetables, meat and meat substitutes, dairy products, and grains). Consult your doctor to confirm your diagnosis.

For hypoglycemia. Low blood sugar often leads to dizziness. Always have a sweet snack handy, such as raisins, juice, chocolate, candy or packets of sugar.

For dehydration. Extremely hot weather, intense physical exertion or the flu can lead to dehydration and dizziness. Rest and drink plenty of liquids, such as water, fruit juice, broth, or sport drinks containing electrolytes (mineral salts).

WHEN TO CONSULT?
- Your dizziness is recurrent or very bothersome.
- It is accompanied by other symptoms (difficulty speaking, pain in one arm, double vision).

WHAT HAPPENS DURING THE EXAM?
The physician interviews the patient and performs a complete general examination, taking the blood pressure, examining the ears and eyes, checking balance and doing neurological tests to determine whether the patient is suffering from dizziness, loss of balance, or vertigo.

The doctor may refer the patient to a specialist for more thorough testing and a precise diagnosis.

WHAT IS THE TREATMENT?

If drugs are causing the dizziness, the doctor will modify the prescription.

Any underlying condition (rapid changes in blood pressure, anemia, hyperventilation syndrome, hypoglycemia or heart disease) will require the appropriate treatment.

Double Vision (Diplopia)

People with diplopia see two of a single object because their eyes cannot properly superimpose the images they perceive.

Diplopia can be vertical (one image above the other), or horizontal (side by side). In 99% of cases, it affects both eyes (binocular diplopia). When only one is affected (monocular diplopia), the double image tends to disappear if the eye is covered. Diplopia can be accompanied by several symptoms, primarily including pain with eye movement and redness. Children with diplopia have a tendency to squint or keep one eye closed because they have not learned to decode the two images.

WHAT ARE THE CAUSES?
Binocular Diplopia
► *Excessive alcohol consuption.*
► *Cyst or tumour behind the eye* can prevent it from moving normally and cause non-symmetrical vision misalignment. Associated symptoms may include exophthalmos (abnormal protrusion of the eyeball), pain with eye movement and, more rarely, a saggy lid.
► *Head or face injury.*
► *Neurological impairment.* In persons over 55, diplopia is usually caused by the paralysis of a secondary cranial nerve after a thrombosis (blood clot in a vessel). Diabetics, smokers, individuals with high blood pressure or elevated cholesterol levels are also more susceptible. In younger persons, it results from the compression of a nerve by a brain tumour. Those affected may have bouts of vertigo, weakness or numbness in the arms or legs, a dilated pupil, or droopy lid.
► *Inflammation of the eye muscle tissue (myositis),* most often accompanied by pain with eye movement, redness and a protruding eyeball.
► *Disease of the eye muscle,* such as myasthenia, often accompanied by a droopy eye.

► *Thyroid gland dysfunction* generally occurs between the ages of 20 and 50 and, in most cases, causes vertical diplopia accompanied by exophthalmos and redness.

Monocular Diplopia
► *Astigmatism.* This is an optical defect that impedes long or close range vision and sometimes causes diplopia.
► *Cataracts* may be accompanied by double vision.
► *Corneal opacity or scar.* Blurry vision and glare (photophobia) are the symptoms.

PRACTICAL ADVICE
See a doctor. Double vision may indicate a potentially serious underlying condition. It is especially important to seek medical advice if a child is affected.

Cover one eyeglass lens. Blocking one lens with a piece of cardboard or gummed paper can provide some degree of relief. If you do not usually wear glasses, buy a pair with clear lenses and cover one side.

Do not walk around like a one-eyed pirate. Although they may help you see better, patches held in place with an elastic band put pressure on the eye and are uncomfortable. They can sometimes even aggravate the problem, further impairing the ability to see with both eyes at once.

Do not place a dressing directly on the eye. The application of any such covering increases the risk of infection.

WHEN TO CONSULT?
► You suspect your child is seeing double. Seek medical attention promptly.
► You see double for more than 24 hours.
► You experience vertigo, dizziness and weakness.
► You have sustained a head injury.
► You experience headache or pain when moving your eyes.

WHAT HAPPENS DURING THE EXAM?

The doctor will initially use prisms and lights to assess the diplopia, then check for redness and, with a special ruler (exophthalmometer), make sure the eye is not abnormally protruding out of the socket. He or she will also look for signs of neurological impairment by conducting a physical examination, particularly of the arms, legs and face.

WHAT IS THE TREATMENT?

Cyst or tumour behind the eye
In most cases, surgical intervention is necessary.

Head injury (fracture or hemorrhage)
The patient will be monitored until the diplopia completely resolves. Residual double vision may be fixed with corrective lenses outfitted with prisms (angles to redirect vision) or by surgery.

Neurological impairment
In the case of thrombosis, pharmacological (drug) therapy amounts only to taking aspirin for the prevention of blood clotting. If the diplopia does not disappear spontaneously, surgery can be performed on the eye muscles or glasses can be outfitted with prisms.

Inflammation of eye muscle tissue
The doctor will prescribe cortisone therapy.

Disease of the eye muscle
Treatment will depend on the cause. For example, myasthenia is usu-ally managed with long-term Mestinon (an anticholinesterase agent) treatment to improve muscle function and help the eye muscles con-tract.

Thyroid gland dysfunction
The doctor will perform a detailed examination of the patient's thy-roid function. Treatment may involve medication (e.g., radioactive iodine), or even surgery in rare cases.

Astigmatism
This optic defect is easily corrected with eyeglasses or contact lenses.

Cataracts
Surgery is the only treatment.

Corneal opacity
Cortisone or antibiotic drops may be prescribed. Surgery is also an option. Laser treatment or a partial or complete corneal transplant can eliminate the scars.

Drowsiness

Drowsiness describes an involuntary and uncontrollable need to sleep during the day that interferes with routine activities. It is not synonymous with daytime fatigue.

WHAT ARE THE CAUSES?

- *Sleep deprivation.* Sacrificing sleep to work late into the night, for example.
- *Overconsumption of stimulants,* such as coffee, tobacco, cola and alcohol.
- *Infections,* such as a cold, flu or other condition that can cause fever.
- *Drugs,* such as antihistamines, muscle relaxants, sleeping pills and painkillers.
- *Difficulty adjusting to the sleep-waking cycle.* Many night-shift workers suffer drowsiness at work and have difficulty sleeping at home. They generally sleep less well and for shorter periods than day-shift employees.
- *Jet lag.* It is always difficult to adjust one's biological clock to a new time zone when travelling. Airline pilots, flight attendants and business people are particularly affected as their work often requires them to travel across numerous time zones.
- *Sleep apnea or hypopnea syndrome.* Apnea and hypopnea are the most common causes of daytime drowsiness: the former describes the cessation of breathing during sleep, the latter a decrease in the breathing rate.
- *Restless legs syndrome* is a neurological condition that disturbs sleep by sometimes causing unbearable tingling in the legs that often forces the sufferer to get up and move about. This sometimes also impedes the sufferer's ability to fall asleep in the first place.
- *Narcolepsy* is characterized by uncontrollable sleep attacks during the day that cause the affected person to take six to eight involuntary naps, even while in the midst of doing something. After a brief five to ten-minute nap, the person awakes rested and

refreshed until the next attack, some two to three hours later. Sufferers also frequently wake up during the night. Narcolepsy is also accompanied by cataplexy, which describes a sudden loss of postural muscle tone that is precipitated by a strong emotional reaction such as anger or laughter. While still conscious, the person slumps over and remains paralyzed for several seconds. Narcolepsy begins at a young age and usually lasts a lifetime whereas cataplexy tends to go away.

► *Idiopathic hypersomnia* is characterized by an uncontrollable urge to sleep that resembles narcolepsy but is not accompanied by cataplexy.

PRACTICAL ADVICE

Get enough sleep at night. Respect your need to recover from daytime fatigue by sleeping seven to nine hours each night.

Avoid consuming too many stimulants. Overindulging in stimulants at any time, not just in the evening, can disturb your sleep.

Do not stay up too late. While a cold shower, listening to rock music, or a breath of fresh air may temporarily wake you up a little, the underlying fatigue will remain. Developing good sleep and hygiene habits is much more beneficial.

Take short naps during the day. Plan short daytime naps, especially if you have narcolepsy. Make sure they are brief to avoid trouble with getting to sleep at night.

Keep regular waking and sleeping hours. Try to go to bed and wake up at the same time throughout the week. Follow the same schedule on the weekend to avoid "jet lag" on Monday morning. If you go to bed and wake up later, it will be more difficult to fall asleep Sunday night and get up Monday morning.

Fight jet lag. If you plan to travel within seven time zones (seven hours difference), try to get some sleep on the plane, expose yourself to light, and adhere to the new time zone when you arrive. If you travel across more than seven time zones, ask your doctor for advice.

Avoid overconsumption of alcohol. Although alcohol initially makes it easier to fall asleep, it disturbs the quality of sleep, causes frequent awakenings during the night, and shortens the length of sleep. Consuming it in large quantities can also have a depressive effect.

Do not go to bed one or two hours earlier than usual unless exceptionally tired. It is very difficult to fall asleep if you go to bed earlier than your usual bedtime. If it is absolutely essential for you to get to sleep, before working the night shift, for example, go to bed considerably earlier than your regular time.

Sleep

At night, sleep occurs in successive cycles, each one lasting an average of 90 minutes. During these cycles, sleep can be light, deep or paradoxal. Paradoxal sleep, during which dreams occur, is characterized by paralysis of the postural muscles, rapid eye movement, ear contractions, and a jerking of the muscles. Deep sleep is more common at the beginning of the night whereas dreams occur more frequently near the end. Sleep is regulated by your internal biological clock and what is known as the "hourglass phenomenon". Both act in concert to produce a good quality of sleep and wakefulness. According to the hourglass phenomenon, the longer one is awake (the fuller the hourglass gets), the greater the need for sleep. That is to say, the hourglass needs to be turned over regardless of the time—day or night—one goes to bed. The internal biological clock causes fluctuations in the need for sleep depending on the time of day, and affects how long it takes to fall asleep and the quality and extent of your rest. The internal biological clock adjusts to its environment primarily according to alterations of light and darkness.

Do not wait for the next sleep cycle. If you missed your usual sleep time, you need not wait two hours before going to bed. Waiting the duration of one cycle will only cause you to lose precious sleep.

WHEN TO CONSULT?

► The drowsiness interferes with your daily activities.
► You have episodes of cataplexy.
► You snore loudly.
► You are unable to tell whether you suffer from fatigue, insomnia or drowsiness.

WHAT HAPPENS DURING THE EXAM?

The doctor will perform a complete physical examination, review your sleep habits, identify the features of drowsiness, and try to identify any specific sleep disorders. It is important to consult your spouse to corroborate the details of your sleeping patterns, particularly in cases of apnea or restless legs syndrome. A consultation with a sleep disorder specialist may also be required. A polysomnography may be used to record brain wave activity during periods of sleep and wakefulness. This test may be administered at home or in hospital.

WHAT IS THE TREATMENT?

In some cases, a mere change in lifestyle or medication will resolve the problem. In cases of apnea or hypopnea, treatment usually involves a CPAP (Continuous Positive Airway Pressure) device, which features a mask attached to a compressor that pushes air into the patient's nose and mouth, keeping the back of the throat open to allow continuous breathing. This machine is available by prescription.

Drugs are available to manage the symptoms of each sleep disorder. Exposure to an inside bright light could possibly improve the work conditions of night-shift workers and accelerate their adjustment to new time shifts.

Dry Skin and Winter Itch

When the skin is dry, it is more delicate and creases become more visible. Dryness—more common on the limbs than the face due to fewer sebaceous glands in these areas—increases the risk of scaling, itching, eczema, cracks, crevices and infection.

As dryness worsens, eczema and often redness may develop, causing scaling and extreme itchiness. Sometimes the skin even cracks, especially on the hands and feet. In the winter, excessive skin dryness is often accompanied by itching. The latter (typically referred to as winter itch) is usually triggered by a temperature change—for example, when one gets out of the day's warm clothes and into fresh pyjamas.

WHAT ARE THE CAUSES

- ► *Dry air.* Dry skin is especially common during the winter months, when humidity outside is low and the heat inside is high.
- ► *Excessive hygiene.* Frequent bathing and showering, as well as the overuse of soap, can cause dry skin. Antiseptic and antibacterial soaps also have a drying effect.
- ► *Drugs prescribed for acne,* like Accutane (isotretinoin), can cause dry skin.
- ► *Air-drying.* Not towelling off and letting yourself drip dry after a bath or shower can contribute to dry skin.
- ► *Overuse of detergents and fabric softeners.* These products remain in the fibres, affecting the skin if excessive perspiration occurs.
- ► *Repeat exposure to chemical products,* e.g., varsol and cleaning agents. Hairdressers, cleaners and dishwashers in restaurants may get eczema and sometimes very painful cracks in their hands.
- ► *Predisposition.* The amount of lipids (fat) on the skin varies from one person to the next. With aging, the skin tends to become drier as the glands become less efficient.
- ► *Allergic reactions.* Allergic eczema can develop from contact with a metal such as nickel, found in some earrings, or from a reaction to certain cosmetics.

► *Systemic illnesses* such as diabetes, kidney failure, malnutrition and, notably, thyroid problems. Dry skin is not the primary symptom for these conditions.

PRACTICAL ADVICE

Take baths rather than showers. Soak in warm water for 20 to 30 minutes or until the skin on your toes starts to wrinkle, occasionally adding bath oil or oatmeal to the water. Wash just before stepping out of the tub to avoid soaking in soapy water.

Avoid frequent baths and overly hot water. Although cleanliness is a personal matter and influenced by cultural differences, a bath or shower once a day is more than enough. Newborns do not need to be bathed every day.

Do not rub the skin. The purpose of washing is to remove dust and grime, not the skin's natural oils.

Do not add foam to the bath water. All bubble-bath products are soap-based. Soaking in soapy water is unadvisable, especially if your skin tends to be dry.

Use a mild soap. Dove brand is recommended, for example, as opposed to strong antibacterial, antiseptic or deodorant soaps.

Apply a moisturizing cream immediately after bathing or showering. This will avoid water evaporation and help the skin retain moisture in compensation for the drying effects of soap and heat. Drinking a lot of water is not enough, as the skin needs to be hydrated from the outside as well. It is especially important to use a moisturizing cream if you are using Accutane.

Use a cream rather than a lotion. Since creams are thicker and contain more fat, they are more effective than lotions. Creams containing urea or lactic acid penetrate the skin better and are therefore more moisturizing. Use an unscented cream on broken or irritated skin.

Avoid calamine. If you already have dry skin, calamine lotion is not advised. Never use Caladryl (a mixture of calamine and antihistamines), as the amount of antihistamine absorbed by the skin cannot be controlled and may cause drowsiness or other side effects.

Use a home humidifier. Dry rooms and dry skin go hand in hand. A humidifier will help remedy the problem.

Wear gloves. Gloves will protect your hands from toxic products like bleach, dish soap and cleaning agents.

Choose cotton garments over wool. Cotton allows the skin to breathe and is easier to wear than wool if you have dry or itchy skin.

As for facial moisturizers, ignore the hype of highly lucrative cosmetics companies. Despite the advertising claims, you require neither the most expensive cream, nor different ones for day and nighttime. If you have sensitive skin, use an unscented non-comedogenic (i.e., does not cause acne), and hypoallergenic product. Whereas young women tend to prefer water-based creams because they do not leave a greasy film on the skin, older women generally opt for the richer variety.

WHEN TO CONSULT?

▶ You have severe itching that persists despite efforts to improve and replenish your skin's hydration.
▶ The symptoms prevent you from sleeping.
▶ You notice redness or sores on your skin.
▶ The skin lesions become infected or inflamed.

WHAT HAPPENS DURING THE EXAM?

The doctor will examine the skin and check for infestation, infection or eczema. He or she will take a thorough history to become familiar with your hygiene and hydration habits and investigate any other possible causes for the dryness.

WHAT IS THE TREATMENT?

Improved skin hydration and reduced exposure to irritating products are often enough to remedy the problem. Menthol creams are also refreshing and provide rapid relief. If necessary, steroid or antihistamine creams can be prescribed to reduce irritation or inflammation caused by dryness.

Earaches and Other Ear Problems

The ear is divided into three distinct parts: the outer ear (the pinna and auditory canal), the middle ear (the eardrum, ossicles and Eustachian tube) and the inner ear (containing the balance and hearing organs). Earaches occur in the outer and middle ear alone because the inner ear lacks the necessary nerve endings.

People often get earaches in airplanes or after coming in from the cold because of re-adjustments to changes in air pressure. The pain is transitory and does not indicate a serious condition. A number of other problems, however, may require medical attention.

WHAT ARE THE CAUSES?

Outer ear

► *Infections.* Most infections of the outer ear are caused by bacteria (swimmer's ear, eczema or psoriasis with a secondary infection, for example). Yeast infections are also common, brought on by heat and dampness in the external auditory canal, or repeated administration of antibiotic drops which can destroy the bacterial flora that normally helps protect the ear canal against infection. In both types of infection, earaches are accompanied by redness, a foul-smelling discharge of pus (often brownish), and itching.

► *Inflammatory diseases.* Eczema, acne or psoriasis can develop in the external ear canal. There may also be inflammation of the cartilage, a condition known as perichondritis. The earache is accompanied by itching, redness and swelling.

► *Frostbite of the pinna.* Cold temperatures cause the blood vessels to constrict. The effects are felt more rapidly in the pinna because of the small number of blood vessels. Earaches are painful and accompanied by redness and swelling.

► *Trauma to the pinna.* A violent blow to the ear can damage the cartilage and lead to a deformity commonly known as "cauliflower ears". Cleaning the ear too deeply with swabs or accidentally penetrating the ear with a foreign object can also cause injury. The trauma causes pain, swelling, bruising and bleeding.

► *Impacted cerumen (wax build-up).* Cleaning your ears with cotton swabs is unnecessary, as the canal usually cleans itself. It can also cause wax to permanently accumulate deep within the outer ear canal, leading to earache and loss of hearing.

► *Sensitivity or allergy to metals.* Metal earrings can cause infections or allergic reactions in the earlobe. In both cases, the pain is accompanied by redness, swelling and a discharge of pus from the lobe.

► *Radiating pain.* Caused by a problem elsewhere in the body, the pain radiates to the ear. The origin may be a toothache, sinusitis, temporomadibular joint (jaw) dysfunction, parotitis (inflammation of the parotid gland, a salivary gland located under the ear), cervical nerve neuralgia (inflammation of the cervical nerves surrounding the ears), or a tumour on the tonsils, the base of the tongue or the nasopharynx.

► *Tumour of the pinna.* The ear is one of the parts of the body most frequently exposed to the sun and, paradoxically, one of the least protected. If an ulcer or tumefaction (lump or swelling) develops on the pinna, it may be painful.

Middle ear

► *Otitis.* Otitis media occurs when the Eustachian tube (the canal linking the mouth and the middle ear) becomes blocked and pressure builds up in the middle ear. This causes irritation of the mucous membrane, leading to secretions that create an environment favourable to the proliferation of nearby bacteria. Earache is accompanied by bleeding, loss of hearing, and if the eardrum breaks, the discharge of foul-smelling pus.

► *Mastoiditis.* This is a severe complication of otitis media, characterized by intense pain, redness behind the ear and sensitivity to the touch.

► *Perforated eardrum.* A broken eardrum is most commonly caused by the accumulation of liquid in the middle ear due to an attack of otitis media. While the perforation frequently heals on its own, this may not be the case in people who suffer from frequent middle ear infections because their eardrums are usually so severely damaged that bacteria circulate freely. Trauma to the ear can also cause dramatic pressure changes that burst the eardrum. The pain experienced at the moment of rupture disappears as the pressure drops, and is followed by a loss of hearing.

► *Barotrauma.* Rapid decompression in an airplane or while scuba diving may perforate the eardrum and cause bleeding, but this will usually heal on its own.

► *Osteospongiosis.* Also known as osteosclerosis, this hereditary illness reduces mobility of the stapes, one of the three ossicles in the middle ear that transmit sound vibrations to the inner ear. If left untreated, it may lead to deafness.

Inner ear

► *Infections,* such as labyrinthitis and vestibular neuritis. These rare infections may affect the balance and hearing organs. Frequently of viral origin (except for labyrinthitis), they are usually accompanied by dizziness or hearing loss, as well as a ringing sound known as tinnitus.

► *Ménière's disease.* This incapacitating disease is still not well understood. Relatively common, it manifests in dizziness, tinnitus and hearing loss caused by congestion and water retention in the inner ear.

► *Trauma caused by extremely loud noise.* This leads to hearing loss and tinnitus.

► *Tumours,* such as a neuroma of the auditory nerve, are accompanied by dizziness, tinnitus and hearing loss.

PRACTICAL ADVICE

Avoid scratching inside the ear. This will only aggravate the irritation or infection.

Never use cotton swabs to clean your ears. The external ear canal is lined with a mucous membrane covered with cilia (small, vibrating hairs) that screen out foreign objects. It does not need to be cleaned.

Cotton swabs (like Q-tips) will only damage the cilia and push the cerumen (wax) deeper into the canal. Use a face cloth or the corner of a wet towel to clean your ears. Remember: never put anything smaller than your elbow in your ear!

Take a painkiller. To ease the pain, take one or two tablets containing 325 or 500 mg of acetaminophen four times a day, up to a maximum of 4 grams a day. Anti-inflammatories are also effective. Follow the manufacturer's instructions. Take both types of medication if the pain is difficult to control.

Relieve itchiness caused by eczema, acne and psoriasis in the external ear canal. Aluminum acetate (Buro-Sol) or 1% cortisone drops, sold over the counter in pharmacies, can provide relief, although their effectiveness is limited because they do not contain antibiotics. In fact, these drops are not recommended if you have an infection, since they can actually make it worse. Consult a doctor before using these products.

Take care of your frostbite. Apply room temperature water compresses for about one hour. Repeat three to four times a day. Hot water or ice should not be used because they can burn the skin. If the pain does not disappear after 12 hours, consult a doctor.

Dislodge a foreign object carefully. If there is a live insect in your ear, tilt your head to the other side and slowly pour lukewarm water into the ear. This will drown the insect and wash it out. If a foreign object has been pushed into the canal, it may fall out by itself if you tilt your head to that side. If it does not, see a doctor immediately.

Take precautions when swimming. People prone to swimmer's ear or suffering from eczema or psoriasis of the ear canal should remember that exposure to bacteria or chlorine in water can trigger an episode of otitis. Prevent the infection by wearing swimmer's ear plugs. Your doctor can also prescribe Buro-Sol or antibiotic cortisone drops, to be administered after you come out of the water.

Dry your ears well. A humid environment is an ideal breeding ground for bacteria, yeast, psoriasis and eczema. After taking a shower or swimming, always dry your ears with a face cloth or the corner of a towel.

Protect your ears from the sun year round. Don't forget your ears when you apply sunscreen! The recommended strength is 15 SPF for adults and 30 SPF for children.

Remove your earrings if your piercing is infected. Do not wear earrings for a few days, and disinfect your earlobes with antiseptic, antibiotic cream or antibacterial soap. Note that rubbing alcohol is not recommended, as it can burn the skin. Ask your pharmacist for advice.

Consult a doctor. If you removed your earrings, cleaned your piercing, and the symptoms persist, visit your doctor. If the symptoms disappear, clean your earrings with antiseptic before wearing them again. If the symptoms reappear, you probably have an allergy, and should wear earrings made of a different type of metal.

Wear good quality earrings. Wearing only gold (minimum 14 karat) or silver earrings is the best way to avoid infections and allergic reactions, though it should be remembered that no metal is completely antiallergenic.

Take care of recently pierced ears. Daily maintenance is necessary to avoid infection. During the two weeks it takes for your body to get used to a foreign object, remove your earrings once a day, clean the stem with antiseptic, and disinfect your earlobes.

Be careful using hair dye. This product will cause severe irritation if it comes in contact with the skin inside the ears.

Protect yourself from excessive noise. People frequently exposed to very loud noise (factory workers, hunters, etc.) should always wear

ear protection. Children and teenagers should never listen to music with headphones at maximum volume.

WHEN TO CONSULT?

- ► The earache or itching is unbearable.
- ► Your earache has lasted more than 12 hours.
- ► There is a red spot behind your ear.
- ► Your ear is bleeding.
- ► You experience hearing loss.
- ► You hear noises in your ears.
- ► You feel dizzy.
- ► There is a persistent infection in your earlobe piercing.
- ► A foreign object is trapped in your ear canal.

WHAT HAPPENS DURING THE EXAM?

Your physician will perform a careful examination of the ear and, if necessary, refer you to an ear, nose and throat (ENT) specialist.

WHAT IS THE TREATMENT?

Outer ear

Outer ear infections are treated with painkillers and drops containing antibiotics and cortisone; yeast infections are treated with antifungal medication; and persistent infections of the earlobe respond well to antibiotics.

If trauma to the ear has caused a hematoma, the blood that has accumulated between the skin and cartilage may be drained.

There are several techniques for removing impacted cerumen, the most common of which involves irrigation with water or a curettage. If an infection has developed, the doctor will use a vaccum procedure.

Tumours on the auricula are easily treated. Treatment should begin immediately.

Frostbite may be complicated by infection or necrosis. In the case of infection, antibiotic drops will be prescribed.

Middle ear

Middle ear infections are sometimes treated with antibiotics, decongestants and painkillers.

If the eardrum remains perforated following repeated episodes of otitis media, minor surgery may be required. The operation involves the attachment of a small piece of sterile paper (resembling a piece of cigarette rolling paper) over the perforation, which holds the skin together to allow healing.

Osteospongiosis usually requires surgical treatment. This minor surgery involves the severing of the ligament attached to the stapes to restore mobility.

Mastoiditis is treated with antibiotics. This condition may require emergency hospitalization to ensure that the inflammation does not spread to the meninges surrounding the brain.

Inner ear

Many inner ear problems (deafness, dizziness, tinnitus) require specialized treatment.

Tumours are treated surgically or with radiation therapy.

Elbow Pain

While the arm is astonishingly resistant and flexible, certain of its structures—notably the elbow—are more vulnerable than others. Perhaps the most common injury affecting the elbow is lateral humeral epicondylitis (tennis elbow), a form of tendinitis (inflammation of the tendons) that afflicts anyone putting repetitive stress on the area, from athletes, to manual labourers, to violinists and sculptors.

WHAT ARE THE CAUSES?

► *Overuse / abuse.* The movement required by certain sports and all types of manual labour can lead to elbow pain and limited function.

► *Trauma.* A fall or blow to the elbow can cause a small piece of bone to detach (sometimes even years later) and interfere with joint movement. In some cases, the elbow remains locked in extension, either with or without pain. The detached piece of bone is known as a "joint mouse".

► *Tennis elbow (lateral humeral epicondylitis).* The pain is concentrated in the outer elbow.

► *Other forms of tendinitis.* Medial humeral epicondylitis (golfer's elbow) results from tendinitis in the inner aspect of the elbow causing pain. Biceps tendinitis, occurring at the point where the muscle and tendon join, can also cause pain in the fold of the elbow.

► *Elbow bursitis.* Small sacs (bursae) between the skin and bone reduce friction during movement. Bursitis occurs when the bursae become inflamed and swell with liquid, sometimes to the size of an egg. This condition, known as "Popeye elbow", is usually painless.

► *Arthritis of the elbow joint.* This inflammatory condition manifests in edema, a sensation of heat, redness, and intense pain in the elbow, reducing the range of movement.

► *Cervical spine problem.* In many cases, a pinched nerve in the neck causes pain in the arms that is sometimes concentrated in the elbow.

PRACTICAL ADVICE

Rest your elbow. Decrease or stop any painful activities.

Use painkillers. Acetaminophen or anti-inflammatories such as aspirin or ibuprofen can be helpful. Take one or two tablets of acetaminophen (325 mg to 500 mg) four times a day, never exceeding 4 grams daily. If taking aspirin or another anti-inflammatory, follow the manufacturer's dosage recommendations. Take both acetaminophen and an anti-inflammatory if the pain is difficult to control. Note, however, that you should never combine aspirin with an anti-inflammatory, as this can lead to stomach ulcers. Taking anti-inflammatories on an empty stomach has the same effect.

Apply an analgesic cream. Zostrix is a non-prescription ointment that blocks the transmission of pain and effectively eliminates elbow pain.

Use a cold compress for tendinitis. Freeze a small plastic bag filled with water. Wrap the frozen bag in a towel (to protect your skin) and apply to the elbow for no more than 10 to 15 minutes at a time, four or five times daily. A bag of frozen peas can also do the job.

Use a hot compress for arthritis. Apply a hot water bottle wrapped in a towel or a heating pad for no more than 10 to 15 minutes at a time, four or five times daily.

Do not lift a heavy briefcase with a straight arm. Also avoid carrying your briefcase in one hand if walking a long distance.

Hold and carry objects carefully. Do not carry heavy objects (like garbage bags) away from your body, using only one arm.

Do not resume activities without rehabilitation. No matter how long you have rested your elbow, do not return to your regular activities before undergoing rehabilitation. Wear an elbow splint two or three centimetres below the painful area while playing sports to absorb some of the shock. This product is available in pharmacies.

Use a good tennis racket. Wood or graphite is preferable, as metal absorbs none of the shock of impact, directing all the pressure into the arm.

Do warm-up exercises. Warm up your muscles before any sports activity.

WHEN TO CONSULT?

- ▶ Your elbow locks and you can no longer bend it. It may be painful.
- ▶ A soft, egg-shaped swelling has appeared on the outside of the elbow. It may be painful and does not disappear on its own.
- ▶ The pain stops you from taking part in many of your regular activities.
- ▶ The pain is accompanied by redness, a sensation of heat, and swelling (possibly caused by arthritis or gout).
- ▶ The pain is accompanied by muscle weakness (possibly caused by a cervical spine problem).
- ▶ Hot or cold treatments and over-the-counter medications (acetominophen or the anti-inflammatories, ibuprofen or aspirin) have brought no relief.

WHAT HAPPENS DURING THE EXAM?

The doctor assesses the symptoms and performs a physical examination. X-rays may be ordered. If the doctor suspects arthritis, he or she will order blood tests to determine the type.

WHAT IS THE TREATMENT?

Physiotherapy is an effective treatment for problems causing elbow pain.

Trauma

If the prescribed medication (anti-inflammatories) and physiotherapy are not helpful, cortisone infiltrations can ease the pain and restore flexibility. Surgery is rarely recommended, although it may be necessary to treat problems resulting from trauma. When the elbow has become locked in extension, for example, the piece of bone blocking movement can be surgically removed.

Tennis elbow

Serious cases that do not improve with medication and rest require local infiltrations of cortisone and, as a last resort, surgery.

Other forms of tendinitis, bursitis and arthritis of the elbow

If the treatments listed in this book are ineffective, cortisone infiltrations often ease the symptoms.

Cervical spine problem

The neck is treated according to the specific problem. Acupuncture, physiotherapy and manipulation may be helpful.

Erectile Dysfunction (Sexual Impotence)

Doctors currently use the phrases "erectile dysfunction" or "erectile problems" to refer to what used to be known as "impotence". These terms describe the inability to achieve or maintain an erection rigid enough for satisfying sexual intercourse. This is not considered to be a significant problem unless it is recurrent and has lasted at least three months. Temporary, isolated incidents do not amount to erectile dysfunction.

Erections are not voluntary. The mechanism relies not only on sexual stimulation (stroking of the genitals, fantasies, etc.), but on a properly functioning nervous system (to transmit signals of excitement), a good circulatory system (to facilitate blood flow to the penis), and an intact penis. Good health, in other words, is crucial for proper erections.

A man with erectile problems (or who cannot achieve erection at all) can still experience desire, have orgasms, and ejaculate, either through masturbation or by rubbing his genitals against his partner's. It is even possible for a man whose erections are not rigid enough for penetration to have children if he ejaculates on his partner's vulva or vaginal opening. However, since having erection is an integral part of the normal sexual response, erectile dysfunction is considered to be abnormal or possibly, the symptom of an underlying illness.

Although still a taboo subject, this problem is very common, with one man in 10 experiencing it at some point in his life. Beginning at age 50, the risk of being affected increases significantly. Erectile dysfunction can have physiological causes, psychological causes, or a combination of both.

Physiological causes
► Rare in healthy men under the age of 50. More common in older men.
► Absence of nocturnal or morning erections.
► Often starts gradually, progressing over months and even years.

► Partial or total inability to achieve or maintain erection, regardless of circumstances.
► Reversible in many cases.

Psychological causes
► Nocturnal or morning erections still occur.
► No problem with erection during masturbation.
► Problem frequently appears suddenly.
► Occurs only in certain circumstances.
► Does not seem to be associated with any illness.

WHAT ARE THE CAUSES?
Physiological
► *Blood vessel abnormality.* Vascular problems in the veins or arteries are responsible for the majority of cases. The most frequent diseases and risk factors include hardening of the arteries (arteriosclerosis), hypertension, high cholesterol, and diabetes.
► *Certain medications.* Antihypertensives, antidepressants, antipsychotics, antiepileptics, cimetidine (to decrease gastric acid secretion) and high doses of anxiety medications (such as Ativan or Valium) can affect the erectile vascular mechanism.
► *Radical Prostatectomy (removal of the prostate gland).* This invasive surgical procedure used to treat prostate cancer may affect the nerves of the penis. Erectile problems occur in 50% to 60% of cases.
► *Smoking.* Smoking is a very significant factor in erectile dysfunction, aggravating arteriosclerosis and causing venous leaks, which prevent the penis from retaining blood.
► *Nerve and central nervous system abnormalities* such as trauma to the spinal cord (causing paraplegia, for example), multiple sclerosis, or Parkinson's disease may be responsible. These disorders can disturb the transmission of nerve impulses from the genital organs to the brain and vice versa.
► *Peyronie's disease.* The abnormal curvature of the penis is caused by hard, palpable scar tissue inside the organ. Erectile difficulties exist only when there is significant deformity.

Psychological causes

- ► *Performance anxiety.* This is the most common psychological cause of erectile dysfunction. The man is afraid he will not be able to achieve or maintain an erection long enough to satisfy himself or his partner.
- ► *Other psychological factors.* Relationship problems or a break-up, hostility toward the partner, lack of interest in sex, poor sexual education, trouble at work, job loss, financial worries, fatigue, a period of sexual abstinence or drug or alcohol withdrawal (after a binge) are just some of the factors that can lead to erectile problems.

PRACTICAL ADVICE

See a doctor. It is important to understand that there is a solution for most erectile problems. Talk to a doctor you trust. If necessary, ask for help from a centre that specializes in erectile difficulties.

Explore fantasies and new stimulation techniques. Concrete steps can be taken to confront psychological causes for erectile dysfunction. Together, couples can improve their communication, indulge in sexual fantasies, increase the duration and intensity of penile stimulation by the partner, try new techniques (such as oral stimulation), or watch erotic movies.

Try not to get too worked up about it. A man faced with erectile dysfunction should try not to worry too much, since performance anxiety (the fear of not being able to "get it up") can short-circuit the mechanism of erection altogether. Instead of focusing on the lack of erection, the man should try to enjoy his sensuality, which may actually help him regain his ability to achieve erections. It is also important for the partner to remember that erectile problems do not necessarily lead to sexual dissatisfaction. In fact, many people tell their doctors that their spouse has become a better lover in the absence of penetration, as the man often starts to explore other aspects of his sexuality.

Adopt healthy eating habits. A high-fat diet can cause as much damage to the penis as to the heart. Arterial or venous vascular problems are responsible for most cases of erectile dysfunction that have a physiological origin. Eat better, lose weight if necessary, and exercise several times a week.

Stop smoking. Smoking disrupts the vascular mechanism of erections by gradually obstructing the small arteries, which reduces the blood flow necessary for erection. It can also cause blood to leak from the veins of the penis during an erection, making it less rigid. Quitting smoking is one of the most important things you can do if you are trying to regain erectile function.

Limit alcohol consumption. One or two drinks relaxes inhibitions and can help a person get "in the mood" for sexual intercourse. Large amounts, however, slow down the nervous system and reflexes, causing erectile problems.

Abstinent? As they get older, circumstances (hospitalization, death of a spouse) may force men to refrain from sexual relations for an extended period of time. Long periods of abstinence such as these may make it more difficult for a man to achieve erection, but the ability can be regained gradually, perhaps over a few weeks of sexual interaction, provided he feels no pressure.

Check your medications. Don't stop taking your medication, even if you fear it might be causing your problem. You should, however, speak to your doctor about replacing your prescription with a drug that does not have this side effect.

WHEN TO CONSULT?
► Your erectile problems have lasted more than three months. Consult sooner if the situation is particularly difficult for you.

WHAT HAPPENS DURING THE EXAM?

Consultation may be lengthy. The doctor takes a complete medical and sexual history to determine whether the erectile dysfunction is primarily physiological or psychological in nature, or both. He or she then performs a specific physical examination to check whether the genital organs, blood vessels, and penile nerves and tissues are functioning normally. Specialized tests such as a penile Doppler (to measure arterial blood flow in the penis) may be used.

WHAT IS THE TREATMENT?

Physiological causes

Blood vessel, nerve and central nervous system abnormalities
If treatment of the underlying disease does not improve the patient's erectile function, the doctor will suggest specific treatments:

► Sildenafil (Viagra). This oral medication dilates the blood vessels of the penis, allowing more blood to flow in. It does not cause an automatic erection nor increase sexual desire; it simply helps a man achieve and maintain erection if he is sexually stimulated. Nearly 80% of users have satisfactory results.

► Intracavernous injections. This treatment consists of injecting prostaglandin E_1 into the side of the penis. The patient must overcome the fear of an injection in this area. With no sexual stimulation, the penis becomes completely rigid within fifteen minutes. The erection lasts for 30 minutes to an hour and is effective in 85% of cases.

► External prosthesis (vacuum pump). This mechanical (not surgical) technique involves an apparatus in the form of a plastic cylinder connected to a pump. The penis is inserted into the cylinder and the air is pumped out, creating a vacuum which forces blood to flow into the cavernous bodies (spongy tissue) of the penis. A ring is placed at the base of the penis to prevent the blood from escaping, and the cylinder is removed. The ring must be removed after 30 minutes to avoid the formation of blood clots. Couples who have mastered the use of this device report that it is effective 80% of the time.

► Transurethral treatment. The Medicated Urethral System of Erection (MUSE) involves inserting a mini-suppository (about the size of a grain of rice) of alprostadil into the urethra (the opening of the penis). The medication is absorbed into the blood and carried to the cavernous bodies of the penis, causing the muscles to relax and the penis to become engorged with blood. The erection occurs within 20 minutes, with or without sexual stimulation, and lasts for about an hour. It is effective in 40% of cases.

► Penile prostheses (implants). There are several types. Silicone prostheses implanted under the skin are totally invisible. Most are inflatable and become rigid by means of a pump located inside the scrotum. In the past, this was the most common way to help men overcome erectile dysfunction. Today, it is a last resort. The implant is irreversible, and only recommended if all other methods have failed to produce results.

It is sometimes necessary to combine medical treatment with sex therapy for the best results.

Radical prostatectomy
The treatments listed above are all applicable to men who have undergone a radical prostatectomy.

Smoking
If the patient has the will to quit smoking, the doctor can prescribe different methods, such as nicotine patches or bupropion (Zyban), an oral medication. Nicotine chewing gum is also available over-the-counter in pharmacies. Quitting for good prevents further damage to the veins and arteries, helping a man regain his erectile capacity.

Peyronie's disease
This condition can disappear spontaneously after six months to two years, with no particular treatment. If the curvature greatly interferes with penetration, some men will resort to surgery after a year and a half or two years.

Psychological causes

The doctor may recommend sex therapy, preferably including the patient's partner. Therapy usually lasts 20 sessions and the success rate is very high.

Excessive Sweating (Hyperhidrosis)

Perspiration is a normal phenomenon that has the essential function of maintaining a constant body temperature.

Two types of sweat glands secrete perspiration: eccrine glands, found everywhere in the skin but particularly on the hands, feet, face and under the arms; and apocrine glands, found in the groin and underarm areas. Eccrine perspiration is largely made up of water and salt whereas apocrine perspiration is rich in organic substances (vitamin C, antibodies, urea, uric acid, ammonia and lactic acid). It is the combination of perspiration and bacteria on the skin that causes an unpleasant odour.

Hyperhidrosis (excessive or profuse sweating) can be general or localized (most often in the hands, feet or underarms). The intensity of perspiration diminishes with age. About 28% of the population suffers from hyperhidrosis.

Besides odour, the signs of profuse sweating include:

► Continually moist hands.
► Hand perspiration that stains paper.
► Underarm perspiration that stains clothing.
► Clothing and shoes that wear out quickly.
► Chilblain on the feet in cold weather.
► Athlete's foot, eczema, blisters, warts and even ingrown toenails.

WHAT ARE THE CAUSES?

► *External factors.* Exercise, heat, alcohol, smoking, spicy foods and caffeine dilate the blood vessels and stimulate the secretion of the eccrine and apocrine glands.
► *Emotional states.* Fear, stress and anxiety can trigger profuse sweating, especially from the palms of the hands, feet and underarms.
► *Illnesses* such as diabetes, heart disease, Parkinson's disease, cancer, pneumonia, thyroid gland disorders, liver or kidney failure (among others), cause excessive general sweating. If profuse

sweating occurs at night, Hodgkin's disease or tuberculosis may be the cause.

► **Hormone imbalance.** During puberty, menstruation and menopause, hormones stimulate the sweat glands even more.

► **Intoxication.** Poisoning from insecticides, herbicides or mercury results in various symptoms, including general profuse sweating. Drug (medicinal and other) and alcohol withdrawal can also give someone the "sweats."

PRACTICAL ADVICE

Observe good personal hygiene. Bathe or shower at least once, but even twice a day. Wash with soap, paying special attention to the hands, feet, underarms, groin area and face. Shaving your underarms will reduce the amount of bacteria—this is true for both men and women who suffer from hyperhidrosis.

Refrain from eating certain foods. Avoid spicy dishes, salmon (which causes blood vessel dilation and stimulates the sweat glands), coffee, tea, cola and chocolate.

Do not go barefoot. You run the risk of catching warts, fungi or bacteria that will increase your foot perspiration problem. Be especially careful in public areas and hot and humid weather – both are ideal conditions for fungi and bacteria.

Know which soap to use. The best option for your problem is a deodorant soap that will halt the action of bacteria. Ask your pharmacist for advice. If perspiration and odour persist, antibacterial cleansers such as Teraseptic or Physohex (available by prescription) are very effective.

Dry off properly. A moist environment is ideal for bacteria and fungi. When you get out of the water, pay special attention to the toes and folds of the skin.

Ward off odour. When the skin is fully dry, sprinkle baby powder, sodium bicarbonate or cornstarch in the underarm area and between the toes. Shaved underarms trap less perspiration.

Know when to use a deodorant or antiperspirant. Deodorants mask underarm odour and leave an antibacterial agent on the skin that destroys odour-causing bacteria. If underarm odour is very pronounced, an antiperspirant will be more appropriate. Antiperspirants contain a substance, aluminium hydrochloride, that blocks perspiration. Some products contain both substances.

Use a stick or roll-on product. Sprays do not last as long and are therefore less effective.

Try different products. If the products described above irritate your skin, try a topical antibiotic cream (available without prescription). Such creams have an antibacterial effect that fights odour. Health food stores and some pharmacies sell crystallized mineral salts to help control bacteria without irritating the skin.

Have a cold bath. Soaking in cold water for 30 minutes will slow down perspiration for approximately three hours. This method can be useful during periods of stress.

Miliaria or Prickly Heat

Miliaria is a skin rash characterized by the appearance of red, pinhead-sized bumps on the face, neck and chest. It is caused by a temporary obstruction of the sweat glands resulting from a rise in body temperature (fever or surrounding temperature). The spots disappear as the temperature drops. This condition is harmless and no treatment is required.

Avoid stress. If stress makes you perspire, learn how to manage it through relaxation techniques or rest.

Choose the right clothing. Cotton absorbs perspiration better than synthetic fibres. Always wear clean undergarments and clothing as they absorb perspiration better. During really hot weather, wear loose-fitting clothing and change regularly.

Wear the right shoes. Leather breathes better than synthetic materials, facilitating the evaporation of sweat. Wear open-toe sandals as often as possible. Do not wear the same shoes two days in a row. Alternate pairs to allow them time to dry out.

WHEN TO CONSULT?
► Perspiration causes problems in your day-to-day life.
► Family and friends notice the odour.
► You have a related health problem.

WHAT HAPPENS DURING THE EXAM?
The examination and possible diagnosis are based on the patient's history, observation of perspiration droplets, traces of moisture on clothing, and wear on shoes. More exhaustive tests are usually not required.

WHAT IS THE TREATMENT?
The doctor may prescribe special antiperspirants. For serious perspiration problems, aluminium chloride-based products dissolved in alcohol or combined with salicylic acid in gel form have good results. Most patients need not use these products for more than 18 months.

The Drionic (available by prescription) is an ion-transmitting device with separate fittings for the hands, feet and underarms that blocks the duct openings of the sweat glands.

Botox (botulinum toxin type A) injections in the underarms, hands, feet, or forehead may be suggested. This will control excessive sweating for about six months.

Expectoration

In theory, a healthy person does not have to cough up sputum. Expectoration (phlegm) is produced by the body's immune system in response to an internal or external attack.

The epithelium (the mucous membrane lining the respiratory tract) consists of cells with thousands of tiny vibrating hairs, known as cilia. When attacked, the epithelium secretes mucus that is expelled by the movement of the cilia, causing the person to cough up phlegm.

Expectoration consists of 95% water and 5% protein. It may be coloured, bloody, or foul-smelling.

WHAT ARE THE CAUSES?

► *Medications.* Angiotensin (used to treat high blood pressure) converts enzyme inhibitors and may lead to coughing. The resulting irritation can cause whitish or coloured (yellowish, greenish, brownish or greyish) expectoration.

► *Foreign body.* If a small object or piece of food becomes stuck in the respiratory tract, it can trigger a dry cough with no expectoration. If the foreign body blocks a pulmonary orifice, it will lead to infection, causing a loose cough, fever, and whitish or coloured phlegm.

► *Infections.* The flu, pneumonia, rhinitis, and sinusitis cause whitish, coloured, or, in some cases, bloody expectoration. Other symptoms include fever, fatigue, headache, nasal congestion, and chills.

► *Acute bronchitis.* The inflammation of the bronchi caused by bacteria or toxins (such as chlorine) causes progressive symptoms, including a loose cough, coloured or bloody expectoration, fever, chills, shortness of breath and chest pain from coughing.

► *Asthma.* This disease can cause dry coughing or a loose cough with expectoration, depending on the degree of exposure to the allergen (substance provoking the allergic reaction). A dry cough indicates irritation of the bronchial tubes, while a loose cough with coloured expectoration is a sign of bronchial inflammation.

Other symptoms of an asthma attack include wheezing, tightness in the chest and the feeling of being smothered.

► *Chronic bronchitis* is most often caused by smoking, although people who work in polluted environments or come into frequent contact with toxic irritants (such as chlorine) are also susceptible. Chronic bronchitis may evolve into emphysema and respiratory failure. It is characterized by a chronic cough accompanied by whitish or coloured expectoration, sometimes containing blood.

► *Emphysema.* This disease most commonly arises in long-term smokers. In the lungs, the alveoli (through which oxygen enters the bloodstream) lose elasticity and progressively deteriorate. The sufferer wheezes and is continually out of breath, with a chronic cough and whitish, coloured or bloody expectoration.

► *Bronchiectasis* causes the dilation of the bronchial tubes, usually due to persistent infections in this area. Certain positions (such as lying down) will cause the sufferer to produce more phlegm than others, depending on the pulmonary lobe affected. Expectoration contains pus and is coloured or bloody. People with bronchiectasis are subject to recurrent attacks of acute bronchitis.

► *Pulmonary abscess.* In most cases, a pulmonary abscess develops when a case of pneumonia remains untreated or is not treated properly. The patient's condition generally deteriorates and he or she begins producing purulent (pus-filled), foul-smelling, coloured or bloody expectoration, accompanied by fever and chills.

► *Pulmonary embolism.* This occurs when a blood clot forms and obstructs a pulmonary artery, causing blood oxygen levels to drop. The patient suddenly begins coughing up coloured or bloody phlegm, becomes short of breath, and experiences intense chest pain. Pulmonary embolisms are fairly common and can be fatal.

► *Cystic fibrosis.* This hereditary disease causes the mucus glands to produce excessively thick, coloured or bloody secretions, which can obstruct the respiratory tract and cause bronchiectasis.

► *Gastroesophageal reflux (GER).* The stomach secretes hydrochloric acid to facilitate digestion, while the sphincter valve between the esophagus and the stomach opens and closes to let food through. If the valve is defective, acid moves up the esophagus and irritates the throat, causing a cough and whitish expectoration.

▶ *Heart failure.* This chronic disease develops when the heart is no longer able to properly pump blood to the body. The symptoms include frothy, coloured and frequently bloody expectoration, fatigue, and shortness of breath upon exertion or at rest (particularly when lying down).

▶ *Lung cancer.* Repeated coughing up of bloody expectoration, rapid weight loss and deformed fingertips (like drumsticks) are strong indicators of lung cancer.

PRACTICAL ADVICE

Quit smoking. Cigarettes are the primary cause of coughing and expectoration. Smoking shortens life expectancy and leads to chronic bronchitis, emphysema, and lung cancer. If you want to quit smoking, talk to your doctor, who can recommend some effective techniques.

Get vaccinated against the flu and pneumonia. If you are over 65 or suffer from heart disease, diabetes or other chronic illness, get a yearly vaccination against the flu and pneumonia in the fall. Two different vaccines are used. Speak to your doctor or ask at your local public health or community health clinic.

Do not ignore the flu. If you do not take care of yourself when you have the flu, your condition will deteriorate. Sleep and rest as much as possible, eat lightly, drink plenty of liquids to avoid dehydration (particularly vitamin-rich fruit juice), and take acetaminophen. If you have a cough but no expectoration, take some cough syrup.

Choose your cough syrup carefully. If you are coughing up phlegm, cough syrups are not recommended. Cough suppressants prevent you from expelling phlegm, leading to an accumulation of secretions in the lungs, and expectorants are ineffective. The best treatment for a loose cough is to stay well-hydrated so the expectoration liquefies and is easier to expel. A cough and expectoration that lasts for three weeks or more may be a sign of a chronic problem.

Take note of your symptoms. If you are coughing up phlegm more and more often, note the colour, odour, and frequency of expectorations. Also note the time of day you tend to expectorate, as well as any other symptoms. Give this information to your doctor, and bring a sample of your expectoration in a clean container to facilitate diagnosis.

Adapt to gastroesophagal reflux. Consume less fatty food, chocolate, mint, alcohol and caffeine. Avoid eating or drinking for two hours before bedtime. Eat smaller, more frequent, meals. Do not wear binding clothes (like a tight belt) that put pressure on the abdomen; this can push the stomach up towards the rib cage and increase GER. When lying down, keep your head raised approximately 20 cm. Quit smoking, and maintain a healthy weight.

WHEN TO CONSULT?

- ► You are coughing and producing sputum for no apparent reason.
- ► You have had a loose cough (with expectoration) for over three weeks. It may be getting worse.
- ► There is blood in your expectoration.
- ► Expectoration is accompanied by chest pain or shortness of breath.
- ► You smoke and have noticed a change in your cough and expectoration.

WHAT HAPPENS DURING THE EXAM?

The doctor interviews the patient and performs a clinical exam. Lung X-rays may be necessary, as well as a culture from the expectoration if infection is suspected. He or she may also order a pulmonary radioisotope scan, which produces an image of the lungs after the injection of a radioactive element.

WHAT IS THE TREATMENT?

Medications

If the cough and expectoration are caused by medication, the doctor will modify the prescription.

Foreign body
The doctor will remove the foreign body from the respiratory tract in a surgical procedure known as a bronchoscopy, which involves the insertion of a tube through the mouth. The procedure is performed in hospital.

Infections and acute bronchitis
The symptoms of a persistent flu are treated with prescription anti-histamines and, in some cases, a cough suppressant. The doctor will prescribe antibiotics for pneumonia, acute bronchitis, chronic bronchitis with secondary infection, and sinusitis or rhinitis with secondary infection.

Asthma, chronic bronchitis, and emphysema
The symptoms are controlled with bronchodilators and anti-inflammatory drugs. If chronic bronchitis is linked to the work environment, the irritant must be identified and every effort made to minimize its effects. This may include better ventilation of the workplace, the wearing of a protective mask, or, in extreme cases, the withdrawal of the patient from the environment altogether. If chronic bronchitis is due to smoking, quitting is the only way to improve the condition.

Brochiectasis and pulmonary abscess
These conditions are treated with antibiotics and postural drainage, whereby the patient lies in an inclined position to clear the phlegm and drain the abscess.

Pulmonary embolism
The patient must be hospitalized immediately and treated with anti-coagulants.

Cystic fibrosis
This condition is treated with bronchodilators, postural drainage, and antibiotics (at the first sign of infection).

Gastroesophageal reflux (GER)

The doctor will prescribe medication to diminish, neutralize, or eliminate acidity in the stomach.

Heart failure

If the cough and expectoration are secondary to heart failure, vasodilators (medications to dilate the blood vessels) and diuretics (medications to increase the volume of urine) are prescribed.

Lung cancer

The appropriate treatment (surgery, radiation therapy, or chemotherapy, depending on the stage of the cancer) is immediately undertaken. Of course, if the patient smokes, he or she must quit.

Eye Fatigue

Eye strain or overuse frequently leads to eye fatigue. Generally not serious, eye fatigue may be a sign of infection in children, or associated with the aging process in people over 50. In rare cases, it is caused by disease or medication.

The symptoms are burning or itchiness of the eyes, heaviness in the eyelids, or pressure on the eye.

In some cases, eye fatigue is accompanied by headache, dizziness, and nausea.

WHAT ARE THE CAUSES?

- *Environment.*
- *Air conditioning.*
- *Heating systems.*
- *Cigarette smoke or air pollution.*
- *Industrial or other forms of dust.*

Certain activities

- *Extended TV or video monitor viewing.*
- *Regular computer work.* Regular work at a computer terminal causes eye fatigue in 15% of people. Twenty minutes of virtual reality causes eye fatigue accompanied by headache, dizziness and sometimes nausea in 60% of people.

Aging

- *Aging.* As the body ages, it secretes less lachrymal fluid (tears) and the eyes become dry. This is the primary reason for eye fatigue in people over 50 years of age.

Deviating or weak eye

- *Latent strabismus (phoria)* causes focusing problems and is characterized by a tendency of the eye to deviate outward or inward. The sufferer has trouble keeping his or her eyes aligned and they may appear crossed.

► **Accommodation spasm** or blurred vision occurs when it becomes difficult for the eyes to focus at either close or long range. It commonly occurs in children under the age of seven or eight who are required to look at the blackboard for extended periods.

► **Convergence insufficiency,** also common in children, prevents the sufferer from sustaining focus in both eyes at close range. The effort required to read, for example, causes blurred vision and headaches.

► **Hypermetropia and astigmatism.** Hypertropia, also known as "farsightedness", is a condition whereby the sufferer has difficulty seeing at close range. Both hypertropia and astigmatism are caused by an irregular curvature of the cornea, which, if left uncorrected, may lead to eye fatigue as the sufferer strains to focus.

Diseases or medication

► **Certain diseases,** such as rheumatoid arthritis, can cause dry eyes.

► **Medications.** Diuretics and antidepressants such as atropine, lithium and bentylol, may also lead to dry eyes.

PRACTICAL ADVICE

For dry eyes. Apply lukewarm wet compresses to the eyelids. Rinsing the eyes with lukewarm water is also beneficial. (Sterilization is not necessary; tap water will do just fine.) Be sure the water is not too hot.

Why do our eyes dry out as we age?

The liquid of our tears (known as lachrymal film) is composed of three layers: the external layer, an oil secreted by the lachrymal gland that prevents the eye from drying out; the middle layer, which is more watery and keeps the cornea oxygenated; and the internal mucinous layer, which secretes a liquid that spreads the tears evenly over the eye. As we age, the number of cells in each of the layers diminishes, causing the eyes to dry out.

Use artificial tears. These non-prescription eye drops can provide temporary relief to sensitive and irritated eyes.

Blink. Staring at a computer monitor or television screen causes you to blink less and dries out the eyes. Make an effort to blink frequently to restore the eyes' normal lachrymal fluid.

Use an air humidifier or place a bowl of water on the heater in your bedroom at night. You will avoid waking up with red, sticky or burning eyes by keeping your eyes hydrated as you sleep.

Take a break from the computer screen. Turn away from the monitor for a few minutes after every hour of work to rest your eyes.

Improve your work environment. Lower the brightness of your computer screen, adjust the contrast levels, or get an anti-glare monitor. The height of your desk should be appropriate to your body size. Place the monitor near the keyboard to avoid eyestrain.

Avoid polluted environments. Smoky rooms, heated cars, air conditioned interiors and dust can cause dry eyes.

Eyelid spasms or twitches

Muscle spasms in the eyelids cause uncontrollable eyelid twitching (blepharospasms). They are associated with fatigue, stress, anxiety, and migraines.

In most cases, the spasms do not last very long and stop on their own. While rest and stress reduction is usually sufficient treatment, doctors may prescribe Botox injections to paralyze the muscle in persistent and bothersome cases. This treatment lasts four to six months and does not impede normal vision or eye movement.

See a doctor. The examination is painless and the remedies effective. Do not hesitate to consult if there is a problem.

WHEN TO CONSULT?

- ► Your eyes are irritated, red, dry, itchy or watery.
- ► Your vision is blurred.
- ► You get migraines when you read.
- ► You see bright spots and zigzagging lights.
- ► You are very sensitive to light.
- ► You suffer from rheumatoid arthritis and have a dry mouth.

WHAT HAPPENS DURING THE EXAM?

The doctor administers the Shirmer or rose bengal test to assess the degree of eye dryness. A small piece of blotting paper is placed in the corner of the eye to absorb tears. After a few minutes, the extent of saturation is measured.

Strabismus and other eye deviations require specialized vision exams.

A complete eye exam is recommended for four-year-old (and sometimes younger) children.

WHAT IS THE TREATMENT?

Standard treatment

In 99% of cases, the doctor recommends artificial tears or lubricants in ointment form. Severely dry eyes may require more specialized medication.

Deviated or weak eye

Eye muscle re-education exercises, performed under the supervision of an orthoptist (specialist in this field) will improve vision in both eyes in cases of strabismus and convergence insufficiency.

In cases of accommodation spasms, the child should rest, change activities, or close his or her eyes for a few moments to regain normal vision. Glasses are advised in cases of hypermetropia and astigmatism.

Eye Irritation

The eye is constantly exposed to irritants such as pollution, smoke, makeup, bacteria, and viruses. The problems that arise are generally mild and respond well to treatment.

One or more of the following symptoms may develop:
- Dryness.
- Irritation.
- Red or bloodshot eyes.
- Pain or burning sensation.
- Tearing or discharge (thick yellowish pus).

WHAT ARE THE CAUSES?

- *Lachrymal gland insufficiency.* Three different glands are responsible for proper eye lubrication and a disorder in these glands causes either dryness, redness or irritation. People over the age of 40 tend to produce fewer tears, probably because of hormonal changes.
- *Blocked tear duct.* An obstruction of the tear ducts (which drain tears behind the eyelid or from the nose) causes excessive tearing.
- *Medications* such as antihistamines, antidepressants, decongestants, diuretics or beta-blockers can affect the eyes.
- *Diseases or infections* such as allergies, conjunctivitis, blepharitis (eyelid infection), keratitis (corneal infection), sinusitis, acne rosacea, viral infections, uveitis (inflammation of the iris), acute glaucoma, arterial hypertension and coagulation disorders can also affect the eyes.
- *Rheumatoid arthritis.* This chronic disease may be accompanied by Sjögren's syndrome, which is characterized by dry skin, mouth and eyes (irritation and absence of tears). Other forms of arthritis are not usually affected by this syndrome.
- *Lifestyle and environment.* Factors such as fatigue, lack of sleep, pollution, computer screen glare, chlorinated water, makeup, alcohol, drugs, air conditioning, excessive heat, prolonged wearing of contact lenses (not specifically designed

for extended use) and intense physical exertion can cause irritation of the eyes.

► **Sunburn.** Ultraviolet rays can burn the surface layer of the eye, causing a burning sensation and excessive tearing.

PRACTICAL ADVICE

Do not ignore redness. Redness is a sign of a problem, particularly when accompanied by pain, discharge and decreased visual acuity. Consult a physician as soon as possible.

Avoid over-the-counter antibiotic eye drops. These can lead the patient to develop a resistance to the antibiotics, resulting in even more serious eye infections and more complicated medical treatment. They may also trigger allergic reactions to the antibiotics.

Avoid vasoconstrictor eye drops ("brighterners"). They decrease eye redness by shrinking surface blood vessels, masking the underlying problem. Once the effect has subsided, the eye usually becomes even redder than before.

Do not rub your eyes. This will aggravate an eye irritation.

Use artificial tears. Especially useful in cases of dryness, these over-the-counter drops relieve eye irritation without damaging the surface of the cornea (epithelium). Apply several times a day, as needed. Avoid products that contain thimerosal, an additive that can cause allergic conjunctivitis.

Apply eye compresses. Warm or cold compresses applied to the eyelids three or four times a day can help diminish eye redness and irritation. Take an analgesic to relieve pain.

Remove discharge. At night, the eyes are at rest and not regularly rinsed by lachrymal fluid. The resulting bacterial proliferation can cause sufferers to awake in the morning with their eyelids crusty and stuck together. Clean them with a Q-tip dipped in baby shampoo (rinse your eyes afterwards) or another product designed for this purpose (for example, Lid-Care). Rubbing your eyes with a damp facecloth can also be effective. Always wash your hands afterwards to avoid spreading the infection to others.

Take antihistamines. If you suffer from allergies or are sensitive to smoke, pollution or other environmental factors, self-medicate with over the counter antihistamines. Always use unscented household products (tissues, soap and detergent).

Don't forget to blink. Certain activities (such as sewing or working for hours on the computer) are so absorbing that we often forget to blink. Be sure to blink to keep your eyes lubricated and prevent irritation.

Rest your eyes. Relieve eye fatigue (caused by staring at your computer screen, for example) by resting your eyes several times during the day. Move your eyes around without focussing on a fixed point, then close them and gently massage your temples. Or, hold a pencil in front of you and follow it with your eyes as you move it in various directions.

Sleep well. If your eyes are frequently dry and irritated in the morning, apply an artificial tear ointment (containing petroleum jelly and mineral oil) before going to bed. Humidifiers are also effective; direct the nozzle towards the ceiling where the air is driest.

Treat a sunburn. Apply cold compresses to the eyes and take an analgesic if you are in pain. To avoid this injury in the first place, wear UV-filter sunglasses that also protect the sides of your eyes. Wear glasses in windy weather, and if boating or skiing, wear polarized sunglasses that reflect the sun's rays.

Replace cosmetic products. Eye cosmetics eventually become contaminated and increase the risk of infection, so replace them every six months. If your eyes are irritated, avoid wearing makeup for a short time and purchase makeup for sensitive eyes.

Ensure proper lighting. If your eyes frequently become irritated for no apparent reason, try adjusting the lighting in your environment. Dim light leads to eye stress, fatigue and irritation. Proper lighting is not harsh, but is bright enough to read comfortably.

Adjust the fit and prescription of your eyeglasses. Glasses that slip down the bridge of the nose make the eye muscles strain to compensate for eye deviation. Your prescription should always be adjusted to your needs; consult your optometrist regularly.

Take care of contact lenses. If your contact lenses are irritating your eyes, stop wearing them for a couple of days and clean them with recommended solutions. Put your makeup on before inserting your contacts, and remove it before taking them out. If your problems persist, consult your optometrist. Because extended-wear contacts can scratch the cornea and cause infection, remove your lenses before bed each night. Dust can become lodged under your lenses and irritate your eyes; if you must spend time in a dusty environment, wear glasses instead of lenses.

WHEN TO CONSULT?

- Artificial tears do not relieve your discomfort.
- Your eyes are sensitive to light.
- You experience pain, persistent yellow discharge and decreased vision.
- You experience a burning sensation, pain or chronic discharge.
- You have swollen, painful or red eyelids.
- You suffer from rheumatoid arthritis and a dry mouth.
- Your contact lenses irritate your eyes.

WHAT HAPPENS DURING THE EXAM?

The physician or optometrist will perform a complete eye exam to determine whether there is a treatable disorder.

WHAT IS THE TREATMENT?

The physician or optometrist may prescribe a different type of artificial tears. In some cases, inserting a microscopic silicone implant into the tear duct ensures consistent eye lubrication. This procedure is quick (five minutes) and painless. The implant is invisible, does not affect your vision and can be worn as long as necessary.

An obstructed tear duct usually requires minor corrective surgery.

Eye infections are treated with antibiotics. Cortisone and medications to dilate the pupil are prescribed for uveitis. Glaucoma is treated with medications that decrease the pressure in the eye or, in some cases, laser surgery (iridotomy).

Treatment for rheumatoid arthritis should also control Sjögren's syndrome.

Fainting

Fainting is defined as the complete loss of consciousness (lasting up to thirty minutes) resulting from decreased blood flow to the brain. Any other symptoms are caused by an underlying condition.

There are several types of fainting, the most common of which are the following:

Simple fainting (vasovagal)
- Most frequent type.
- Accompanied by slack muscles and a pale face.
- Often preceded by two or three minutes of heat sensation, dizziness, weakness, sweating and blurred vision.

Fainting due to heart disease
- May be preceded by heart palpitations or chest pain.
- Often accompanied by sweating and a pale face.
- If the person is not lying down, he or she may experience brief convulsions (rhythmic spasms of one or more parts of the body).

Fainting secondary to an epileptic fit
- Fainting occurs without warning or is preceded by an aura (visual, auditory or olfactory hallucination), numbness, or convulsions.
- In most cases, a number of other symptoms manifest: the affected person suffers convulsions and generalized stiffness of the body lasting 30 to 60 seconds; the eyes roll back and the face turns reddish or bluish; the person froths at the mouth and may bite his or her tongue; sphincter muscles relax and the person urinates involuntarily.

Fainting secondary to lower blood pressure (orthostatic hypotension)
- Occurs only from a standing position, especially in the morning or at night (when getting up to go to the bathroom, for example).

► May be preceded by a few minutes of dizziness and blurred vision.

Fainting secondary to childbirth, cough, or defecation
► Quite rare.
► Usually lasts only a few seconds.

WHAT ARE THE CAUSES?
Simple fainting (vasovagal)
► *Intense emotion,* extreme pain, heat, prolonged standing, stress, hunger, fatigue, alcohol consumption.
Classic migraine (migraine with aura), in rare cases.

Fainting due to heart disease
► *Arrhythmia or infarction.* Fainting may occur during or after physical exertion or, in some cases, spontaneously.

Fainting secondary to epileptic fit
► *Neurological problems.* Epileptic fits usually occur spontaneously, but may be triggered by rapidly fluctuating lights.
► *Withdrawal from medications or alcohol.*

Fainting secondary to low blood pressure (orthostatic hypotension)
► *Medications.* This type of fainting is particularly common in elderly people taking a number of different medications such as antidepressants, antihypertensives, or antiparkinsonian drugs.
► *Diabetes or polyneuritis.*

Fainting secondary to childbirth, cough, or defecation
► *Precise cause unknown.* It is believed that the respiratory effort (particularly, the Valsalva maneuver) increases pressure in the thorax and reduces blood flow to the heart, causing fainting.

PRACTICAL ADVICE
Lay the affected person on the floor. Do not hold an unconscious person in an upright or seated position.

Keep the person's mouth clear. Do not try to force an unconscious person to swallow anything, whether it is liquid, medication, or nitroglycerine. If the person is having convulsions, avoid putting anything in his or her mouth (including fingers or pencils).

Do not get up too quickly. If you have just revived from a faint, wait a little while before getting up.

Do not look for the ideal place to lie down. If you are feeling faint, you have only a few seconds before you lose consciousness. Lie down on the floor where you are.

Avoid breathing too deeply and quickly. This can bring on hyperventilation, which can lead to fainting. Breathe normally.

Avoid prolonged standing, excessive heat, dehydration and alcoholic beverages. Particularly if you suffer from frequent fainting spells.

Know how to help. If you witness someone fainting, do the following: make sure the person is lying on his or her back with legs raised and apply a cold cloth to the forehead. If this fails to rouse the person, check breathing and the pulse and use cardiopulmonary resuscitation (CPR), if necessary. If the person is vomiting or drooling, turn the head to the side. Protect the head during convulsions, and try to turn the sufferer onto his or her side.

Call 911. If a person remains unconscious for more than two or three minutes, is having convulsions, faints repeatedly, has chest pain, is paralyzed on one side, or has an intense headache, this is an emergency.

Help prevent fainting due to low blood pressure (orthostatic hypotension). Make sure a person with low blood pressure gets up very slowly in the morning, resting on the side of the bed for a few minutes before standing up.

WHEN TO CONSULT?

► You have recently fainted.

► You have suffered a trauma in the last 48 hours; you are having convulsions; you experience prolonged or repeated fainting; you have chest pain or an intense headache; you are paralyzed. This is an emergency. Consult immediately.

WHAT HAPPENS DURING THE EXAM?

At the doctor's office

The doctor will need to know what happened before, during and after the fainting spell, so someone else who witnessed the event should accompany the patient. All medications and health records should also be brought to the doctor's office. The type and thoroughness of the examination depends on the possible causes and the patient's age and medical history. The doctor may make recommendations about the patient's job and whether or not he or she should drive a car.

At the emergency room

First, the patient is stabilized and any serious causes (such as arrhythmia or infarction) ruled out. The doctor then performs a complete physical, cardiac or neurological exam. He or she may also assess heart activity and blood pressure or order blood tests, an electrocardiogram or an electroencephalogram. In some cases, oxygen is administered and the patient is attached to an intravenous drip. If more thorough testing is required because the cause is still unclear or a serious underlying condition is suspected, the patient is hospitalized.

WHAT IS THE TREATMENT?

Simple fainting (vasovagal)

This is seldom serious. In very rare cases, the doctor will prescribe medication (such as beta-blockers).

Fainting due to heart disease

Arrhythmia can be controlled with drugs or a pacemaker.

Fainting secondary to epileptic fit
Antiepileptic agents are prescribed.

Fainting secondary to low blood pressure (orthostatic hypotension)
This can be prevented by modifying the patient's medication, adding salt to his or her diet, and raising the head of the bed by 15 cm (use boards or bricks to ensure the bed is raised evenly).

Fatigue

Fatigue is the body's response to excessive energy expenditure and is most frequently caused by unhealthy lifestyle habits or psychological problems. It is a warning sign that something is not right. Sufferers may feel extremely fatigued when they wake up in the morning, or become worse as the day progresses.

WHAT ARE THE CAUSES?

Unhealthy lifestyles

► *Unhealthy diet.* People who skip meals or are constantly on a diet deprive themselves of energy. Poor nutrition and high sugar or fat diets do not provide the body with its required nutrients.
► *Lack of physical exercise.*
► *Lack of sleep,* due to jet lag or shift work, for example.
► *Substance abuse.* Substances such as coffee, tobacco, alcohol and drugs can disturb sleep, lead to addiction, or cause lethargy after their stimulating effects have worn off.

Overwork

► *Too many jobs.*
► *Perfectionism.* Society encourages people to strive for peak performances every time they do a job, which leads to perfectionism and the risk of professional burnout.

Psychological problems

► *Excess stress.* Fatigue can be caused by tension at work, financial worries, marital difficulties or family problems.
► *Adaptational problems.* Adapting to a new school, town, boss, or recent divorce are all situations that can lead to fatigue.
► *Anxiety, depression, and other mental problems.*
► *Boredom or lack of stimulation.* People who are unemployed or under-stimulated by their occupation may feel fatigued.

Medication
▶ *Certain medications,* such as sleeping pills, anxiolytics, antihypertensives, and antihistamines can cause fatigue. Taking too much medication may also have this effect.

Physical diseases
▶ *Anemia, diabetes, arthritis, hypothyroidism, infections, cancer, heart failure, chronic fatigue syndrome, etc.* In these cases, fatigue is generally accompanied by other symptoms. Chronic diseases like diabetes or heart disease cause fatigue because the body requires a great deal of compensatory energy.

PRACTICAL ADVICE
Eliminate possible causes. Before worrying that a physical disease is at the root of your fatigue, eliminate any other possible causes. You may need help to precisely determine the origin, particularly if there is a serious underlying problem.

Eat three meals a day. The human body is like a car and needs regular refuelling to keep going. Eat enough healthy food to give you the energy you need.

Eat a well-balanced diet. Eat lean meat, fish, poultry and legumes, as well as large servings of fruit and vegetables. Choose whole wheat bread and cereals, as well as low-fat dairy products.

Avoid strict diets. Diets that impose too many restrictions on the type of food you can eat may lead to fatigue.

Avoid fat and sugar. Food with high fat or sugar content delivers many calories but very little nutritive value. Very sweet food, particularly when eaten with coffee (which maintains a higher blood sugar level), triggers an increase in insulin production. When insulin levels drop, the body reacts with fatigue.

Avoid coffee, tea, and tobacco. These substances are stimulants and can therefore disturb your sleep, which leads to fatigue.

Avoid drugs. Marijuana lowers energy, while stimulants like cocaine throw the body off-balance and cause fatigue after the immediate effects have worn off.

Avoid abusing medications. Even non-prescription medications can cause side effects such as fatigue.

Exercise. Choose a sport you enjoy and do it regularly. Regular participation in low-impact sports is preferable to occasional participation in rough high-impact sports. Daily exercise is also important. Do some gardening, use the stairs, walk to the bus stop, etc.

Get enough sleep. Do not sleep less so that you can work more.

Do not devote all your energy to your work. If your work becomes an obsession and drains all your energy, you will become fatigued and likely not perform as well.

Choose a relaxation technique. If you are stressed, choose an exercise or activity that helps you relax. Try not to worry so much; the petty problems of daily life can sap your energy and are ultimately not worth it.

Find an interest. If life seems drab and boring, try finding an activity—work or recreation—that brings you some satisfaction.

Set some time aside for leisure. Keep some room in your life for relaxation and fun. Do not wait for vacations to organise events or activities with friends or family.

Know your limits. Do not feel obliged to do more than you reasonably can. Think of yourself first.

Be patient. Improving your lifestyle and habits will take time and patience.

WHEN TO CONSULT?

► You are so fatigued that you are unable to take part in your usual activities.

► Your fatigue is causing you distress (this may be a sign of depression).

► You have changed your habits, but still feel tired.

► Your fatigue is accompanied by changes in your stool, fever, weight gain or loss, heavy menstrual bleeding, intense thirst, or any other symptom.

WHAT HAPPENS DURING THE EXAM?

The doctor interviews the patient to determine whether the fatigue is due to an unhealthy lifestyle, excess tension, medication, or disease. A complete physical exam and blood tests may also be necessary.

WHAT IS THE TREATMENT?

The cause determines the treatment. Modifying lifestyle habits can make a significant difference in the patient's level of fatigue and improve his or her quality of life. In some cases, modifying prescribed medication is effective. If the fatigue is caused by persistent psychological tension, the doctor may refer the patient to a mental health professional (psychologist, guidance counsellor, social worker, or psychiatrist). If necessary, antidepressants are prescribed. If the fatigue is secondary to a disease, the treatment will correspond to the underlying cause.

Fever

When the body fights off infection, leukocytes (white blood cells) secrete pyrogenic (heat-releasing) substances that stimulate the hypothalamus (the area of the brain regulating body temperature), causing fever (an increase in body temperature).

Normal body temperature fluctuates throughout the day. The average is 37 °C when recorded with an oral thermometer and 37.5 °C when taken rectally.

Fever should not be confused with hyperthermia. Although the latter also involves an increase in body temperature, this is due to external factors such as intense physical exertion or an extremely hot environment.

A fever manifests in the following ways:

► Oral temperature of 38 °C or higher.

► Rectal temperature of 38.5 °C or higher.

► May be accompanied by chills, aches, extreme fatigue, or generally poor condition.

WHAT ARE THE CAUSES?

► *Infection.* Viruses, bacteria, yeast and parasites are responsible for a number of diseases (flu, ear infections, pneumonia, bronchitis, urinary tract or liver infections, gastroenteritis, etc.). This is the most frequent cause of fever.

► *Medications* in combination, or certain types (for example, thyroid medication or central nervous system stimulators such as Ritalin) at doses too high for the patient can cause fever.

► *Acute attacks of inflammatory diseases* such as arthritis or Crohn's disease.

► *Certain types of cancer* can cause a persistent fever.

► *Illicit drugs* such as ecstasy, cocaine, or amphetamines (speed).

PRACTICAL ADVICE

Be patient. A fever is one of the body's defense mechanisms and does not require treatment as long as body temperature remains between

38 °C and 39 °C. Bring the fever down if it rises above 39 °C orally or 39.5 °C rectally, or if you are very uncomfortable.

Do not use rubbing alcohol. A rubdown with this product can cause the skin to absorb the alcohol and lead to poisoning. It also does very little to relieve the fever.

Choose your thermometer carefully. Thermometers that stick to the forehead are not effective, as they only record skin temperature. Use mercury or electronic thermometers, either oral or rectal (rectal are the most reliable). Precise readings with a mercury thermometer take two minutes rectally and five orally. If using an electronic thermometer, follow the directions.

Get some rest. Your body is fighting off an attack and needs its strength. Stay in bed, or at the very least, slow down.

Take medication. To lower the fever, take one or two acetaminophen tablets (325 mg to 500 mg), four times a day, never exceeding 4 grams daily. Anti-inflammatories are also helpful; follow the manufacturer's dosage recommendations. Take both medications if the fever persists. Ibuprofen, an anti-inflammatory, should be administered with caution, particularly to a child. Give a child acetaminophen first, calculating the dose at a maximum of 15 mg per kilogram of body weight, every four to six hours, up to 5 doses daily. If this is not effective, administer ibuprofen, never exceeding 30 mg per kilogram of body weight per day. Spread this amount out over three or four doses at five to eight-hour intervals. Never give ibuprofen to a dehydrated child, as this can cause kidney damage.

Never give aspirin to a child. Even baby aspirin should be avoided. In the presence of a viral infection (particularly, but not exclusively, chickenpox), aspirin can cause Reye's syndrome (a serious neurological kidney and liver disease primarily affecting children). As fever is a frequent symptom of infection, aspirin should be avoided in all cases. Acetaminophen is the recommended medication. After the age of 14 the child can be given aspirin if he or she has had chickenpox or been vaccinated.

Drink plenty of liquids. Drink at least eight glasses of liquids a day (water, fruit or vegetable juice, bouillon, soft drinks, coffee, caffeinated or herbal tea). If children refuse to drink, offer them frozen fruit juice "popsicles".

Cool down. Take a cold bath or shower, use a fan, apply cold compresses, or take a dip in a pool to lower your body temperature. Since young children should not take cold baths, use lukewarm water or compresses, changing the latter regularly.

Sponge baths. Evaporation can help reduce body temperature, so give the fevered person a soothing sponge bath, applying cold water on the areas of the body producing the most heat (groin or armpits).

Get comfortable. Fever causes chills followed by intense heat. Cover yourself lightly to bring down your body temperature.

Eat lightly. Drink plenty of liquids and eat only if you are hungry. Light snacks are best.

Record your symptoms. Before visiting the doctor, take your temperature and make a note of any other symptoms to help the doctor arrive at a diagnosis.

WHEN TO CONSULT?

- ► An infant under three months old or an elderly person is suffering from a fever.
- ► Your body temperature has remained higher than 39 °C for over 48 hours, despite medication.
- ► Your fever is accompanied by a stiff neck and headache.
- ► You have a fever, your condition deteriorates, or other symptoms appear, such as fatigue, listlessness, or vomiting.

➤ You suffer from a chronic disease (for example, heart disease or diabetes).

WHAT HAPPENS DURING THE EXAM?

The doctor will collect the necessary information from the patient and perform a physical exam. Blood tests, urine analysis and other tests may be ordered. In some cases, diagnostic tests require hospitalization.

WHAT IS THE TREATMENT?

A fever is symptomatic of the body fighting off some kind of attack, so the cause determines the treatment.

Finger Deformities

There are two types of finger deformities. The first, known as gnarled fingers, is caused by nodules in the joints and leaves the fingers more or less straight and aligned. The other is characterized by cubital deviations (curvature towards the baby finger), which is very painful, though extended periods of remission do occur. Both types are unattractive as well as incapacitating.

WHAT ARE THE CAUSES?

▶ *Osteoarthritis.* Most common in men over the age of 55, this disease is caused by wear and tear on the joints due to aging. It is frequently accompanied by nodules on the joints, and in rare cases, deformities. The condition may be painful, particularly in its early stages, but does not usually prevent sufferers from going about their daily activities.

▶ *Rheumatoid arthritis,* the most frequent cause of finger deformities, primarily afflicts women over the age of 30. It is an inflammatory autoimmune disease (this term describes diseases that occur when the body's immune system cannot distinguish its own cells from foreign agents). It affects one or several joints, stimulating the development of antibodies that attack the joint lining, sometimes to the point of boring a hole in the bone or causing it to crumble. The joint becomes unstable, leading to deformities in the fingers. The attacks are progressive and very painful, followed by more or less extended periods of remission.

▶ *Unnoticed subluxation (minor dislocation) or fracture* can cause the fingers to deviate.

PRACTICAL ADVICE

Modify or reduce manual work. Stop doing any activity that causes too much discomfort. Respect the limits set by the pain.

Avoid picking up heavy objects. Unstable joints cannot withstand the stretching this activity requires and may fracture or become dislocated.

Keep your fingers warm. Chronic pain is soothed by humidity and heat. Wrap your hand in a hot wet towel covered with a dry towel to preserve the heat. Dipping your hand in a hot paraffin bath is even more effective. As it dries, the paraffin soothes the fingers.

Wear finger splints overnight. This will rest your joints and help correct deviations. Use only under doctor's recommendations.

Adapt your environment to your condition. Occupational therapists specializing in the hand can give you advice on helpful changes you can make (to door handles, utensils, tools, and your clothes, for example).

Take anti-inflammatories. Take these medications with meals, as they may cause ulcers when swallowed on an empty stomach. Follow the manufacturer's dosage recommendations carefully.

WHEN TO CONSULT?

- ► You wake up with joints that are swollen, red, hot and painful, for no apparent reason.
- ► Your fingers are beginning to deviate or you notice a nodule on a joint.
- ► Your finger is swollen, locked or deformed after a trauma (the finger suffered a blow or you broke a fall with your hands, for example). You are unable to move the finger normally.

WHAT HAPPENS DURING THE EXAM?

Early diagnosis greatly improves prognosis. X-rays help determine the stage of the disease and the appropriate treatment. Blood analysis is used to test for rheumatoid factor and, if necessary, to detect the intensity of inflammation and the patient's tolerance for prescribed medications.

WHAT IS THE TREATMENT?

Osteoarthritis

The pain can be controlled. Treatment begins with acetaminophen, after which mild anti-inflammatories (such as aspirin or ibuprofen) may be recommended. In severe cases, narcotic medication is used for serious pain control to preserve finger mobility, and ultimately, safeguard the sufferer's autonomy. Immobilization (using splints or moulded supports) can also help control pain.

Occupational therapy helps sufferers get over everyday hurdles.

Reconstructive surgery is strongly indicated in cases of osteoarthritis of the thumb. A thumb deformity can cause serious incapacity as it threatens the ability to grasp objects.

Rheumatoid arthritis
If the inflammation is caught early and properly controlled, the development of deformities can be delayed or prevented. This requires continuous medical supervision. Treatment begins with anti-inflammatories. Some cases require cortisone (administered in pills or local infiltration), gold compounds, or medications such as methotrexate to soothe the inflammation. New drugs for rheumatoid arthritis will soon be available.

Immobilizing the fingers in a straight position can help control pain and prevent deformity.

Reconstructive surgery is recommended when deformities severely impede normal hand function. It can restore finger alignment and function, or replace a joint with a prosthesis.

Occupational therapists teach sufferers exercises and help them learn new ways to go about their daily activities.

Unnoticed subluxation (dislocation) or fracture
In cases of incapacitating deformity, the patient will undergo reconstructive surgery.

Food Cravings

It is well known that pregnant women often have sudden food cravings, but they are not the only ones. Everyone, at some time or other, has felt an irresistible urge to eat a certain type of food. This is generally entirely normal and in no way cause for concern. In some cases, however, cravings can occur so frequently they become a problem; in others, they can be symptomatic of a disease. (Please note that this chapter does not address serious food disorders such as bulimia.)

Cravings can be described in the following way:
- A sudden, irresistible urge to eat a particular type of food, particularly something sweet or greasy.
- May be preceded by dizziness or weakness.
- May occur after a meal (postprandial hypoglycemia).

WHAT ARE THE CAUSES?

Organic causes
- **Diseases causing hypoglycemia (low blood sugar)** such as diabetes, pancreatic tumours, and pituitary or adrenal gland disorders. People who suffer from postprandial hypoglycemia (drop in blood sugar levels after meals) feel better if they eat something sweet.
- **Intestinal parasites** such as taenia (an intestinal worm). This is very rare.

Psychological causes
- **Boredom.**
- **Stress.**
- **Joy.**
- **Sadness.**
- **Depression.** A recent theory has linked seasonal affective disorder with changes in eating habits. Mood is regulated by serotonin (a neurotransmitter), which can be affected by certain foods. For example, caffeine (found in coffee and chocolate) creates euphoria, which explains why people with seasonal depression may crave it. Serious depression usually causes loss of appetite.

Hormonal causes

► *Pregnancy, premenstrual syndrome, oral contraceptives.* Oestrogen generally stimulates the appetite. This is believed to occur because it causes a drop in serotonin, which controls the urge to consume sweets. Hormonal causes may explain why women tend to get the munchies more often than men.

Other causes

► *Unbalanced diet.* A balanced diet contains protein, fats and carbo-hydrates. A diet lacking one of these groups leaves the body dis-satisfied, even if the person has consumed an adequate number of calories. This is particularly true if carbohydrates are lacking.

PRACTICAL ADVICE

Eat a balanced diet. Mix foods from the three main groups: proteins, fats, and carbohydrates. This will help lessen your craving for sweets.

Avoid refined sugar. Eat sugar that takes longer to digest, such as can be found in pasta or bread.

Avoid temptation. If you know you have a tendency to snack while watching TV, change your habits, or keep raw vegetables within arm's reach.

Exercise regularly. This helps control your appetite.

Ask for help. Speak to a therapist or dietician if you are becoming worried about how much you snack.

If you're pregnant, don't worry. Remember, your cravings are temporary.

Indulge yourself every once in a while! Eating is one of the great pleasures of life. Giving in to your cravings every now and then is good for you.

WHEN TO CONSULT?

► You are snacking excessively.

WHAT HAPPENS DURING THE EXAM?

The doctor takes a history and may ask the patient to keep a journal of the cravings to help determine whether they are caused by an organic or psychological condition, or tend to occur after meals. If an organic cause is suspected, the appropriate tests will be ordered.

WHAT IS THE TREATMENT?

Organic causes

The underlying condition will be treated: the patient's diabetes will be controlled, a pancreatic tumour removed, or hormones prescribed to correct pituitary or adrenal gland insufficiency.

Psychological causes

If recommended diets are not enough, psychotherapy may be recommended, perhaps in combination with medication or light therapy (for seasonal affective disorder). Behavioural therapy may be used to modify the patient's association of certain emotions with eating.

Hormonal causes

Food cravings that occur during pregnancy generally disappear after the child is born. If they are linked to premenstrual syndrome, there is usually no need for treatment, although PMS may be treated if it causes other, more serious symptoms. If the cravings are caused by the birth control pill, the prescription may be modified.

The foot is a complex mechanism that supports and absorbs body weight, acts as a propulsion lever, and adjusts as your body makes contact with the ground. It is also one of the most neglected body parts—that is, until a problem develops.

There are a number of types of foot pain:
- Pain in the toes or soles of the feet.
- Pain in the heel (caused by calcified bone tissue in the heel, known as a heel spur), or diffuse pain beginning in the heel and radiating towards the toes (plantar fasciitis, frequently associated with heel spurs).
- Pain due to the inward deviation of the big toe (hallux valgus or bunion).
- Pain due to the upward deviation of the second toe (hammer toe).
- Pain due to the downward deviation of the toes (claw toes). In many cases, both feet are affected.
- Pain due to an overly high arch (hollow foot)
- Pain due to flat feet.

WHAT ARE THE CAUSES?

- **Excessive pressure or friction from footwear.** People who wear very narrow or high-heeled shoes, stand for long periods of time, are obese, or take part in rigorous physical activity may experience pain and develop bunions, heel spurs, plantar fasciitis, hammer toes or claw toes.
- **Hereditary or anatomical predisposition.** Foot deformities such as bunions, hollow foot, or flat feet are often hereditary. Hollow feet often co-exist with claw toes, while flat feet are often accompanied by bunions. Hammer toes are common in people whose second toe (beside the big toe) is longer than the others.
- **Diabetes.** As the disease progresses, it may cause inflammation of the nerves (polyneuritis) leading to desensitization of the feet (and therefore frequent foot injuries), as well as deformities such as hammer toes, claw toes, and hollow foot. These conditions are

frequently accompanied by poor circulation in the lower extremities and bluish discoloration of the toes.

► **Rheumatoid arthritis** is a chronic and progressive disease characterized by joint inflammation (particularly in the hands and feet), resulting in deformities such as bunions or flat feet. Bad shoes, prolonged standing, and intense physical activity aggravate the problems. The disease also causes pain (usually more intense at night), as well as redness, sensations of heat, joint swelling, and morning foot stiffness.

► **Vascular disorders.** As the blood vessels age, circulation becomes less efficient, sometimes causing the toes and feet to develop a bluish tinge.

► **Osteoarthritis and osteoporosis.** These diseases are associated with aging and make the feet more susceptible to pain and fractures. Osteoarthritis describes the natural erosion of the joints, causing the tissues to lose flexibility. Osteoporosis describes a lack of calcium in the bones, which causes them to become fragile and vulnerable to fracture.

► **Certain neurological diseases.** Parkinson's disease prevents certain muscles from relaxing, resulting in limb stiffness that leads to claw toes and hollow foot. Multiple sclerosis affects areas of the nervous system that control pain and muscles, frequently resulting in pain in the feet and involuntary muscle contractions that make walking difficult. Friedreich's ataxia (a hereditary degenerative disease affecting the cerebellum and the nerve fibres running down the spinal cord) can also cause foot deformities (hollow foot).

► **Lumbar spine problems or calf muscle tension** can cause pain that radiates to the feet.

PRACTICAL ADVICE

Proper footwear is the best prevention. Wear shoes made of cloth or soft leather with laces and a large toe box. The absolute best choice for stability is a pair with a wedged sole to absorb body weight and shocks. There are a variety of styles available in any shoe store. Solid wide heels no higher than 5 cm with a firm back to stabilize the foot are also recommended. Walking or sports shoes are excellent choices – be sure to wear those specifically made for your activity.

Choose the right shoe size. Make sure there is enough space between the big toe and the tip of the shoe to prevent rubbing. Buy your shoes at the end of the day when your feet are slightly swollen from walking and standing. Never buy shoes that are uncomfortable when you first try them on, as it is unlikely they will ever fit properly and may damage your feet.

Make adjustments for comfort. Buy padded insoles or lifts to absorb body weight.

Lose weight. Your feet need to support you as long as you live. Treat them well and maintain a healthy weight.

Ease the pain. Rub ice on a sore heel and take painkillers as needed. Whirlpool footbaths (sold in department stores and pharmacies) warm up and massage sore feet. You should generally soak your feet for fifteen minutes at a time, but if you have sores on your feet or suffer from diabetes or serious circulation problems, speak to your doctor first.

Massage your feet and do exercises. Massage a sore foot with your hands, using oil or cream (avoid irritating products). Massaging the calves and stretching the feet gently will provide even greater relief. Sit in a chair and roll a small ball (like a tennis ball) under the foot for ten minutes. If you suffer from plantar fasciitis, flex your toes as though you were trying to catch something with them.

Decrease physical activity. At least for a few days.

Avoid wearing shoes without socks. This increases friction.

WHEN TO CONSULT?
► Your foot pain persists.
► Your feet or toes are misshapen.

► You limp.
► Your feet are easily injured.
► You notice redness, swelling, or skin discoloration on your feet.
► Your lower limbs feel stiff in the morning or painful at night.
► Your feet have become insensitive or you have cuts that do not heal.
► You feel pain in the lower back or calves, as well as your feet.

WHAT HAPPENS DURING THE EXAM?

The doctor will examine your feet and, if necessary, perform a thorough physical examination. He or she may order further tests, such as blood tests, X-rays, a CT scan or a bone radioisotope scan.

WHAT IS THE TREATMENT?

Heel pain

Heel spurs can be treated with lifts (small strips of shock absorbent material inserted in the shoe under the heel), painkillers, anti-inflammatories, moulded orthopedic soles (plantar orthotics), or cortisone injections in the heel.

Plantar fasciitis responds well to anti-inflammatories and physiotherapy.

Foot or toe deformities (bunions, hammer toe, claw toes, hollow foot, flat feet)

Plantar orthotics are usually recommended for deformities, although in certain cases, the patient may be required to undergo surgery. There are three types of orthopedic soles: preventive, to avoid the development of deformities; corrective, to rectify already-existing deformities while the foot is still flexible; and palliative, to provide comfort if the deformity cannot be corrected.

Diabetes, rheumatoid arthritis, vascular disorders, osteoarthritis, osteoporosis, neurological diseases, lumbar spine problems, and calf muscle tension

The doctor will treat the ailment responsible for the foot pain and prescribe orthopedic soles or special shoes.

Foreskin Conditions

The foreskin is the fold of skin on uncircumcised men that covers the glans (tip) of the penis. Circumcision is the complete or partial surgical removal of the foreskin for religious, personal, or in rare cases, medical reasons.

The relative benefits and disadvantages of circumcision—with respect to urinary or sexually transmitted infections, cancer of the penis, and sexual pleasure—are still controversial. Speak to your doctor.

Foreskin infection
► Redness and itching of the glans and foreskin.

Phimosis
► Abnormal tightness of the foreskin.
► The skin closes over and tightly binds the glans.
► Often present at birth.
► May cause pain with erection or difficulty urinating.

Paraphimosis (or strangulation of the glans)
► Foreskin is stuck at the base or back of the glans and cannot be drawn back to its original position.
► Constriction and edema of the glans.
► Extremely painful condition. Requires emergency hospital consultation due to the risk of cyanosis and tissue necrosis.

WHAT ARE THE CAUSES?
Foreskin infection
► *Poor hygiene.*
► *Diabetes.* Excess sugar in the body creates an environment favourable to the development of yeast, especially in moist warm areas, such as under the foreskin.
► *Antibiotic therapy,* either long-term or repeated. Antibiotics destroy bacteria, but in the long run, the absence of bacteria creates a breeding ground for yeast, which is impervious to antibiotic treatment.

Phimosis and paraphimosis
► *Often occurs spontaneously.*
► *Infections.* In most cases, phimosis and paraphimosis follow recurrent infections or tears in the foreskin.
► *Lack of treatment.* Strangulation of the glans (paraphimosis) can sometimes develop if phimosis is left untreated.

PRACTICAL ADVICE

Foreskin infection
Maintain good hygiene. Slowly retract the foreskin and gently wash with a neutral, unscented soap. Strong soaps will burn the skin, only making the problem worse. Rinse thoroughly, dry well, and carefully draw the foreskin back over the glans.

Never pull or stretch the foreskin. Always be careful when retracting or drawing the foreskin forward, whether bathing or engaging in sexual activity.

Never forcibly retract the foreskin of a child. This may cause permanent damage. Let a doctor evaluate the situation.

Phimosis and paraphimosis
Remain calm. If there is edema, compress the swollen area for a few minutes, then push it under the top of the foreskin and try to draw the foreskin over the glans. If successful and the foreskin remains in this position, apply a cold compress for 15 to 20 minutes every two hours.

WHEN TO CONSULT?
► The glans and foreskin are red and itchy.
► The foreskin cannot be retracted and you have trouble urinating.
► You are unable to draw the foreskin over the glans, which is swollen, very painful, and bluish in colour. This is an emergency!

WHAT HAPPENS DURING THE EXAM?

Foreskin infection

An analysis of the secretions under the foreskin may be necessary. The process of taking a sample is painless: the doctor simply touches the area very lightly with a sterile cotton swab.

Phimosis

The physician takes a history and performs a clinical exam to make a prognosis.

Paraphimosis

The doctor performs a visual examination to assess the situation.

WHAT IS THE TREATMENT?

Foreskin infection

The usual treatment is good hygiene and antibiotic cream (anti-bacterial or antifungal). Circumcision is a last resort.

Phimosis

In most cases, circumcision is the only treatment. The sclerosed foreskin is removed under local or general anesthesia to free the glans.

Paraphimosis

The area can be anesthetized and the foreskin replaced manually. In certain cases, an incision is made where the foreskin has narrowed in order to allow it to slide more easily. If these measures are unsuccessful, the doctor will proceed with a circumcision.

Frequent Urge to Urinate

The bladder is a muscular bag-shaped organ lined with mucous membrane located in the pelvis. Urine enters the bladder from the kidneys through ducts called the ureters. During urination, the bladder contracts, the sphincter between the bladder and the urethra (the canal leading out of the body) opens, and the urethra dilates to expel urine.

The urge to urinate usually occurs when the bladder contains approximately 250 to 300 millilitres of liquid (a little over a cup). Humans generally eliminate one to two litres of urine, six to eight times a day and once during the night (although many people do not go at all at night). Unless you have consumed an unusually large amount of liquid, going to the bathroom more often may indicate a problem.

The frequent need to urinate does not necessarily mean the sufferer's bladder fills up more quickly than others. It may be a symptom of an aging or overactive bladder (characterized by frequent or inefficient contractions), tissue inflammation/irritation, or a blocked or dysfunctional urethra that prevents the bladder from emptying completely. Certain diseases can also be responsible. It should be noted that a frequent urge to urinate is not the same as urinary incontinence.

This problem can have a significant impact on a person's quality of life, often leading to sleep disturbance, reduced sexual activity, diminished self-confidence, embarrassment, shame, and social withdrawal. Wary of their inability to control their bladders, sufferers need to be near a bathroom at all times to avoid soiling their clothes and smelling of urine. The constant fear of public humiliation forces them to limit their activities, and embarrassment and lack of knowledge of available treatments commonly prevents people from seeking medical help.

The frequent urge to urinate can take the following forms:

► Need to urinate more than eight times during the day and twice at night.

- ► Urgent need to urinate.
- ► Difficulty controlling the bladder.
- ► Urinary flow may be normal but can diminish, even to just a few drops.

Children and the frequent urge to urinate

Young children have small bladders that fill up quickly. Children therefore go to the bathroom more often than adults; an 18-month-old, for example, will urinate about ten times a day. This is a normal part of the bladder's maturing process: as the child grows, the bladder's capacity increases and the individual gains more control over the sphincters.

A child's bladder is mature by the age of five. Until then, it is entirely normal for the child to struggle a bit with control.

Here are a few tips to help children control their bladders:

- ► Daycare rules often allow children to go to the bathroom at set times during the day only. However, because their little bladders fill up more quickly and they have yet to gain complete control, they should be allowed to go whenever they feel the need. Insist upon this with your daycare and ask for a doctor's note, if necessary.
- ► Children at play may ignore the signal telling them their bladder is full and go only at the last minute, sometimes causing leakage. Remind them regularly to use the bathroom and listen to their body.
- ► Preventing constipation is also important. A child's intestine takes up a lot of space in the pelvic area, leaving very little room for the bladder to fill up completely. A diet rich in fibre (grains and whole-wheat bread, fruit and vegetables) will help keep them regular and avoid excessive urges to urinate.
- ► In North America, parents usually try to have their children completely toilet-trained by the age of two or earlier. This is a little early for a lot of children. Two and a half or three years old is a more reasonable expectation, particularly with respect to bed-wetting. Children learn gradually and are better able to gain control when they are a little older.

WHAT ARE THE CAUSES?

▶ *Habits and lifestyle.* People who drink large quantities of water have to urinate more often. Coffee or tea has a diuretic (causing increased output of urine) and irritating effect on the bladder; more than five cups a day can significantly increase urination. Alcohol (particularly beer) also acts as a diuretic, as do certain natural products like glucosamine and so-called "system-cleaning" and "slimming" herbal supplements.

▶ *Unknown causes.* In most cases, even a complete physical examination reveals no specific cause.

▶ *Aging.* As they age, both men and women experience a decrease in muscle tone (in the sphincter, for example). The brain therefore receives signals to empty the bladder more often, affecting the capacity of sufferers to retain urine for long periods of time.

▶ *Diabetes.* Diabetics who are unaware of their condition or do not adequately control their blood sugar levels experience excessive thirst and drink large amounts of liquid, leading to a frequent need to urinate.

▶ *Bacterial or viral urinary tract infections* cause inflammation and irritation of the lining of the bladder, leading to an increased need to urinate that may also be accompanied by pain, burning with urination, blood in the urine and, in rare cases, fever.

▶ *Sexually transmitted infections.* Gonorrhea, chlamydia, herpes, and condyloma (genital warts) cause inflammation of the bladder's mucous membranes, leading to an increased need to urinate and, in some cases, burning with urination, itching, and blood in the urine.

▶ *Interstitial cystitis* is similar to an ulcer and characterized by a lack of glycosaminoglycans, the tissue lining the bladder. In the absence of a lining, urine comes into direct contact with the mucous membrane of the bladder wall, causing irritation and the need for repeated emptying. Lower abdominal pain that disappears with urination is symptomatic of the problem. For reasons not yet understood, this condition primarily affects women (nine women to every one man).

► **Benign prostate hypertrophy.** The prostate is a walnut-sized male gland located under the bladder and crossed by the urethra. For no known reason, the prostate begins to grow after the age of thirty and can eventually become large enough to compress the urethra and prevent the bladder from emptying normally.

► **Obstructed urethra.** Trauma to the urinary tract or pelvic region can obstruct the urethra, increasing the urgency and frequency of the need to urinate. This can result from surgical scarring, catheter implantation, or bike and motorcycle accidents. It can also happen if a foreign object gets caught in the bladder (kidney stones or anything coming in through the urinary meatus - the opening through which urine is expelled).

► **Detrusor muscle hyper-reflexibility.** The detrusor, the main muscle of the bladder, stretches to accommodate urine and contracts to expel it. Certain neurological ailments (multiple sclerosis, spina bifida, cerebrovascular accidents, or spinal cord trauma) can damage or destroy the nerves controlling the bladder, causing detrusor spasms (sudden muscle contractions) when the bladder is empty.

► **Overactive urethra (neurological causes).** Neurological damage suffered by quadriplegics can cause the urethra to close instead of dilate during urination. This disrupts the coordination between the urethra and bladder, causing spasms in the latter. Sufferers experience a frequent need to urinate and the flow of urine may be abnormal.

► **Sensitive bladder.** For unknown reasons, some people are particularly sensitive to the presence of urine in their bladders and need to urinate frequently as a result. This generally occurs in people who do not drink much liquid and whose urine is quite concentrated.

PRACTICAL ADVICE

Change your habits. Moderate your consumption of liquids and do not drink before going to bed at night. Be sure, however, to stay well hydrated: the minimum requirement for water is eight 250-millilitre glasses per day. Take medications or natural products with diuretic effects in the morning. Control your consumption of coffee, tea, and alcohol.

Re-train your bladder. A simple exercise can help you re-educate your bladder muscles. For the first week, try to refrain from urinating for one minute when the urge strikes. During the second week, wait two minutes, and during the third, hold off for three. Continue increasing the amount of time weekly, until the urges diminish.

Train your bladder to contract at the proper time. A biofeedback technique involves going to the bathroom at set times during the day (every three hours, for example), and holding it in until the next scheduled time. When urinating, expel urine until your bladder feels empty. To be sure, stand up, sit back down, and try to urinate again.

Plan for accidents. Elderly or sick people frequently have reduced mobility and are unable to get to the bathroom often or quickly enough. A chamber pot or specially made absorbent undergarments can be very useful.

Keep a journal. Prepare yourself for your doctor's appointment. A week before, start writing down how often you urinate during the day and at night. Take note of the flow (normal or diminished), as well as any leakage. This will help your doctor get a complete picture of your problem and put you one step ahead in the diagnostic process.

WHEN TO CONSULT?

► You go to the bathroom more than eight times a day, for no apparent reason.
► Your urges to urinate make you get up more than twice during the night.
► You have stomach pain that is relieved when you urinate.
► Your symptoms negatively affect your quality of life.

WHAT HAPPENS DURING THE EXAM?

The doctor takes a complete history and performs a physical exam. He or she may also do a urine analysis (to check for blood in the urine as well as sugar and protein levels), a urine culture (to screen for bacteria), a urinary cytology test if there is blood in the urine (to analyze the cells in the urine), and an endo-urological exam (in-depth examination of the bladder), if necessary. For men, the physical examination will include a digital rectal exam to assess the size of the prostate gland.

WHAT IS THE TREATMENT?

In most cases, anticholinergic agents are the treatment of choice. These medications inhibit bladder contractions, delaying the perceived need to urinate. Ditropan, Ditropan XL, Detrol, and Unidet are the most commonly prescribed products, and are generally taken over the long-term (for months or years).

Unknown causes

Aside from modifying any behaviour that may be contributing to the problem, the doctor may prescribe an anticholergenic agent. If ineffective, low doses of tricyclic antidepressants (such as amitriptyline) can inhibit an overactive bladder. These drugs also require long-term prescriptions.

Aging

The doctor will recommend modifying any behaviour that may be contributing to the problem. A lifetime prescription to anticholinergic agents may also be required.

Diabetes

Once the disease is diagnosed and blood sugar levels stabilized, the patient's extreme thirst should dissipate.

Urinary tract infections and sexually transmitted infections (STIs)

These ailments are treated with antibiotics.

Interstitial cystitis

The doctor will prescribe medication (such as Elmiron) to help rebuild the tissue lining the bladder. This is a long-term prescription.

Benign prostate hypertrophy

In half the cases, pharmaceutical treatment can solve the problem. The doctor can prescribe alpha-blockers (such as Flomax) to relax the prostate muscle (allowing the bladder to empty more completely) or, if ineffective, Proscar, to prevent the prostate from enlarging. Both of these drugs are prescribed for life and can be used with anticholinergenic agents to inhibit bladder contractions. In some cases, surgery is required to remove the swollen area of the prostate and anything obstructing the bladder and urethra.

Obstructed urethra

If there is a foreign object in the bladder, surgery under local anaesthesia is required to remove it. A trauma to the urinary apparatus or in the pelvic area may also require endoscopic surgery to repair any damage or plastic surgery to rebuild the urethra. In most cases, the frequent need to urinate can be controlled.

Detrusor muscle hyper-reflexibility

If possible, the doctor will prescribe medication to treat the underlying disease. If there is no treatment available, he or she will use anticholinergenic agents to deal with the overactive bladder.

Overactive urethra (neurological causes)

Anticholinergenic agents are prescribed and a urinary catheter is used to empty the bladder. Regular follow up is required to prevent kidney problems (a damaged bladder may cause urine to overflow back into the kidneys).

Sensitive bladder

In 50% of cases, drinking more liquids solves the problem. In other cases, the doctor prescribes anticholinergenic agents.

Gum Disease

A number of underlying problems can cause gum disease. The most severe types of gum disease eventually destroy the periodontium (supporting tissue connecting the teeth to the maxilla or jaw bone). This degeneration is gradual and usually begins after a case of gingivitis has gone untreated. Symptoms generally include bleeding gums, bad breath, an unpleasant taste in the mouth, and in some cases, pain.

A list of the different types of gum disease follows:

Gingivitis
- Mild infection of the gums.
- Can lead to an irritation of the gums causing inflammation, swelling, redness, discharge and bad breath.

Trauma caused by dental prosthesis (dentures)
- Irritation of the gums.
- Sometimes accompanied by pain and bleeding.

Yeast infection
- Redness and white blotches on the palate.
- Bad breath.

Periodontitis
- Progressive destruction of the bone supporting the teeth.
- Displacement of the teeth either forward or backward, creating new spaces between the teeth.
- In some cases, increased sensitivity of the teeth and gums.

Aphtha (canker sores)
- Small, painful ulcers. In many cases, canker sores are recurring.

WHAT ARE THE CAUSES?

Gingivitis

► *Poor dental hygiene.* This leads to an accumulation of bacteria that forms an invisible film (known as bacterial or dental plaque) over the teeth and gums and thickens over time if not removed.

► *Heredity.*

► *Smoking.* Nicotine attacks the tissues of the mouth, increasing the risk of gum disease.

► *Hormonal changes* due to pregnancy.

► *Lowered immunity.* Stress, fatigue or any illness affecting the immune system leaves the body open to bacterial infection, thus encouraging the development of periodontal disease.

Trauma caused by dentures

► *Poorly fitting dentures.*

► *Food fragments* or seeds caught beneath the prosthesis.

Yeast infection

► *Permanent dentures.*

Periodontitis

► *Poor dental hygiene* causing gingivitis. If left untreated, gingivitis may cause periodontitis.

Aphtha (canker sores)

► *In 80% of cases, the cause is unknown.* The ulcers may be viral in origin (and therefore contagious) or caused by bacteria and

---

Home Recipes

Mouthwash: Mix hydrogen peroxide (3% H_2O_2 per 10 volumes) with equal parts water for an antibacterial mouthwash.

Toothpaste: Mix small amounts of sodium bicarbonate (baking soda), hydrogen peroxide and water to form a paste, for a traditional recipe with antibacterial properties.

a genetic predisposition. Possible trigger factors include fatigue and stress, as well as iron, folic acid, vitamin B_{12} and zinc deficiencies. Canker sores may also develop from oral trauma (after a dental procedure, for example), inflammatory digestive tract diseases (such as Crohn's disease), certain drugs (barbiturates and antiepileptics), or the fluctuations of the menstrual cycle.

PRACTICAL ADVICE

Maintain good oral hygiene. Be sure to remove bacterial plaque daily. Brush your teeth carefully after every meal and before going to bed. Use dental floss and an antibacterial mouthwash at least once a day, preferably at bedtime.

Don't stop brushing your teeth if your gums bleed. On the contrary, brush more often than usual, but more gently. Bleeding is a sign of inflammation caused by bacterial plaque, but note that it can also indicate that you are brushing too vigorously.

Take painkillers. One or two acetaminophen tablets (325 mg to 500 mg), four times a day will help ease the pain. Never take more than four grams a day. Anti-inflammatories are also helpful. Follow the dosage recommended by the manufacturer. If the pain is difficult to control, take both types of medication.

Never apply crushed aspirin directly to mucous membranes to relieve pain. The acid in the aspirin tablet may burn your gum tissues.

Do not try to remove tartar on your own. You may injure yourself. See a dentist for a cleaning.

Use a soft toothbrush and fluoride toothpaste. Don't forget to replace your toothbrush every three to four months.

Brush the sensitive area with lukewarm water. Receding gums expose the roots, leaving them unprotected and more sensitive.

Wait for the ulcer to heal. Ulcers disappear on their own within seven to ten days. In the meantime, never apply salt directly to a sore. This will only increase the burning sensation and may aggravate the problem. Rinsing your mouth with salt water, however, may provide some relief. Take a painkiller before meals to ease the pain and make it easier to eat. Over-the-counter anaesthetics (Orabase or Amosan) are also effective. Avoid viscous Xylocaine (for example, Oragel); this topical analgesic numbs the reflexes and may cause choking when you eat. Avoid excessively hot, spicy or salty foods, as they can exacerbate the pain. Remember that ulcers may be contagious. Don't take any chances: avoid sharing your glass, cup, eating utensils and toothbrush, and refrain from kissing anyone while you have the ulcer.

See your dentist regularly. Have your teeth cleaned at least every six months.

Consult a dentist even if you do not feel pain. Pain is often a sign of advanced periodontitis.

WHEN TO CONSULT?

► You have one or more of the following symptoms: bleeding gums, bad breath, unpleasant taste in the mouth, pain.
► A canker sore persists for more than ten days.

WHAT HAPPENS DURING THE EXAM?

The dentist examines the gums for any change in shape or colour, checking to see whether they bleed upon contact with the instruments. He or she then uses a periodontal probe—a precise measuring instrument calibrated in millimetres—to determine whether any spaces have appeared between the gum and tooth. The larger the space, the more likely it is that the periodontium is degenerating. Finally, X-rays are used to assess the degree of bone disintegration.

WHAT IS THE TREATMENT?

Gingivitis
Tartar removal and rigorous oral hygiene will resolve the problem.

Trauma caused by dentures
The direct cause—prosthesis, food fragments, seeds, or any other irritant—must be removed. If the dentures don't fit properly, they can be modified. Once the cause has been eliminated, the wound will heal on its own.

Yeast infection
Dental prostheses or dentures should not be worn overnight, as they prevent gum tissue from breathing. This type of infection is treated with specific antifungal medications (either topical or oral). The lesions will usually heal in seven to ten days.

Periodontitis
This problem requires very specific treatment. The periodontist must remove any bacterial plaque and irritating factors, and may prescribe antibiotics. Reconstructive surgery may be necessary, depending on the case and the state of the periodontium. Periodontitis must be treated immediately to stop its development, since the damage it causes is irreversible.

Aphtha (canker sores)
The cause determines the treatment, but many therapies may include the prescription of a cortisone-based medication (such as Kenalog Orabase) to relieve inflammation. The doctor may also ask the pharmacist to prepare a medicated mouthwash (containing antihistamines, antifungals, cortisone and antibiotics).

Hair Loss

Everyone loses approximately 100 hairs every day in the third phase of the hair's life cycle. There are four stages in all: the growth stage (known as anagen, lasting two to four years, affecting eighty-five per cent of your hair at any given time); the resting, or non-growth stage (known as catagen, lasting one month, affecting five per cent); the falling out stage (telogen, lasting approximately three months); and the re-growth stage, where the cycle begins again. Different strands go through the stages at different times, which explains how the hair maintains its volume.

Various types of hair loss (alopecia) can affect the appearance and volume of the hair.

Pattern baldness (androgenic alopecia)
- Ninety-five per cent of men are affected to some degree.
- First signs appear in the man's twenties.
- Hair loss begins at the temples, proceeds to the forehead, and then to the top of the head.
- Missing hair is replaced with soft, downy hair.
- Five per cent of women are affected. In these rare cases, hair loss occurs on the top of the head, leaving the hairline at the forehead and temples unaffected.

Telogen effluvium
- The resting period is prolonged.
- Shed hair has transparent bulbs at the end.
- In most cases, no more than 50% of the hair is affected.
- Hair loss is evenly spread over the scalp.
- There is no inflammation.
- Hair loss begins suddenly and continues for two to four months.

Anagen effluvium
- Affects the hair in its growth stage.
- Shed hair is thicker at one end, with bulbs often appearing at the tip.

- It affects up to 90% of the hair.
- Hair loss is evenly spread over the scalp.
- There is no inflammation.
- Hair loss begins suddenly and continues for one to four weeks.

Tinea (ringworm)

- This problem is most common in children.
- Hair breaks near the root.
- Patches appear on the scalp.
- Patches are rough and may be itchy or flaky.

Alopecia areata

- In most cases, hair loss is localized in one area.
- Causes circular patches of baldness generally the size of a dime or quarter, but sometimes larger.
- The condition may be diffuse, total (affecting the entire scalp), or universal (affecting the rest of the body).

Hirsutism

- This problem affects only women.
- The hairline recedes around the forehead and temples.
- This may be accompanied by other signs of virilization (development of typically male characteristics), including body hair, acne, deeper voice, amenorrhea (absence of menstrual period), hypertrophy (enlargement) of the clitoris, and decreased breast size.

Trichotillomania

- Compulsive disorder causing sufferers to obsessively pull or twirl their own hair.
- Hair does not grow back after it has been torn out.

Traction alopecia

- Occurs in individuals who wear certain hairstyles (such as a pony tail) that exert pressure (or traction) on their hair; develops over a number of years.

Scarring alopecia
► Scarring on the scalp prevents hair growth.
► Bald patches resemble those of alopecia areata.

Seborrheic alopecia
► Gradual hair loss.
► Accompanied by scalp redness or dandruff.

WHAT ARE THE CAUSES?

Pattern baldness (androgenic alopecia)
► *Genetic predisposition.*
► *Male hormones (testosterone).*

Telogen effluvium
► *Intense stress or illness* such as major surgery, childbirth, high fever, hypo/hyperthyroidism, among others.
► *Excessively strict diets* can lead to vitamin deficiency (generally rare in Western countries) or iron deficiency.
► *Medications* such as anticoagulants, heart medication, excessive amounts of vitamin A (over 5000 units daily), acne medication (Accutane), or psoriasis treatments (in rare cases).

Anagen effluvium
► *Chemotherapy and radiation therapy.* Hair loss begins suddenly and lasts from one to four weeks, even though the treatment may last longer. Hair grows back after therapy ends.
► Poisoning.

Tinea (ringworm)
► *Fungal infection* transmitted from humans or animals.

Alopecia areata
► *Immune system reaction,* whereby the body produces antibodies to fight its own hair.
► *Rare immune disorders* such as lupus or lichen planus.

Hirsutism
Without signs of virilization:
► *Mediterranean ancestry.*
► *Pregnancy, menopause.*
► *Medication,* male hormones, cortisone, birth control pills containing progesterone.

With signs of virilization:
► *Ovarian tumours.*
► *Adrenal gland disorders.*

Trichotillomania
► *Psychiatric problems.*

Traction alopecia
► *Traction* (caused by hairstyle) over a number of years, preventing the hair from growing back.

Scarring alopecia
► *Old wound or injury.*

Seborrheic alopecia
► *Skin conditions* (eczema, hives, contact dermatitis) that cause inflammation, resulting in the skin's inability to hold the hair.

Other causes
► *Rare diseases* such as lupus or lichen planus.

PRACTICAL ADVICE
Wash your hair every day, particularly if it is greasy. Contrary to popular belief, this is not damaging.

Use mild, unscented, clear shampoo to help your scalp retain its natural defenses. Trust results, not labels, and remember that the most expensive shampoo is not necessarily the best. Avoid shampoos that strip the hair of their natural oils, as this will cause excessive dryness.

Beware of miracle tonics. Do not trust the promises of companies selling re-growth lotions and creams. They are a waste of time and money.

Do a strand test before using permanent or semi-permanent hair colour. These products can cause allergies (contact dermatitis) as well as irritation or chemical burns.

Ask your doctor to check your medication. A number of prescription drugs can affect your hair.

Find a good hairdresser. He or she can show you tricks for camouflaging thinning hair. Hair weaves provide a natural look, but require frequent touch-ups as the hair begins to grow out. Consult a cosmetician for advice about a toupee or wig.

Avoid low-protein and low-iron diets. They can cause hair loss.

Do not give yourself a permanent and dye your hair at the same time. This can cause a peroxide burn on the scalp.

WHEN TO CONSULT?
▸ You have localized hair loss.
▸ You have diffused and abundant hair loss.
▸ Your scalp is irritated, flaky, or itchy.

WHAT HAPPENS DURING THE EXAM?
The doctor performs a dermatological examination, possibly using a microscope or fluorescent Wood's light. A mycological culture or biopsy may be sent to the laboratory for analysis. A trichogram samples a small amount of hair for examination to determine whether it is in the growth or resting stage. The doctor may also order blood tests to detect diseases, vitamin deficiency, and hormone levels.

WHAT IS THE TREATMENT?

Pattern baldness (androgenic alopecia)

Propecia is a medication that can stabilize 60% to 70% of hair and stimulate cosmetic re-growth by up to 10%. It is a lifelong treatment that costs $60 a month and is not usually covered by medical insurance. In 2% to 3% of cases, it affects sexual function. Propecia is contra-indicated for women who are pregnant or planning to become pregnant. Hair transplants (moving hair from thicker to thinner areas) provide a permanent, if expensive, solution. Three or four sessions are required for full treatment.

Telogen and Anagen effluvium

The cause (medication, vitamin deficiency, thyroid problems, stress, etc.) must be identified and eliminated. There is no other treatment.

Tinea

The doctor prescribes oral antifungal medication and special shampoo (for example, Nizoral).

Alopecia areata

Abnormal immune system reactions to the hair are usually temporary and nine out of ten cases of alopecia areata resolve on their own within six to twelve months. If the condition persists longer, cortisone lotion or local injections may be effective. If there is considerable hair loss, the doctor may consider immunotherapy or phototherapy.

Hirsutism

If blood tests reveal a high level of male hormones, the doctor will prescribe hormone therapy (Diane 35) in combination with other medications. Cosmetic techniques and laser diode treatments can help get rid of unwanted hair.

Trichotillomania

Psychiatric therapy or psychotherapy may help the sufferer control this compulsive disorder.

Traction alopecia

In many cases, changing hairstyles will allow the hair to grow back.

Scarring alopecia

Because there are no veins in scar tissue (it is not vascularized), hair cannot grow back. Hair transplants, therefore, cannot take root on the scar tissue itself, but can be grafted onto the area just beside the scar to camouflage the bald spot.

Seborrheic alopecia

Shampoos such as Nizoral or Selsun can help reduce scalp inflammation. In most cases, treating the underlying skin condition will resolve the hair loss problem. In severe cases, hair transplants are necessary.

Hallucinations

A hallucination is defined as an alteration of one or more of the senses (most commonly sight or hearing), leading sufferers to see or hear things that are not actually there (like noise in a completely silent room). In some cases, the sense of smell, taste, or touch is affected, making sufferers believe someone has brushed by them in an empty room, for example, or that food is cooking when it is not.

Hallucinations occur when the brain cannot accurately receive and interpret stimulus from the environment. Unfortunately, the sufferer is not always aware that his or her perceptions are false and is unlikely to consult a physician.

It is important to distinguish normal hallucinatory phenomena that occur when the brain is preparing for sleeping or waking cycles from abnormal hallucinations that require medical consultation. Having visions of fleeting movement as you fall asleep, or waking up to an imagined phone ringing in the middle of the night, are common examples of normal hallucinations.

Although the causes are multiple, hallucinations can be grouped into three broad categories: those related to mental health problems, those due to organic or physical causes, and those caused by drugs, alcohol or certain medications.

WHAT ARE THE CAUSES?

- ► *Mental illness.* Schizophrenia, major depression, profound grief or emotional shock, and mania (pathological mental condition manifesting in grandiose ideas or compulsive and excessive spending, for example) are the most common psychiatric disorders responsible for hallucinations. Forms of dementia (such as Alzheimer's disease) can also provoke hallucinations.
- ► *Organic disease.* A number of organic pathologies, including cataracts, epilepsy, renal failure, heat exhaustion, loss of hearing, and severe dehydration (causing the sufferer to see a mirage in a desert, for example) can alter the senses.

- *Drugs and alcohol.* Certain drugs (LSD, cocaine, marijuana, magic mushrooms) can cause transient hallucinations. Prolonged drug or alcohol abuse may also entail chronic hallucinations that persist long after the psychogenic effect of these substances has dissipated.
- *Medications.* Several medications, including antihistamines (for allergies), antidepressants, anxiolytics (for anxiety), and hypnotics (sleeping pills), can cause hallucinations, particularly if consumed in high doses or in combination with other medications or alcohol.

PRACTICAL ADVICE

Consult a physician. Put aside your embarrassment and confide in a physician to help determine the cause of your hallucinations.

Be observant. If you believe a person close to you is suffering from hallucinations, watch for unusual behaviour. Is he or she seeing, hearing, or smelling things that do not exist or speaking to the air? Ask the individual directly to confirm your suspicion and then suggest a medical consultation. Accompany your loved one to the doctor's office, as he or she may not be fully aware of the situation.

Seek help. A number of community organizations provide information, counselling and support for people afflicted with mental illness, dementia or substance abuse.

Do not listen to the "voices". Auditory hallucinations can take the form of commands compelling the sufferer to do specific things (open the door, go to the basement, phone someone). In some cases, the orders are dangerous (the sufferer may be told to commit suicide, attack someone, or set fire to the house, for example). If someone close to you tells you he or she is hearing voices, find out if they are ordering the sufferer to hurt anyone and treat this as an emergency, particularly if the voices have only recently appeared and the person is not used to dealing with them. It is crucial for the sufferer to consult a doctor as soon as possible.

WHEN TO CONSULT?

► You see or hear things that others do not.

► Your hallucinations do not disappear when you stop consuming drugs or alcohol.

WHAT HAPPENS DURING THE EXAM?

Reviewing your medical history, as well as a complete physical and psychological examination is often enough for your doctor to determine the cause of your hallucinations. Complementary examinations (such as a CT scan) are often necessary for a precise diagnosis.

WHAT IS THE TREATMENT?

Treatment is possible only if the patient admits he or she has a problem. The doctor will encourage the patient to question the hallucinations and help him or her differentiate fact from fiction. One of the most important steps in treatment occurs when the patient realizes the hallucinations are symptoms.

Mental Illness

If the hallucinations are caused by mental illness, the doctor prescribes specific drugs to treat the primary disorder, which should reduce or eliminate the hallucinations.

Organic Disease

In cases of organic (physical) disease, the appropriate treatment is undertaken and the hallucinations should disappear.

Drugs and alcohol

The patient is advised to abstain from drugs or alcohol. In cases of severe addiction, the patient must undergo a supervised detoxification program.

Medication

The prescription is modified.

Hangover

Almost every adult has lived through the "morning after" a night of revelry and drinking at one time or another. Hangovers are harmless unless consumption is frequent or excessive. In extreme cases, the sufferer may fall into a coma. Certain medical studies have shown that hangovers can lead to behavioural abnormalities, although there are a number of contradictory studies.

Tolerance for alcohol varies from one individual to another. In general, men should not have more than three drinks a day and women should have no more than two, unless of course they are pregnant when they should have none at all. One drink equals one glass of beer or wine.

A hangover is a period of discomfort characterized by the following symptoms:

► Sleep disturbance (in most cases, the individual falls asleep rapidly and wakes up after a few hours).
► Thirst.
► Headache.
► Moroseness.
► Irritability and nervousness.
► Nausea and vomiting.
► Dizziness.
► Irritation of the esophagus.
► Irritation of the stomach.
► Acidic breath and body odour (caused by the acetone being released by the body).
► Slowed reflexes.
► Amnesia (commonly called a "black out", where the individual forgets what happened during the binge).
► Trembling.
► Vomiting blood.
► In serious cases: heart palpitations.
► In extreme cases: coma.

WHAT ARE THE CAUSES?

► *Dehydration.* Alcohol has a dehydrating effect when consumed in excess.

► *Diminished vitamin C.*

► *Electrolyte imbalance.* Electrolytes (phosphorus, potassium, calcium) are the body's mineral salts, allowing the transmission of nerve impulses to the muscles. Excess alcohol disturbs the balance of these substances, slowing the reflexes.

► *Hypoglycemia (low blood sugar).* Alcohol increases the body's production of insulin, lowering blood sugar levels.

► *Acidosis.* The body's pH levels become more acidic due to alcohol consumption or a disease such as diabetes. This condition compounds electrolyte imbalance, further slowing the reflexes.

► *Esophageal irritation or hemorrhagic gastritis.* Inflammation of the stomach due to the toxic effects of alcohol that can cause the sufferer to vomit blood in extreme cases.

► *Toxins.* Hangover headaches may be caused by a toxic substance (acetaldehyde) released as alcohol is broken down in the blood. Headaches may also be due to the additives or impurities in certain drinks.

PRACTICAL ADVICE

Drink plenty of liquids. One of the main causes of a hangover is the dehydration induced by alcohol. Drink a lot of water before going to bed and when you get up. Gatorade sports drinks or a salty broth (beef, chicken or vegetable) will replace the mineral salts (particularly sodium). Drinking replenishing liquids while you drink alcohol, as well as the morning after, will prevent you from getting too drunk, help you avoid headaches, and make recuperation easier.

Avoid acidic food. This is not a good time to drink orange juice!

Avoid coffee. As an irritant and diuretic, coffee will only make you feel worse.

Avoid aspirin and acetaminophen. Aspirin can increase blood-alcohol concentration and irritate the stomach, while acetaminophen (found in Tylenol, for example) can do harm to the liver if taken with excess alcohol.

Don't trust home cures. "Hair of the dog" (such as beer and tomato juice) will only aggravate the problem. If you feel the need to have a drink the next day to ease the trembling, this may be a sign that you are addicted to alcohol and are going through withdrawal.

Call in sick. Hangovers diminish fine motor coordination skills and affect performance, so if you are responsible for people's safety in your job (bus driver or airline pilot, for example), the lives of your passengers may be at risk.

Take vitamin C. Alcohol reduces the amount of vitamin C in your body. Take small doses (vitamin C is an acid, and should generally be avoided in your state). Vitamin B complex (particularly the thiamin it contains) can also be helpful.

Take antacids as needed. This will soothe your upset stomach and any pain in the esophagus.

Avoid certain food as you drink alcohol. Chips or other salty snacks like pretzels only make you thirstier, encouraging you to drink more. (This is why many drinking establishments offer free snacks.) Salty food also speeds up dehydration.

Avoid smoky environments. The combination of tobacco smoke and excessive alcohol should be avoided. Both contain acetaldehyde, which has a particularly toxic effect on the liver, thus aggravating the hangover. Antidepressants, neuroleptic drugs and sedatives can also make a hangover much worse.

WHEN TO CONSULT?

► You have followed the advice in this chapter, but your hangover has persisted over 36 hours.

WHAT HAPPENS DURING THE EXAM?

The doctor performs a clinical examination. He or she may order specific tests if diabetic acidosis is suspected. In some cases, blood electrolytes, venous pH levels, and blood sugar levels are analyzed.

WHAT IS THE TREATMENT?

The patient is advised to follow the practical advice in this chapter. The doctor may also prescribe an antacid and proton pump inhibitors (to prevent the production of stomach acids). In very serious cases (vomiting blood, black stool), the patient should go to the emergency room for thorough testing.

Headaches take various forms, from migraines, to those caused by tension, skull trauma, cervical spine problems (cervicogenic headaches), and specific diseases. They may be episodic or chronic, the latter having a severely negative effect on the sufferer's quality of life.

Migraines are the most devastating type of headache. Only 16% of women and 6% of men are affected. Few headaches are truly migraines. The pain is often accompanied by nausea, watery eyes, vomiting, or intolerance to light or noise. Although precise causes are not yet known, there may be a genetic factor, as a family history of migraines exists in 60% of cases.

Headaches manifest in a variety of ways. Migraines, in particular, are characterized by intolerable throbbing or hammering pain. Headaches may also be concentrated in specific spots on the skull, feel like a tight band wrapping around the head, radiate up from the neck to both sides of the head, or be experienced as continuous, shooting pain.

There are also many different trigger factors. Migraines, for example, may be caused by a dilation of the arteries at the base of the brain, accompanied by inflammation of the artery walls. Muscle spasms around the skull and nape of the neck contribute to the pain of tension and cervicogenic headaches.

WHAT ARE THE CAUSES?
Migraine
- ► *Hormonal fluctuations in women* caused by puberty, ovulation, menstruation, pregnancy, childbirth, and menopause. The estrogen and progestogens in oral contraceptives or hormone replacement therapy can also be responsible.
- ► *Stress* caused by the death of a loved one, family problems, a recently developed disease, financial difficulties, or work problems, for example.
- ► *Certain food or drinks.*
- ► *Strong odours* such as tobacco smoke, perfume or industrial pollution.

▶ *Cold.* Eating ice cream or leaving the head exposed in cold temperatures may trigger a migraine.

▶ *Concentrated effort* due to physical exertion (during demanding sports activities such as running, playing football, tennis, or lifting weights), orgasm, or intellectual work.

Tension headaches
▶ *Intense anxiety.*
▶ *Depression.*

Cervicogenic headaches
▶ *Bad posture* due to prolonged immobilization, non-ergonomic computer work stations, repetitive movement, sleeping on the stomach, inadequate pillows (too thick/thin), or spinal deviation.

Headaches due to skull trauma
▶ *Blows to the head* can injure the cervical spine or shake the brain.

Toxic or withdrawal headaches
▶ *Alcohol abuse.*
▶ *Caffeine withdrawal.*
▶ *Carbon monoxide poisoning.*

Metabolic headaches
▶ *Irregular or skipped meals.*
▶ *Hypoglycemia.*
▶ *Lack of oxygen* (high altitude headaches).

Medication-induced headaches (rebound headaches)
▶ *Repeated use of certain medications* (such as aspirin, acetaminophen, tranquilizers, Viagra, sedatives, and ergotamine) can increase the frequency and, in some cases, intensity of headaches.
▶ *Certain medications* used to treat cardiovascular diseases such as nitroglycerine and calcium channel-blockers.

Headaches due to vascular problems
- *Very high blood pressure.*
- *Brain aneurysm* (dilation of the artery).
- *Brain hemorrhage.*

Infection-induced headaches
- *Fever.*
- *Infections* such as meningitis or sinusitis, among others.

PRACTICAL ADVICE

Do not over-medicate. While one or two aspirin or acetaminophen tablets are indicated for occasional headaches, overuse of this type of medication decreases its effectiveness and can actually increase the frequency and, in some cases, intensity of headaches. When the medication is constantly present in the bloodstream, the body develops a tolerance, causing each dose to last a shorter time and have progressively less analgesic effect. Sufferers will also frequently experience rebound headaches upon waking as the levels of medication decrease during the night. Taking another painkiller, however, only temporarily relieves the pain and actually triggers the return of the headache when the effects wear off.

Avoid oral decongestants. Although they can relieve sinusitis and its accompanying headaches, they must not be used as a treatment for

---

Cluster headaches and smokers

Cluster headaches (also known as Horton's cephalalgia) affect five to eight men (generally heavy smokers) for every one woman. They manifest as intense pain behind the eye or in the temple, accompanied by redness, tearing of the eyes, nasal congestion, and facial sweating. Smoking is one of the main trigger factors for cluster headaches, making it essential for sufferers to undergo a treatment program to quit. Other trigger factors must also be eliminated.

headaches because they contain pseudoephedrine, which contracts the blood vessels as it helps decongest, leading to high blood pressure in the medium-term. Speak to your pharmacist.

Avoid excessive physical exertion. If you suffer from neck pain, avoid physically demanding work (renovations, spring cleanings, etc.) during your treatment.

Seek out quiet. Too much noise can cause tension, triggering a headache.

Eat at regular hours. Have your meals at the same time every day.

Get some rest. Headache sufferers often feel compelled to take a break from their activities and lie down for a few hours, which is beneficial as sleep has been shown to help cure headaches.

Adopt a healthy lifestyle. A healthy diet, regular light physical activity (such as walking) and neck and back exercises can all help prevent headaches.

Deal with stress as it appears. Don't let your frustrations build up. Deal with conflicts as they arise and set aside time to relax every day.

Keep busy. If you are bored or under-stimulated, increase your daily activities. This will keep your mind occupied and distract you from your headache.

Keep a journal. To help find ways to prevent headaches, keep a record of them, noting when they occur and what foods or other factors seem to act as triggers.

Take care of your neck. If you suffer from cervicogenic headaches, do neck stretching exercises in a warm shower (raise your shoulders, hunch them forward, pull them back, and rotate your head, or extend it back with your chin in the air). Stop immediately if you feel any pain. At night, use a pillow that is neither too thick nor too thin to fit in the crook of your neck (not under your head). Do not carry backpacks, bags with shoulder straps, or heavy briefcases.

Avoid foods that trigger headaches. A number of foods and food additives have been shown to trigger migraines in some people. A partial list includes alcohol, red wine (due to the tannin it contains), tyramine (in strong or aged cheese, marinated or smoked fish, chicken livers, and citrus fruit), chocolate, nitrites (in wieners and cold cuts), monosodium glutamate (an additive often found in Chinese cuisine), large amounts of caffeine (in coffee, tea, cola, and chocolate), nuts, onions, and aspartame (in diet soft drinks). Take note of the food items consumed in the two days before developing the migraine. Eliminate any suspected triggers and observe how this affects the frequency and duration of your headaches. Re-introduce or permanently eliminate any foods, as appropriate.

Change your method of contraception. The birth control pill can either increase the risk of migraines or aggravate them in women who already suffer these debilitating headaches. Not all birth control pills are contra-indicated, however—the "mini-pill" (progestin-only oral contraceptives), for example, does not cause migraine. Talk to your doctor about alternative methods.

Slow down. Whatever kind of headaches you suffer from, you will not get rid of them unless you slow down, as your hectic pace may very well be the triggering factor.

Consult a physician. If your headaches disturb your daily activities, see a doctor for a precise diagnosis and appropriate treatment. Recurrent headaches are not normal.

There is hope. You do not have to live with the pain. Medical understanding of headaches is progressing rapidly, so the diagnosis you received five years ago may no longer be accurate. New medications to combat migraines and other severe headaches have also appeared in recent years, making effective relief possible now in 90% of cases.

WHEN TO CONSULT?

➤ You have never suffered from headaches before.
➤ Headaches disrupt your daily activities or cause you to miss work.
➤ Your headaches are becoming increasingly frequent and intense.

WHAT HAPPENS DURING THE EXAM?

The doctor takes a detailed personal and family history and performs a complete physical examination (including an assessment of the nervous system, cervical spine, and sinuses). In rare cases, the physician will refer the patient to an emergency room in order to withdraw some lumbar spine fluid and rule out the possibility of a ruptured blood vessel, which indicates a brain hemorrhage. Depending on the diagnosis, the doctor will either treat the patient directly or refer him or her to the appropriate specialist (physiatrist, neurologist, ophthalmologist, ENT specialist, dentist, etc.).

WHAT IS THE TREATMENT?

Standard treatment

Standard treatment for headaches includes lifestyle changes, the elimination of trigger factors, and the correction of bad sleeping or working posture. Medical treatment is individualized and based on the diagnosis, as well as the intensity and frequency of headaches.

Mild to moderate tension headaches are effectively treated with over-the-counter or prescription analgesics such as aspirin, ibuprofen, codeine, or anti-inflammatories. To avoid rebound headaches, they should not be taken more than twice a week.

For acute migraine or cluster headaches, the doctor prescribes serotonin receptor antagonists such as ergotamine tartrate or DHE (dihydroergotamine). The physician may also prescribe one of the new triptan drugs, a new class of medication with greater efficacy and fewer side effects that has revolutionized migraine treatment. In some cases, medication can be used to prevent headaches. Tricyclic antidepressants, beta-blockers and calcium channel blockers can also be used as preventive treatment.

If there are significant psychological elements underlying the sufferer's headache, the treatment may involve behavioral psychotherapy (whereby doctor and patient analyze stress factors and identify solutions) and relaxation techniques (for example, biofeedback).

Medication-induced (rebound) headaches

The patient is weaned off the over-the-counter or prescription drug. The process requires the full cooperation of the patient as well as medical supervision. Once the patient is no longer dependent on the medication, he or she will be better able to identify the initial source of the headache, which can then be treated.

Cervicogenic headaches

Physiatrists (or physical medicine specialists) are the best qualified to assess and treat this type of headache. Depending on the specific case, the specialist will prescribe physiotherapy, heat or cold therapy, cervical traction, massage therapy, therapeutic neck exercises, spinal manipulation, or anesthetic or cortisone injections in the occipital nerve. Osteopathic treatment can also be very effective. The effectiveness of acupuncture and chiropractic treatment has not been scientifically proven.

Hearing loss and deafness can be defined as a decrease in auditory acuity or the quality of the sounds heard. In other words, the terms describe a loss of auditory perception or comprehension. The most common type of irreversible hearing loss involves the higher frequencies (such as the sound of a flute or jet engine). Middle-frequency sounds are those we hear most often (such as the sound of the voice), and low-frequency sounds are deep (such as thunder).

People in the sufferer's immediate environment are usually the first to notice the problem, as they are forced to repeat themselves or speak loudly.

Deafness can be unilateral (only one ear is affected) or bilateral (both ears), reversible or irreversible, sudden, gradual, or stable.

There are different kinds of deafness or hearing loss:

Conduction deafness

► Caused by a problem in the external ear canal, from the tympanum (eardrum) to the middle ear.

► Autophonia (sufferer hears his or her own voice more loudly in the affected ear).

► In most cases, this condition is reversible.

Cochlear deafness

► Caused by a problem with the cochlea, the organ in the middle ear responsible for sound perception.

► May manifest as bilateral high-frequency deafness in the elderly or people who have been exposed to very loud noise.

► May manifest as unilateral low-frequency deafness in patients with Ménière's disease.

► May manifest as loss of perception of all sounds in cases of deafness caused by heredity factors or infection.

► In rare cases, manifests as a loss of perception of normal, middle-frequency sounds corresponding to the human voice.

► In most cases, progression is gradual and irreversible.

► In rare cases, deafness develops suddenly.
► Does not cause pain.

Nerve deafness (caused by damage to the auditory nerve)

► Unilateral or bilateral loss of all hearing.
► Primary symptom is difficulty following conversations (loss of auditory speech comprehension).
► In most cases, damage is irreversible.
► Usually a gradual progression; in rare cases, develops suddenly.
► Does not cause pain.

WHAT ARE THE CAUSES?

Conduction deafness

► **Wax build-up or foreign object** in the outer ear canal.
► **External otitis.** This form of otitis (sometimes known as "swimmer's ear") causes acute pain, swelling of the outer ear canal, and pus.
► **Otitis media.** This infection of the middle ear causes fluid to build up behind the tympanum (eardrum), acute pain, fever, and sometimes pus.
► **Middle-ear trauma** is caused by the difference in air pressure between

---

The Dangers of Walkmans

When you use a portable cassette or CD player (commonly known as Walkmans), you should always be able to hear the person next to you. If you cannot, the volume is too high. These machines easily reach 95 to 100 decibels, but safety dictates avoiding anything louder than 85 decibels. Listening to very loud music on your Walkman can lead to irreversible cochlear deafness. Moreover, listening to a Walkman while riding your bike, in-line skating, or even walking can be dangerous, since it blocks out the sounds around you, making you less attentive to your environment.

the middle ear and the external environment. Sports like snorkeling or skydiving, as well as ear trauma caused by a blow to the head or the insertion of a foreign object into the ear (a cotton swab, for example) may perforate the eardrum, sometimes causing bleeding.

► *Otosclerosis* (also known as otospongiosis) is a hereditary disease causing the immobilization of the stapes, a bone in the middle ear. The condition occurs in 0.4% of the population and is particularly common in women.

► *Tympanosclerosis.* This thickening of the tympanum (ear drum) may be hereditary or caused by repeated middle-ear infections. It causes irreversible deafness.

Cochlear deafness

► *Aging of the ear,* in most cases.

► *Hereditary or congenital conditions* (causing people to be born deaf).

► *Repeated exposure to very loud noise.* Noise from a factory, gunshots, loud music, or a piercing scream in the ear can lead to gradual hearing loss. See box insert.

► *Improper use of a portable cassette or CD player (walkman).* (*See box insert.*)

► *Viral infections* such as shingles (developing when the chicken pox virus is reactivated) or herpes can lead to vesicles or sores around the ear, causing deafness that is reversible only in rare cases.

► *Ménière's disease.* This chronic disease manifests in frequent and sudden attacks of vertigo, accompanied by a humming in the ears, deafness, and sometimes nausea and vomiting. It also increases the pressure of the endolymph (liquid in the inner ear).

► *Infectious diseases.* In rare cases, syphilis, measles, rubella (German measles), or even chlamydia can cause deafness if the infection reaches the middle ear.

► *Cochlear otosclerosis* (otospongiosis) causes abnormal growth of middle-ear bones and is particularly common in young adults.

▶ *Certain antibiotics* in the aminoglycoside family, such as gentamicin and tobramycin, used to treat serious infections.

▶ *Bacterial infections* of the inner ear or the spreading of toxic substances produced by bacteria through the middle ear.

▶ *Trauma, tumour, extremely loud noise.* Sudden deafness is usually caused by bleeding in the ear resulting from trauma, such as a blow to the ear. Sudden cochlear deafness may also be the result of a tumour in the ear (in the cochlea) or exposure to extremely loud noise (such as a cannon shot or an exploding bomb).

▶ *Unknown causes.* Some cases of sudden deafness are unexplained, although the cause appears to be vascular or infectious. In 50% to 75% of cases, the loss of hearing is reversible.

Nerve deafness (caused by damage to the auditory nerve)

▶ *Severing of the auditory nerve* caused by a skull fracture. In almost all cases, the loss of hearing is irreversible.

▶ *Benign tumours* pinching the auditory nerve. In many cases, the loss of hearing is reversible.

▶ *Aging* can cause gradual and irreversible hearing loss.

▶ *Unknown causes,* in some cases.

PRACTICAL ADVICE

Clean your ears gently. As long as you do not have a perforated eardrum, wax build-up can be cleaned out with three drops of body-temperature mineral oil (sold in pharmacies), olive oil, almond oil,

---

What the ears can take

A person working in a factory or any other loud environment should never be exposed to noise levels over 85 decibels for eight hours. The amount of exposure time should be halved for every increase of three decibels. At 88 decibels, therefore, maximum exposure time should be four hours per day; at 91 decibels, two hours is the maximum and should be followed by 16 hours of quiet; at over 120 decibels, the ears will begin to hurt, which is a warning sign against any further exposure.

or Baby's Own. Wait 15 minutes before removing the softened wax. Do not use cotton swabs, as they will only push the wax deeper into the canal, possibly causing irritation or leaving small pieces of cotton lint behind. Repeat this process daily to unblock your ears, or once a month to prevent build-up.

Apply heat. If you think your child is suffering from otitis media, give him or her painkillers and apply heat to the ear to ease the pain. Use a hot towel or hold the child's ear to your chest. Consult a doctor.

Do exercises to control vertigo. If you suffer from Ménière's disease, exercises involving slow head movements will reduce the intensity of vertigo.

Protect yourself from loud noises. If you work in a noisy environment, wear special earplugs that reduce noise levels by 30 to 40 decibels. Ear protectors that cover the entire ear and filter out loud noise while still allowing you to hear can also be useful.

Beware of quinine. Occasionally prescribed to prevent malaria during trips to certain countries, quinine can cause tinnitus and, in rare cases, hearing loss. Speak to your doctor before taking it.

Pay attention to your children's hearing. If you suspect your child is hard of hearing, take him or her to the doctor. Early detection and treatment can prevent learning problems.

Avoid dangerous situations. Be alert: alarms or other signs of immediate danger can go unnoticed by people who are hard of hearing or deaf. If you have Ménière's disease and are having an attack, avoid work that requires an intact balance system. Although vertigo does not occur all the time, it may come on suddenly.

WHEN TO CONSULT?

➤ You believe you have an ear infection or your child's ear is sore.
➤ You have noticed rapid hearing loss in one ear.

- ► You frequently need to ask people to repeat themselves, or are told you are speaking loudly.
- ► Hearing loss is interrupting your regular activities.
- ► You feel nauseous and have vertigo.
- ► You fear that your child is hard of hearing.
- ► Even if the situation does not seem urgent, consult a doctor.

WHAT HAPPENS DURING THE EXAM?

The doctor takes a history and performs a physical exam, including an ear examination. If the patient has balance problems, the doctor checks for abnormal (jerky) eye movement that may indicate a disease affecting the balance centre. The patient is also asked to perform specific movements to check the cranial nerves and rule out any brain condition (such as a tumour).

If the problem is straightforward (such as wax build-up), the patient is treated immediately. More complex problems require a more detailed examination, including hearing tests, an assessment of the patient's balancing apparatus (inner ear), X-rays, and a neurological consultation.

WHAT IS THE TREATMENT?

Conduction deafness

Wax build-up or foreign object

The foreign object or wax blockage must be removed. To remove wax, the doctor may pour warm water in the ear canal or use a curette.

External otitis or otitis media (middle ear)

External otitis is treated with a local antibiotic, while otitis media requires oral antibiotic treatment. In some cases the doctor may make a small insertion in the tympanum to relieve pressure. If the patient's ear infections are recurrent or resistant to medication, the doctor may insert a tube through the tympanum.

Middle ear trauma

In the case of a perforated eardrum, the doctor will provide treatment for infection if there is pus in the ear or the perforation occurred in a potentially contaminated environment (for example, while diving underwater). If there is a danger of hearing loss or serious infection, the eardrum may be repaired with a graft (tympanoplasty). If the middle ear bones are damaged and there is severe hearing loss, the bones will be repaired.

Otosclerosis
Surgery to replace the stapes with a metal or plastic prosthesis is necessary.

Tympanosclerosis
Tympanoplasty, the reconstruction of the eardrum and middle ear bones, is the only possible treatment, although it is rarely performed because the chances of recovery are very small.

Conduction deafness
Congenital cochlear deafness or that due to aging cannot be treated. If the sufferer is unable to understand conversation at a normal level, he or she will be given a hearing aid.

Viral infection
Anti-viral agents may be prescribed.

Ménière's disease
Some treatments may reduce the auditory effects. A low-salt diet and diuretics may be prescribed to stabilize endolymph pressure; if necessary, the doctor may administer the antibiotic gentamicin through the eardrum to reduce the symptoms. This procedure is usually performed under local anesthesia and is well-tolerated. Surgery to sever the vestibular nerve will also have the same effect.

Infectious diseases
There is no treatment for cochlear deafness caused by infectious diseases.

Cochlear otosclerosis (otospongiosis)

The progression of this disease can be halted with fluorine treatment.

Certain antibiotics

There is no treatment to reverse the auditory effects of certain antibiotics. In most cases, hearing loss is permanent.

Bacterial infection

The doctor will prescribe an antibiotic. The length of treatment is determined by the severity of the infection. In some cases, an ear or blood culture is required to identify the bacteria responsible.

Trauma, tumour, extremely loud noise

Deafness may be reversible, depending on the severity of the damage and whether treatment is possible.

Unknown causes

If the cause cannot be determined, the doctor may prescribe strong doses of vasodilators, cortisone, and anti-inflammatories.

Deafness due to auditory nerve damage

Severing of the auditory nerve

A severed auditory nerve cannot be surgically repaired. If the nerve is completely severed, deafness is irreversible.

Benign tumour

A tumour does not always require treatment. If it stops growing on its own, the hearing problem may not get better, but it will at least stop worsening. In other cases, local radiation therapy can be used to stop tumour growth, or it can be removed surgically. The latter treatment is the most likely to restore hearing.

Hiccups

Hiccups are caused by the sudden and involuntary contraction of the respiratory muscles (intercostal and diaphragmatic), closing the epiglottis to produce the characteristic "hic" sound anywhere between four and sixty times a minute. Hiccups are more common in men than women.

Surprising though it may seem, the human body does possess a hiccup centre (located between the third and fifth cervical vertebrae); when nerve impulses traverse it, hiccups are provoked. Unlike the cough, sneeze and vomiting reflex, hiccups appear to have no practical or protective function.

There are three types of hiccups:

Benign hiccups
- Brief and intermittent.
- Last several seconds to several minutes.

Persistent hiccups
- Last 48 hours or longer.
- Recur frequently.

Refractory or intractable hiccups
- Last months or years.
- May cause weight loss or fatigue (due to difficulties eating).
- May cause insomnia.

WHAT ARE THE CAUSES?

Benign hiccups
- ***Stomach distension.*** A large meal, rapidly swallowed solids or liquids, carbonated beverages or aerophagia (air swallowed while eating) can provoke stomach distension. Doctors believe that gastric distension irritates the diaphragm, or stimulates stomach nerves that run to the hiccup centre.
- ***Sudden temperature change.*** Very hot or cold beverages, or moving suddenly from a hot to cold environment (and vice-versa) can activate the hiccup centre.

► *Excessive absorption of alcohol* can cause stomach distension and neutralize natural hiccup inhibitors in the brain.

► *Heavy smoking* (over a pack a day). Coughing irritates the diaphragm.

► *Psychological factors.* For unknown reasons, changes in stress levels and mood can cause the hiccups.

Persistent and refractory hiccups (generally caused by a disease pinching or irritating the phrenic nerve which innervates the diaphragm)

► *Gastrointestinal disorders,* such as gastro-esophageal reflux, esophageal inflammation or obstruction, thoracic tumours, or disorders of the stomach, pancreas or gallbladder.

► *Central nervous system disorders,* such as Parkinson's disease, tumour, and cerebral thrombosis or hemorrhage.

► *Toxic or metabolic disorders,* such as diabetes, kidney failure, or alcoholism.

► *Irritation of the diaphragm* caused by a heart attack, sub-diaphragmatic abscess, hiatus hernia or distension of the spleen.

► *Infectious diseases,* including influenza, meningitis, pharyngitis, laryngitis, pneumonia, pleurisy, or bronchitis.

► *Medications* (tranquilizers such as Valium or Librium) can induce the hiccups.

► *General anesthesia.*

► *Abdominal surgery.*

► *Severe psychological disturbances.* For unknown reasons, anxiety and personality disorders can cause the hiccups.

► *Family history.* If other members of your family tend to get the hiccups, you may be predisposed.

PRACTICAL ADVICE

Do not take medications. Contrary to popular belief, tranquilizers do not eliminate the hiccups. In some situations, they can even be dangerous (*see What is the Treatment?*).

Do not induce vomiting. Although provoking nausea can be effective, avoid vomiting, since there is a high risk of inhaling the vomitus.

Do not ingest noxious substances. Ignore traditional home remedies, and absolutely avoid inhaling or ingesting noxious substances such as ammonia, vinegar or ether.

Stimulate the pharynx. Stimulating the palate modifies nerve impulses to the hiccup centre, eliminating the problem. This can be done in a number of ways:
- Pull vigorously on your tongue until the hiccups cease.
- Drink one or more glasses of ice water.
- Consume one tablespoon (15 ml) of granulated sugar, without water. For infants or children, dissolve one half teaspoon of sugar in 125 ml water.
- Suck on an ice-cube or hard candy.
- Provoke a sneeze (inhale a small amount of pepper).
- Induce nausea (press on the back of your throat with your finger).
- Gargle with ice water.
- Drink a glass of water upside down (bend forward and drink from the opposite rim of the glass).
- Eat a piece of dry bread.

Distract the sufferer. Forgetting that you have the hiccups is often enough to get rid of them.
- Surprise the sufferer.
- Tickle children.
- Bet the person that he or she cannot stop the hiccups in the next five minutes.

Modify your breathing to inhale the maximum amount of carbon dioxide, which decreases the frequency of hiccups.
- Hold your breath as long as possible.
- Breathe out as slowly as possible.
- Breathe in and out of a brown paper bag at least ten times, as quickly and deeply as possible. Do not let any outside air enter the bag.

Compress the diaphragm. Stop the contractions causing the hiccups:
► Bend forward for several minutes while sitting on the ground or a chair with your knees pulled up to your chest.
► Place a bag of ice on the diaphragm, just below your rib cage.

Stimulate the uvula (small piece of tissue that dangles from the back of the throat), if the hiccups persist for more than 60 minutes:
► Rub the palate with a finger, tongue depressor or cotton swab (Q-tip).
► Raise the uvula slightly using a spoon.

Breathe slowly. Rapid and shallow breathing is often recommended, but is in fact useless and potentially dangerous, as it decreases the level of carbon dioxide in your lungs, thereby increasing your hiccups. It also causes light-headedness and, sometimes, loss of consciousness.

WHEN TO CONSULT?
► The hiccups have lasted over 48 hours.
► Hiccups recur intermittently (for example, every week).
► You are also experiencing chest or stomach pain, indigestion or difficulty swallowing.

WHAT HAPPENS DURING THE EXAM?
The doctor will interview the patient and perform a physical examination. Chest X-rays, stomach exams and blood tests may be ordered to help detect disorders such as diabetes or kidney failure.

WHAT IS THE TREATMENT?
In 90% of refractory or persistent hiccups cases, a disease is responsible and the treatment will correspond accordingly. The other 10 % of persistent cases are treated in a number of ways:

Behaviour modification
It is important to eat slowly, chew well and avoid large meals. Sufferers should also limit consumption of soft drinks, alcohol and tobacco.

Alternative therapies

Cases with psychological origins and those that do not respond to conventional therapy may be treated with hypnosis or acupuncture.

Medications

If other treatment is unsuccessful, tranquilizers or psychotropic medications may be prescribed (anticonvulsants, muscle relaxants, or antidepressants).

High Blood Pressure (Hypertension)

High blood pressure, or hypertension, results from an increased force of the blood within the arterial network. Blood pressure measurements are based on two variables: systolic pressure, referring to the pressure in the vessels when the heart contracts; and diastolic pressure, describing the level of pressure between contractions. Hypertension occurs when either or both of these values increase.

A blood pressure reading of around 120/80 mm Hg (millimetres mercury) is normal (the top number refers to the systolic pressure, the bottom to the diastolic pressure). Anything higher than 140/90 mm Hg is a problem. For diagnostic purposes, an abnormally elevated blood pressure reading must be recorded on roughly three separate occasions with intervals of a few weeks or months. In general, no symptoms accompany hypertension, though localized headaches at the nape of the neck occurring very early in the morning can sometimes be a warning sign.

Hypertension falls into two categories: essential, or primary hypertension, which has no clearly identifiable cause in 85% of cases; and secondary hypertension, the cause of which can generally be clearly determined.

WHAT ARE THE CAUSES?

Essential or Primary Hypertension

► *Hereditary factors* are often responsible, along with aggravating factors such as stress and obesity. While stress leads to an overproduction of adrenaline that increases blood pressure, it is not yet well understood why obesity is a factor.

Secondary Hypertension

► *Renal impairment* (blockage of a renal artery or any other kidney disease).
► *Endocrine (hormone) impairment* (adrenal glands, thyroid).
► *Certain drugs,* such as anti-inflammatories and decongestants.

PRACTICAL ADVICE

Do not do exercise that requires heavy lifting. Weight-lifting, for example, can raise your blood pressure. Do aerobic exercise instead.

Avoid excess salt intake. Salt causes water retention in the arteries, contributing to increases in blood pressure. You should therefore stop eating high-salt foods such as deli or cured meats, potato chips and even some canned soups or other goods. As well as allowing you to reduce your pressure with little sacrifice, any drugs you might be taking to help lower blood pressure will become more effective.

Avoid gaining weight. Maintain a healthy weight. If you are overweight, ask your doctor to recommend a diet.

Do not consume more than two ounces of alcohol daily. Too much alcohol (more than three ounces daily) can have a harmful effect on your pressure. As a guideline, one ounce of alcohol is roughly equivalent to two beers or two large glasses of wine.

Stop smoking. Smoking can aggravate blood pressure related problems and cause serious heart ailments. Tobacco causes the arteries to contract and harden over the long term, increasing pressure.

Do not take your pressure too often. Although monitoring your pressure is advisable, checking it too often has no benefit, can become compulsive, and increase stress and therefore blood pressure. Check it approximately once every two weeks, or whenever you experience discomfort.

Do not dismiss the diagnosis. It is never pleasant to discover one has an illness, whatever it is. Ignoring the symptoms or failing to follow the prescribed treatment, however, could have serious consequences. Talk to your doctor if you think you have high blood pressure as this is a problem that can be successfully managed with little impact on your regular routine.

Purchase a device to measure blood pressure at home. First have it checked at a clinic or pharmacy (most have on-site blood-pressure monitoring devices) to ensure it gives accurate results. If you choose to buy one, be sure to follow the instructions to avoid obtaining a distorted reading. Check your pressure regularly, about once a week or every two weeks, recording your readings each time so you can discuss them with your doctor at your next appointment. Remember that a systolic pressure greater than 140 mm Hg and a diastolic pressure greater than 90 mm Hg are higher than normal. You should also have your pressure checked by a doctor at least once a year as a precautionary measure.

Eat more fruit. The potassium found in fruit is good for you and may help lower blood pressure.

Eat garlic. While the virtues of garlic are not supported by any hard-core scientific evidence, it is known to act as a vasodilator (agent that expands blood vessels) to some degree. While sometimes effective, it should be noted that it is not a recognized medical treatment for high blood pressure.

Avoid stressful situations. Try not to fret about the little things, or as the saying goes, "don't sweat the small stuff." While not necessarily a causal factor, stress can contribute to increased blood pressure.

Practice relaxation techniques. Methods such as transcendental meditation and yoga are excellent techniques for some people, but must be practiced regularly (at least two or three times a week) for the full benefits to be appreciated.

Exercise. Taking a brisk 45-minute walk about three or four times a week can help lower pressure.

WHEN TO CONSULT?

► If your systolic pressure is 200 mm Hg and your diastolic pressure is 120 mm Hg or higher, see a doctor immediately.

▶ Your systolic pressure is above 140 mm Hg and your diastolic pressure is above 90 mm Hg.
▶ You have localized headaches at the nape of your neck upon waking in the morning.
▶ You are short of breath after only mild exertion.

WHAT HAPPENS DURING THE EXAM?

The doctor will check your blood pressure and if it is high, check it again on several different occasions with various intervals. He or she will also take a thorough history to determine if high blood pressure, cardiovascular disease or kidney disease runs in the family. He will then perform a complete physical examination and possibly order a blood work-up and urine test. An electrocardiogram may also be administered, as will a lipid (cholesterol, triglyceride) assessment.

WHAT IS THE TREATMENT?

While hypertension is not curable, it can generally be managed with drugs. In most cases, the patient is required to take a number of different medications at the same time. Note that if you discontinue the treatment, the risk of rapid regression is high.

Essential or Primary Hypertension

When your pressure is only slightly elevated, the doctor will recommend a better diet and an exercise or weight-loss program. If blood pressure remains high, he or she will prescribe a drug treatment, which can be increased or decreased according to the requirements of the patient. For pronounced hypertension, the doctor will initiate drug treatment immediately.

Secondary Hypertension

Treating the cause will effectively manage the problem.

The pelvis is often confused with the hip. Terms like "wide-hipped" or "hip measurements" in fact refer to the part of the body formed by the iliac bones of the pelvis on either side of the trunk, to which the lower limbs (legs) are attached.

In reality, the hip is the joint linking the thigh bone (femur) to the pelvis. It is a deep joint, where inflammation is not easily visible. Pain originating in the hip is not felt locally and manifests in the following ways:

► Pain in the inguinal (groin) area.
► Pain in the outer thigh, near the buttocks.
► Limping.
► Stiffness in the thigh (impeding certain flexing movements).

WHAT ARE THE CAUSES?

► *Bursitis of the hip.* Intense or unusual physical activity can lead to this benign condition.
► *Hip fracture.* This is a serious problem suffered mostly by the elderly that frequently results from taking a fall in the home.
► *Osteoarthritis.* People generally begin to feel normal aging of the joints, including the hips, around the age of 50. Hip dysplasia is a rare genetic deformity that increases the risk of osteoarthritis in middle-aged adults.
► *Arthritic diseases.* Rheumatoid arthritis is one example of an arthritic disease causing inflammation of the joints. In most cases, several joints are affected.
► *Septic arthritis.* This condition occurs when a bacterial infection in the blood penetrates the hip.
► *Cancer.* Bone tumours or metastatic cancers can infiltrate the hip bones.

PRACTICAL ADVICE

Ease the pain. If pain develops after intense or unusual physical exertion, take painkillers: two acetaminophen tablets (325 mg to 500 mg) four times a day, never exceeding four grams daily. Anti-inflammatories can also be helpful; follow the manufacturer's dosage recommendations.

Take both medications at once if the pain is difficult to manage. Wrap some ice in a towel and apply for 20 to 30 minutes, several times a day. Do not apply heat—this will only increase the inflammation.

Avoid resting your weight on the hip or forcing the damaged joint. This can worsen the condition, so use crutches or a cane.

Prevent hip fractures. Reduce the risk of falling at home. Follow your prescription to the letter to avoid dizziness or vertigo and get rid of small rugs or mats that raise the risk of tripping and sliding. Install hand-rails in the hallway and bathroom, as well as an anti-slip mat in the bathtub. Wear anti-slip shoes. Do not store anything higher than eye-level as climbing up to get something in a high cupboard increases your risk of falling. And of course, avoid stairs, if possible.

WHEN TO CONSULT?
► You feel pain in the groin.
► You are limping.
► The pain that appeared after physical activity has not diminished after 48 hours.
► You have suffered a trauma (falling, accident).

WHAT HAPPENS DURING THE EXAM?
The doctor will interview the patient and perform a complete exam. Hip X-rays may be necessary to check for fracture.

WHAT IS THE TREATMENT?
Bursitis of the hip
If anti-inflammatories, rest and cold compresses are not effective, the doctor may prescribe a local cortisone infiltration.

Hip fracture
Surgery is required to repair or replace the hip. The patient may continue to limp after surgery.

Osteoarthritis and arthritic diseases

Anti-inflammatories are usually prescribed and a cane or crutches may sometimes be required. The patient may also be advised to modify his or her activities by taking shorter walks or avoiding stairs, for example. Complete hip replacement is a last resort.

Septic arthritis

Antibiotics are required, as well as a surgical procedure to drain the pus. The infection may lead to the disintegration of the hip a

---

Children and hip problems: medical emergency

A child with hip problems will complain of pain in the groin, stiffness and even knee pain. He or she will also have a high fever and feel generally under the weather. Toddlers may refuse to move their leg or stop walking suddenly. Consult a doctor immediately.

The child may be suffering from septic arthritis (bacteria infecting the hip joint) and require antibiotics and an operation to drain the pus. If left untreated, the condition can have serious consequences, including the partial destruction of the hip, chronic limping, or even hip replacement. Hip infections are rare in children over the age of four.

If the symptoms develop a few weeks after a cold or flu, there is a strong likelihood that the child is suffering from a case of synovitis (inflammation of the synovial membranes lining the joint cavity). This condition lasts a few days and is generally not serious. Full recovery usually only takes ten days of complete rest and anti-inflammatory treatment. Consult a doctor to confirm the diagnosis.

Legg-Calvé-Perthes disease is a much rarer condition that occurs in children between the ages of four and eight. It involves the inflammation of the cartilage and bone of the hip joint. Most of the time, effective treatment consists of physiotherapy, a brace, and bed rest. In severe cases, hip surgery to correct a deformity may be necessary.

few years later, in which case complete hip replacement is necessary.

Tumours
Surgery, radiation therapy or chemotherapy is indicated, depending on the case.

Hoarseness

Dysphonia signifies a change in the voice, whether in timbre, strength or range. Such modifications can be caused by any condition affecting one of the three essential elements of the voice: the lungs, vocal cords (in the larynx), or resonators (located above the vocal cords).

The term "hoarse" usually describes a change in timbre, when the voice becomes husky and rough. In some cases, sufferers lose their voice altogether (aphonia). Hoarseness and laryngitis should be distinguished, the former being only a symptom, while the latter is a disease.

WHAT ARE THE CAUSES?
- *Nodes.* Small, benign growths on the vocal cords (known as singer's nodes) generally caused by overuse of the vocal cords.
- *Benign or malignant tumour* on the larynx.
- *Vocal cord paralysis.*
- *Throat trauma* caused by a blow to the throat in a car or sports accident, for example.
- *Psychological or emotional shock.*

Laryngitis (inflammation of the larynx)
- *Infection,* such as a cold or flu. Laryngitis can also result from over-extending the voice (while screaming at a sports event or singing at the top of your lungs, for example).
- *Inhalers,* such as those used by asthma patients, can cause yeast to develop, leading to laryngitis.
- *Gastroesophageal reflux* can cause posterior laryngitis.
- *Smoking.* Tobacco is extremely irritating to the vocal cords and can cause chronic smoker's laryngitis, also known as Reinke's edema. The voice becomes gravelly and limited in range, the vocal cords swell, and the mucous membranes slacken. These changes can even be observed in teenagers who started smoking very young.

PRACTICAL ADVICE

Keep quiet. Refrain from speaking for 24 hours or longer to rest your vocal cords. Avoid whispering. Whispering creates tension in the upper respiratory tract and dries out the vocal cords.

Breathe in steam. Two or three times a day, hold your head over a bowl of hot water for 10 or 15 minutes, or take a long hot shower.

Maintain humidity at 40%. Use a humidifier or open a window.

Drink plenty of liquids. Even if you do not feel thirsty, drink plenty of liquids to stay hydrated. Water, herbal teas, or lemon-based drinks will liquefy your secretions.

Gargle after using cortisone inhalers. Asthma sufferers who use pump inhalers containing cortisone-based medication should gargle with water each time after using them. This will remove any traces of cortisone from the mucous membranes and prevent yeast infections that cause laryngitis.

What causes a scratchy throat?

If the larynx is dry, the vocal cords are not properly lubricated, which may create the need to clear the throat.
- Seasonal allergies cause inflammation of the mucous membranes in the nose and sinuses. Secretions are thick, viscous, and dry.
- Stress.
- Excessively dry environment.
- Medications that dry out the mucous membranes.
- Dairy products and chocolate make the saliva more viscous. Chocolate, coffee and mint can aggravate gastroesophageal reflux and change the quality of the secretions. Avoid these food items before any event requiring you to use your voice (such as a public speech or singing recital).

Swallow slowly. Swallow your saliva slowly instead of clearing your throat.

Take a lozenge. If the inflammation is acute, a cough drop can stimulate saliva and help soothe the throat. Do not eat lozenges or candies continuously, however, as this can provoke gastroesophageal reflux.

Prevent hoarseness or a scratchy throat.
► Avoid screaming or forcing your voice. Do not try to speak above ambient noise (for example, in a car with open windows or at a dance club). Do not overextend your voice by using it in an unusual way (by doing an impersonation, for example).
► Avoid singing when you have a cold or sore throat.
► Breathe normally. If you speak too quickly without taking the time to breathe, or hold your breath before speaking, you will not be able to produce sound efficiently.

Do not smoke. There are a number of methods to help you quit.

Avoid decongestants containing antihistamines. These medications dry out the mucous membranes. If you must take them, be sure to drink plenty of liquids.

Control your consumption of alcohol. Alcohol dilates the blood vessels, which can inflame the pharynx. It also lowers inhibitions, possibly causing you to scream more than you should.

Take acetaminophen instead of aspirin or anti-inflammatories. Aspirin is excellent for relieving pain and lowering fever, but its anticoagulant properties can cause a vocal cord hemorrhage if the speaker makes a sustained or strenuous effort with his or her voice. Ibuprofen anti-inflammatories have a similar effect. Take one or two acetaminophen tablets (325 mg to 500 mg) four times a day, never exceeding four grams daily.

WHEN TO CONSULT?

► Your voice has been hoarse for the last ten days.

► It is somewhat difficult to swallow, especially if you are suffering from gastroesophageal reflux.

► Your voice has become very hoarse or you have lost it altogether after being hit on the head or in the throat.

► You are a heavy smoker, your voice is deteriorating, you are suffering from permanent hoarseness, or have a persistently sore throat.

WHAT HAPPENS DURING THE EXAM?

The doctor may order a throat culture, lung X-ray (particularly if a vocal cord is paralyzed) or biopsy (if a tumour is detected).

An otorhinolaryngologist (ear, nose and throat specialist) may be consulted for a thorough examination of the vocal cords. He or she will administer a number of painless techniques that vary in complexity. The simplest exam involves shining a light beam onto a mirror in the throat to make the vocal cords clearly visible. More involved techniques include the use of a small telescope linked to a camera and television, and an endoscopy, whereby fibre optics are inserted into the throat just above the vocal cords.

WHAT IS THE TREATMENT?

Rest your vocal cords, inhale steam, and drink plenty of liquids—this is often enough to clear up a case of hoarseness. In most instances, medication is not required. Good vocal hygiene can prevent the problem from recurring. If the hoarseness is chronic, orthophonic re-education techniques can help. Surgery is sometimes required, particularly in the case of resistant singer's nodes or a tumour.

Hot Flashes

Hot flashes occur when blood vessels near the surface of the skin dilate (vasodilation), causing a sudden increase in the temperature of the epidermis and the sensation of intense heat.

Hot flashes come on suddenly and can last up to thirty minutes or more. During this time, red blotches usually appear on the skin, and the thorax, neck and face feel hot. In some cases, the sufferer will break into a cold sweat.

WHAT ARE THE CAUSES?

► *Menopause.* One of the consequences of the gradual decrease in female hormones, usually beginning around the age of forty, is the unpredictable dilation of the blood vessels. Hot flashes are normal symptoms of menopause, with 50% to 70% of menopausal women experiencing them several times a day. They are often accompanied by increased perspiration.

► *Rosacea.* This is the second most common cause of hot flashes after menopause. A chronic skin condition of unknown origin, rosacea most frequently develops in people with light complexions over the age of thirty. The symptoms include red blotches and intermittent temperature increases of the skin on the cheeks, nose, chin and forehead. Lesions resembling acne pimples, visible red veins on the surface of the skin, and a bulge on the nose caused by an excess of tissue (rhinophyma) are also symptomatic. In some cases, the condition causes eye irritation and redness.

► *Hyperthyroidism.* The thyroid is a small gland located at the base of the neck that secretes essential hormones. Hyperthyroidism (overactive thyroid) can develop for a number of reasons and describes a condition that increases the metabolic rate, thereby producing extra heat, which is then purged through the skin. In addition to hot flashes, people with overactive thyroids also experience rapid weight loss, increased appetite, trembling, and accelerated heartbeats. The development of a goiter, a lump in the neck caused by an enlarged thyroid, is also symptomatic.

► **Mastocytosis.** This rare disease affects the mastocytes or mast cells (a type of skin cell) and leads to an overproduction of certain chemicals that stimulate skin surface vasodilation. The other primary symptoms are diarrhea, heart palpitations and abdominal cramps.

► **Tumour of the suprarenal gland (pheochromocytoma).** These tumours are benign in 90% of cases. Located in the kidneys, they stimulate the production of chemicals causing vasodilation. The patient may experience other symptoms, such as nausea, dizziness, vomiting, heart palpitations and high blood pressure.

► **Cancerous tumours.** Very rare intestinal tumours cause an overproduction of serotonin, a chemical that stimulates the dilation of blood vessels on the skin surface. The symptoms of this type of cancer include hot flashes, sweating, abdominal cramps, diarrhea, and difficulty breathing.

PRACTICAL ADVICE

Avoid trigger elements. People suffering from rosacea and menopausal women should take certain precautions. Avoid consuming hot and spicy food, alcohol, coffee and tea as much as possible. Sudden changes in temperature (from an air conditioned room to outside during a heat wave, for example) should also be avoided, as well as very hot baths, showers and saunas, all of which encourage the dilation of the blood vessels at the skin surface. For certain people, intense emotions and stress (nervousness before a public speaking engagement, for example) can provoke hot flashes.

Wear natural fibres. Synthetic fibres trap heat and perspiration during a hot flash, making the symptoms worse. Cotton, wool or linen lets the body breathe so that excess perspiration can evaporate more easily.

Cool down. A hand-held or battery-operated fan, spray water bottle or wet towels should be kept handy for easy access during a hot flash.

Eat more frequently. Five or six snacks a day keep the metabolism working at a steady, continuous rate, and avoids the sudden increases in temperature caused by eating fewer larger meals.

Drink plenty of water. Drinking six to eight glasses of water a day also helps keep the body from sudden temperature spikes.

Protect yourself from the sun. Over time, exposure to the sun's rays or tanning lamps causes the blood vessels to dilate, intensifying the symptoms of rosacea. Avoid tanning salons and use a sunscreen with a minimum of SPF 15 protection.

Cover up red blotches. Foundation make-up specially created for this purpose is available. Ask a cosmetics expert.

Avoid abrasive cleansers or washcloths. If you suffer from rosacea, use a gentle unscented soap with water to clean your face. Rinse well and dry your face with a soft towel. Apply a prescription medicated cream to control red blotches and lesions.

WHEN TO CONSULT?

➤ Although most cases of hot flashes are benign, there is still a remote possibility that they indicate a more serious problem. Don't take any risks: consult your doctor.

WHAT HAPPENS DURING THE EXAM?

The doctor will ask relevant questions and perform a complete physical exam. If needed, he or she will order further evaluations, such as blood or urine tests and X-rays.

WHAT HAPPENS DURING THE TREATMENT?

Menopause

Hot flashes can be controlled with hormone replacement therapy.

Rosacea

Betablockers will considerably reduce red blotches and hot flashes. A medicated cream will also help control red blotches, pustules and pimples. Because rosacea is a chronic condition, these are long-term treatments.

If the surface of the skin is marked by fine blood vessels, the doctor may suggest erasing them with electrodesiccation, a treatment involving small electric shocks to burn the dilated vessels that can be done right there in the doctor's office. Laser treatment is another effective treatment, but also quite expensive and, unlike electrodessication, is usually not covered by government health insurance. Rhinophyma (an excess of tissue causing a bulge on the nose) requires plastic surgery to remodel the nose.

Hyperthyroidism
There are various different causes of hyperthyroidism and each one requires a specific treatment. Once the thyroid begins functioning normally again, the hot flashes will stop.

Mastocytosis
This disease requires medical or surgical treatment, depending on the form in which it appears. Hot flashes will disappear over the course of treatment.

Tumour of the suprarenal gland and cancerous tumours
Both types of tumours must be surgically removed. In the case of cancerous tumours, chemotherapy, radiation therapy and drug treatments can control or eliminate the symptoms.

Insomnia

Insomnia is defined as a sleep disturbance affecting the quantity or quality of sleep, the effects of which are felt the following day. It is important to remember that not everyone needs to sleep seven or eight hours a night to be well rested; some people function perfectly well on only a few hours.

Daytime consequences include fatigue, drowsiness, irritability and difficulty concentrating. The onset of insomnia can be sudden (due to changing time zones while traveling, for example) or insidious and without an identifiable cause. Insomnia can be acute (causing problems for less than two weeks), subacute (present for two weeks to six months) and chronic (persistent for over six months).

There are three categories of insomnia:

Sleep onset (initial) insomnia
► The sufferer has difficulty falling asleep in under 30 minutes after going to bed.

Sleep maintenance (middle) insomnia
► The sufferer wakes up frequently during the night and is awake for longer than 30 minutes in total.

Terminal insomnia
► The sufferer wakes up at least 30 minutes before the desired time.

WHAT ARE THE CAUSES?
► *Stress, anxiety and depression.*
► *Restless leg syndrome* causes an irresistible urge in the sufferer to constantly move his or her legs, making sleep difficult.
► *Sleep apnea,* a decrease in the frequency of breathing during sleep, can cause a feeling of suffocation that partially wakens the sufferer. This disorder is most common in overweight, middle-aged men.
► *Periodic or repetitive movements* of the lower limbs during the night may cause someone to wake up.

▶ *Pain.* Chronic pain, or that caused by arthritis, is a frequent cause of sleeplessness.

▶ *Digestive problems* such as heartburn or acid reflux.

▶ *Nocturia,* the need to urinate during the night.

▶ *Cardiac or respiratory disorders* can cause shortness of breath, preventing restorative sleep.

▶ *Itchiness.*

▶ *Stimulants* such as coffee, nicotine, alcohol and drugs, as well as medications for hypertension, angina pectoris or asthma can contribute to insomnia; anti-inflammatories, antidepressants and, in some cases, anti-parkinsonian medications, can also be contributing factors.

▶ *Circadian rhythm disturbances* such as jet lag, night shifts, or constantly changing shift work are common examples. Changes in the sleep-waking cycle (going to bed unusually late or early) can also have this effect.

▶ *Environmental factors* such as noise, light, an uncomfortable mattress or room temperature, or noisy sleeping partner.

▶ *Poor sleep habits,* such as an irregular schedule or extended daytime napping.

▶ *Emotional distress,* such as problems at work, divorce, illness, or the death of a loved one.

▶ *Major lifestyle changes* caused by a newborn baby or the death of a relative, for example.

PRACTICAL ADVICE

Avoid sleeping pills. Do not take over-the-counter sleeping pills. Never use pills prescribed for another person. Try to treat your insomnia with the methods outlined in this chapter. If you feel that you absolutely require sleeping pills, consult your physician.

Go to bed when you are tired and ready to sleep. Do not go to bed too early, no matter what the excuse.

Avoid stimulating physical and intellectual activity just before bedtime. Avoid sports, studies or computer games at least one hour before bedtime.

A bed is for sleeping. Sleeping can become a problem if the bed is associated with a number of other activities such as reading, watching television or eating. Other activities should take place in the living room. (Note: sexual activity is the only exception to the rule!)

Do not eat just before bed. This advice is particularly important for individuals who suffer from digestive troubles or obesity. If you are hungry, eat a light snack.

Wait 20 minutes. If you have been trying to sleep for 20 minutes without success, get up and go to another room. Wait until you are tired and able to sleep before returning to bed.

Alcohol is not a sleep aid. Although alcohol can help a person fall asleep, it disturbs the quality of sleep.

Get up at the same time every day. Do not get up at six o'clock during the week and sleep in until noon on weekends. Getting up late on Sunday morning can make it difficult to get to sleep Sunday night. Sleeping more than one hour past your normal time can disrupt your sleep patterns.

Try to relax. Take a hot bath or get a massage.

Do relaxation exercises. There are a number of effective methods, including yoga, progressive relaxation, visualization, and meditation. Choose the one most suited to you and practice it regularly.

Avoid napping. If you must sleep during the day, be sure to do so before three o'clock in the afternoon and for no more than 45 minutes.

Adopt a healthy lifestyle. Avoid coffee, alcohol, and cigarettes before going to bed. An active lifestyle including regular, daily exercise (walking, swimming) promotes a better quality of sleep.

Sleep in a tranquil, quiet environment. Your bedroom should be quiet. Purchase a comfortable mattress and blinds or curtains that block out the light. Decorate with calming colors.

Reset your clock by getting up a little earlier or later every day. Consult a sleep clinic for a detailed and specific program, if necessary.

WHEN TO CONSULT?

► You have suffered from insomnia for several days.
► You feel anxious about falling asleep (this may be a symptom of depression).
► You have insomnia and feel depressed.
► Your sleep disturbance has an impact on your daily activities (causing fatigue, severe drowsiness, difficulty concentrating, or mood swings).
► You are using alcohol or sleeping pills to sleep.
► You suffer from respiratory difficulty or restless leg syndrome.
► Your partner is worried about your irregular breathing during the night (sleep apnea) or informs you of your incessant movement (periodic leg movements).
► You wake up suddenly in the middle of the night with a feeling of suffocation (sleep apnea).

WHAT HAPPENS DURING THE EXAM?

The doctor takes a complete history of your insomnia and attempts to identify the physical, psychological, pharmacological, or environmental causes at the root of the problem. Lab tests are sometimes required. If sleep apnea is suspected, a sleep clinic consultation may be indicated. The patient may be referred to an Ears, Nose and Throat specialist for an assessment. The doctor may request that the patient maintain a journal documenting sleep over a two to three week period.

WHAT IS THE TREATMENT?

In many cases, the practical advice outlined in this chapter will correct the factors responsible for the sleep disturbance.

If restless leg syndrome or periodic leg movements are severe enough to disrupt sleep, the doctor may prescribe medication.

Sleep apnea can be treated with medication, a home respiratory device (CPAP), and in some cases, corrective surgery.

In cases of resistant insomnia, a psychological consultation may be helpful. The physician will prescribe a hypnotic (sleeping pill) if he or she feels it is warranted. In general, however, sleeping pills are not recommended for periods longer than one or two weeks, as they are addictive and become less effective as the sufferer's drug tolerance increases.

Intermittent Claudication

Like angina pectoris, intermittent claudication is caused by poor circulation. Leg pain develops during physical activity, causing the sufferer to limp, but dissipating after a few minutes of rest. The time it takes for the pain to develop remains constant in one individual, but varies from person to person. It is frequently accompanied by cold feet, slow-healing sores, and cold patches on the legs.

WHAT ARE THE CAUSES?

- *Poor arterial circulation* deprives the muscles of oxygen during basic exercises such as walking. The cramps disappear when the legs are at rest.
- *Risk factors* are identical to those for heart disease: smoking, diabetes, hypercholesterolemia, high blood pressure, and aging.

PRACTICAL ADVICE

Avoid hot compresses. People suffering from intermittent claudication tend to get cold feet. Hot water bottles should be avoided, however, because circulation in the extremities is insufficient to move heat out of the area and skin damage can result. Wear wool socks instead.

Walk. Walking encourages circulation in the legs and prevents the development or progression of the disease.

Take aspirin. One tablet of aspirin (325 mg) every second day or one "baby" aspirin (80 mg) every day decreases the likelihood of developing blood clots that further impede circulation. Be sure to find out from your doctor whether aspirin interacts with any other medication you are taking or is contra-indicated.

Quit smoking. Smoking is the number one risk factor. The death rate is 25% five years after diagnosis for people who continue smoking, and 10% to 12% for those who quit. The risk of amputation is 10% for smokers five years after diagnosis. It is significantly lower for non-smokers.

Decrease your consumption of alcohol. Over the long-term, alcohol consumption leads to arteriosclerosis (cholesterol deposits in the arteries), reducing blood flow and causing circulation problems and intermittent claudication.

Take care of your heart. Whatever is good for the heart is good for the arteries in the legs. Quit smoking, exercise regularly, lose weight, and eat less fat.

WHEN TO CONSULT?

► Your legs hurt when you walk.
► Sores on your feet become infected or heal very slowly.

WHAT HAPPENS DURING THE EXAM?

After interviewing the patient to determine the nature of the pain, the doctor assesses the state of arterial circulation by using a stethoscope to check the pulse at different locations on the body (groin area, ankle, etc.).

The doctor also examines the legs for possible sores or cold patches (two signs of poor circulation). A Doppler ultrasound test may be ordered to determine whether there has been any narrowing of the arteries, and if so, to what extent.

If bypass surgery or arterial dilation is necessary, the doctor orders an arteriography exam, a diagnostic test involving the injection of coloured fluid into the arteries to make any narrowed areas visible by X-ray. In some cases, arteriography is performed with magnetic resonance imaging (MRIs) or axial tomography.

WHAT IS THE TREATMENT?

Regular walking is the best treatment, but risk factors must also be eliminated. Quitting smoking will stop or slow the progression of the disease in smokers, who constitute 80% of sufferers. Diabetics (representing 16% of cases) must control their blood sugar levels. People suffering from high blood pressure (23% of cases) or high cholesterol must be treated for these conditions. People carrying excess weight must go on a diet.

The doctor will prescribe a low dose of aspirin to thin the blood.

In more advanced cases, pain is experienced even while at rest, gangrene develops, and the sufferer's livelihood and quality of life are severely affected. The treatment for this is arterial bypass or dilation (whereby inflatable balloons are inserted into the artery), a procedure that is also used for failing arteries surrounding the heart.

In approximately 80% of cases, the disease will stabilize or improve over the five years following diagnosis, provided the sufferer quits smoking and controls all other risk factors.

Involuntary Weight Loss

This chapter does not address weight loss due to voluntary diets or anorexia nervosa, but rather the involuntary, unexplained loss of 10% to 15% of an individual's regular body mass. For example, unexplained weight loss is noteworthy when individuals weighing 55 kilograms (120 pounds) lose 5 to 8 kilograms (11 to 18 pounds), or those weighing 70 kg (155 pounds) lose 7 to 10 kg (15 to 22 pounds).

When weight loss is caused by an underlying illness, there are usually other symptoms such as loss of appetite, fatigue, blood in the stool, difficulty swallowing, and abdominal pain.

WHAT ARE THE CAUSES?

- *Extreme stress* can prevent a person from eating or sleeping well.
- *Change in diet* (switching to vegetarianism, for example).
- *Malnutrition and poverty.*
- *Depression* due to the death of a loved one, job loss, heartbreak, or financial worries, for example. Depression may also accompany a physical disorder.
- *Isolation of the elderly.* Elderly people who are alone frequently lose the desire to prepare food and eat.
- *Certain medications* (for example, certain antibiotics and cancer drugs) can suppress the appetite, change the taste of food, or provoke nausea and vomiting. Drug interactions may also cause the patient to lose his or her appetite.
- *Alcoholism.* Alcoholics sometimes eat little and poorly.
- *Intestinal parasites* caught during a trip abroad, for example.
- *Gastroenteritis.* Acute diarrhea causes water loss and rapid weight loss.
- *Chronic or recurring abdominal pain* caused by gallstones, for example.
- *Inflammatory diseases of the digestive tract* such as Crohn's disease, ulcerative colitis, chronic pancreatitis, or celiac disease.
- *Inflammatory diseases* such as rheumatoid arthritis or systemic lupus erythematosus.

- ▶ *Diseases affecting the vital organs* such as kidney, heart, lung, orliver failure, diabetes, or hyperthyroidism.
- ▶ *Infectious diseases* such as tuberculosis, AIDS, or pneumonia.
- ▶ *All types of cancer,* particularly cancer of the lung, stomach, intestine, or blood (lymphoma or leukemia).
- ▶ *Alzheimer's disease.* In advanced stages, patients forget to eat.

PRACTICAL ADVICE

Consult a doctor immediately. Although the cause may be serious, it is a mistake to let fear of the unknown stop you from seeing your doctor. If a serious disease like cancer is responsible for your weight loss, the earlier it is diagnosed and treated, the better your chances are of beating it.

If you are suffering from extreme stress. Set aside some time for rest and relaxation and make a point of eating properly. Be sure not to replace meals with cigarettes and coffee. Quitting smoking can help you avoid several diseases that often cause weight loss.

If you are suffering from viral gastroenteritis. Be sure to drink plenty of liquids if you are losing weight due to acute diarrhea.

Consult your family doctor regularly. Regular medical check-ups are recommended. Go to your family doctor as he or she is familiar with your case and keeps records of your weight, family and personal medical history, previous lab test results, and so on. If you do not have a family doctor, get one. Drop-in clinics are meant for minor emergencies.

Avoid isolation. Ask your local community support organization for help if you need it.

Limit alcohol consumption. An aperitif may whet the appetite, but too many drinks will suppress it.

If a disease has already been diagnosed. If you suffer from diabetes or lung failure, for example, follow the doctor's orders and continue taking your prescribed medications. If you find it very difficult to follow your treatment, speak to your doctor.

WHEN TO CONSULT?

► You have lost between 10% and 15% of your normal weight.
► The weight loss is accompanied by fatigue, blood in the stool, abdominal pain, or difficulty swallowing.
► You feel depressed and you have lost weight.
► A child or adolescent has lost weight. This in itself is cause for concern.
► You are pregnant and have lost weight. This in itself is cause for concern.

WHAT HAPPENS DURING THE EXAM?

The doctor takes a history and performs a complete physical examination, ordering blood and other lab tests. Radiological exams may be necessary, particularly lung X-rays for smokers.

WHAT IS THE TREATMENT?

Treatment varies according to the cause. If the patient is losing weight due to depression, antidepressants may be prescribed. A consultation with a psychologist or psychiatrist may also be recommended.

Inflammatory diseases and heart or lung failure can be treated with effective medications.

Antibiotics are prescribed for bacterial infections.

Diabetics may be required to modify their diets, practice regular exercise, and, if necessary, take medications to control the disease. If the patient is suffering from cancer, a number of treatments are possible, including surgery, chemotherapy, or radiation therapy.

Irregular Heart Beat (Arrhythmia)

The term "arrhythmia" describes an irregular heartbeat (contractions of the heart muscle) that may or may not be dangerous.

Normal heart rate in a body at rest is 60 to 80 beats per minute and can be measured by the pulse. Arrhythmia refers to any change in heart rhythm, including accelerations (tachycardia) and decelerations (bradycardia).

Heart palpitations are the primary symptom of arrhythmia, although they are not always apparent (causing some sufferers to remain unaware of the problem). They may arise spontaneously (in the absence of any heart problem) for those who are extremely sensitive or suffering from anxiety.

There are different forms of arrhythmia, the most common of which are listed below:

► Extrasystole. This term describes a premature or surplus heartbeat, which is experienced as an erratic or skipped beat. The sufferer may also cough lightly and feel like the heart is rising into the throat. This is the most common type of arrhythmia and frequently goes unnoticed. In most cases, it represents a harmless irregularity in an otherwise healthy heart and is not accompanied by any other symptoms. Extrasystole is sometimes accompanied by brief dizzy spells, but these are no cause for concern.

► Bradycardia. This medical term (literally meaning "slow heart") has a number of of possible causes and describes a slowing of the heart rate to less than 60 beats per minute. While medical attention is required in some cases, a slower heart rate is considered normal in people with no other symptoms. In some cases, bradycardia causes people to tire quickly and become breathless or dizzy.

► Atrial (or auricular) fibrillation describes rapid and erratic contractions of the atria (the two upper cavities of the heart) that propel blood toward the ventricles (the two lower sections).

The right atrium sends blood to the right ventricle, which in turn pumps it to the lungs, while blood from the left atrium is pumped to the left ventricle and then the rest of the body. When the atria are in a state of fibrillation, they do not contract adequately, possibly leading to an irregular heartbeat. Atrial fibrillation may go unnoticed as sufferers do not necessarily experience palpitations and there are no other symptoms. Although blood continues to be pumped to the ventricles, the inadequate force may cause it to accumulate in certain parts of the ventricle. This can lead to the formation of a clot that can block an artery and even lead to a cerebrovascular accident, if the clot moves to the brain.

► Ventricular tachycardia describes rapid ventricular contractions (faster than 100 beats per minute) that may or may not be regular. This form of arrhythmia is more rare and indicates poor ventricular function. Sufferers feel generally unwell, experience heart palpitations, and their skin becomes pale and clammy. In cases of extremely rapid heart rate, sufferers become dizzy and faint.

► Paroxysmal tachycardia. This form of arrhythmia occurs primarily in younger individuals and manifests in sudden attacks brought on by abnormal electric signals in the heart. This causes a rate increase of up to 200 beats per minute that lasts a few minutes or even hours. The heart rate returns to normal just as suddenly as it accelerates. Paroxysmal tachycardia is usually accompanied by palpitations and may occur spontaneously or be triggered by mild physical effort (bending over to retrieve an object, for example), emotional stress, or extrasystole.

► Ventricular fibrillation. This acute form of arrhythmia is characterized by small, quick, irregular and inefficient contractions of the ventricles that stop blood flow to the lungs and rest of the body, leading to loss of consciousness. It generally occurs in the first stages of myocardial infarction (heart attack).

WHAT ARE THE CAUSES?

Extrasystole

► **Sudden stress, fever, anemia.**

► **Stimulants,** such as caffeine, alcohol, tobacco, or cocaine.

► *Overdose of certain drugs,* such as thyroid medication or diuretics.
► *Large meals,* particularly when combined with alcohol.

Bradycardia
► *Calmness, rest, peak physical condition.*
► *Physical reaction to unpleasant stimuli* ("vagal" reflex).
► *Certain coronary disease or high blood pressure medications.*
► *Hypothyroidism,* slowing the functions of the entire body.
► *Serious conditions,* such as critical hypothermia and anorexia.
► *Congenital abnormalities.*
► *Sinus node disease.* The sinus node, located in the atrium, regulates heart rate. If it malfunctions, bradycardia may ensue.
► *Heart attack.* In the early stages of certain types of myocardial infarction, the heart rate may slow down noticeably.

Atrial (or auricular) fibrillation
► *Coronary artery disease.* Auricular fibrillation may be the result of an earlier infarction.
► *High blood pressure.*
► *Valve (particularly the mitral valve) problems,* caused by ailments such as emphysema or chronic bronchitis.
► *Hyperthyroidism.* An overactive thyroid gland leads to an accelerated heart rate and may cause atrial fibrillation.
► *Alcohol abuse.* Drinking large amounts of alcohol in a short period of time can also cause atrial fibrillation.
► *Aging.* Atrial fibrillation is more common in elderly people and increases in frequency as people get older (particularly after the age of 65).

Ventricular tachycardia
► *Heart attack.* Ventricular tachycardia occurs in people with heart muscle abnormalities, most commonly caused by a previous myocardial infarction.
► *Heart failure.* Ventricular tachycardia almost always occurs in people with weakened hearts due to such problems as coronary artery disease, high blood pressure, and valve problems.

- ***Congenital deformity.*** Ventricular tachycardia may occur in young individuals with a heart deformity.
- ***Stimulants,*** such as alcohol, tobacco, coffee, and illicit drugs.
- ***Medications,*** such as diuretics and pseudoephedrine (found in decongestants).

Paroxysmal tachycardia

- ***Excess electrical impulses to the heart.*** Some individuals develop surplus electrical conduction mechanisms that can lead to a kind of "short circuiting".
- ***Emotional hypersensitivity.***
- ***Hyperthyroidism.***
- ***Lung disease.***

Ventricular fibrillation.

- ***Acute myocardial infarction (heart attack)*** resulting from the sudden obstruction of an artery by a blood clot is the most common cause of ventricular fibrillation. This type of arrhythmia is the most common cause of sudden death in North America.

PRACTICAL ADVICE

Emergency measures. If you have heart palpitations and feel as though your heart is rising to your throat, you may be suffering from extrasystolic arrhythmia. Get up and walk around slowly (provided, of course, you are not feeling dizzy). If the palpitations come on suddenly and are very rapid, sit down and breathe deeply. If they are accompanied by dizziness and weakness, lie down and call for help. It is very important to remain in a lying position, as standing up can further lower your blood pressure and cause you to lose consciousness.

Provide cardiopulmonary resuscitation (CPR). If someone has lost consciousness and you cannot detect a pulse on the person's wrist, provide artificial respiration and cardiac massage (CPR) until medical assistance arrives. This will control the arrhythmia and keep the person alive.

Do not take nitroglycerine unless you are experiencing chest pain. Nitroglycerine lowers blood pressure, which can cause you to lose consciousness.

Always warm up before intense physical activity. Particularly if you are susceptible to arrhythmia.

Avoid stimulants. Such as caffeine (in coffee, tea, cola, or chocolate), tobacco, alcohol (particularly strong drinks like cognac), and illicit drugs (especially cocaine).

WHEN TO CONSULT?

► Your heart palpitations are accompanied by dizziness, loss of consciousness, chest pain, or shortness of breath. Consult immediately.

► You have heart palpitations and suffer from heart disease. It is particularly important to consult if you have high blood pressure or have previously had a myocardial infarction.

► You experience palpitations and have risk factors for cardiovascular disease such as a family history of hypercholesterolemia or smoking.

► Your heartbeat at rest is irregular and faster than 100 beats per minute.

WHAT HAPPENS DURING THE EXAM?

The doctor takes a history of the symptoms and discusses the patient's lifestyle and family medical history. Various tests are administered to identify the type and seriousness of the arrhythmia. An electrocardiogram (E.C.G.) is used to measure the patient's current heart activity, while a Holter monitor records it over a 24-hour period. The latter (activated by a simple button) is a small device (about the size of a Walkman) featuring electrodes that attach to the skin. The patient is required to take note of the symptoms and relay this information to the doctor. The physician may also order an exercise electrocardiogram to check the state of the heart during physical exertion.

To detect an occasional arrhythmia, the patient may be asked to wear a transtelephonic monitor for a few days or weeks. This device records the heart rate for one minute at a time and is activated by the patient manually whenever symptoms arise.

Blood tests and heart ultrasounds may also be ordered.

WHAT IS THE TREATMENT?

Extrasystole
Most cases of extrasystole are harmless and generally require no treatment beyond a change in lifestyle.

Bradycardia
If the condition is caused by medication or an ailment, the doctor will modify the patient's prescription or treat the underlying disease. In serious cases, a pacemaker may be installed to ensure a minimum heart rate and avoid the appearance of symptoms.

Atrial (or auricular) fibrillation
A variable heart rate can be slowed down and regularized with medication. In some cases, a normal heart rate can be achieved only through electrical cardioversion (applying electrical currents directly to the heart). This technique is also used for emergency defibrillations, although much higher electrical currents are required to restart the heart. Atrial fibrillation requires daily doses of anticoagulants to prevent the formation of blood clots.

Ventricular tachycardia
In serious cases of arrhythmia, the heart rate can be stabilized with anti-arrhythmic drugs or, in particularly hard-to-treat cases, electrical cardioversion therapy (*see above entry*). It is now also possible to treat this type of arrhythmia by implanting a defibrillator device (a sort of sophisticated pacemaker that administers internal electrical shocks to control the arrhythmia).

Paroxysmal tachycardia

A special fulguration treatment using microwaves may be administered to "burn" the focal point of the arrhythmia. The process involves inserting a catheter equipped with a probe and tiny electrical wire into the heart via a blood vessel.

Ventricular fibrillation

If left untreated, death is imminent. Resuscitation procedures must begin as soon as possible. Medical attention involves the use of a heart defibrillator (the administration of electrical shocks to restart the heart).

Jaundice

Jaundice is characterized by a yellow discoloration of the skin and mucous membranes. Perhaps the most obvious sign of the condition is yellowing in the whites of the eyes (the sclera). Jaundice requires medical attention.

The change in skin coloration occurs when the tissues become permeated with bilirubin, a greenish-yellow bile pigment produced during the normal process of red blood cell destruction at the end of their 120-day life-span. The pigment is then chemically transformed by the liver, stored in the gallbladder, and directed towards the intestine for digestion. When the level of bilirubin in the blood is too high, the liver cannot transform it at an adequate pace, resulting in jaundice.

Jaundice can be accompanied by fever, chills, nausea, vomiting, loss of appetite, weight loss, unusual pain in the upper abdomen, pale stools and dark urine (coffee or tea coloured).

Jaundice itself is not serious, but the disease triggering it can be. It is therefore important to consult a doctor to determine the underlying cause. In most cases, early diagnosis leads to a better prognosis.

WHAT ARE THE CAUSES?

► *Disorders that create an excess of bilirubin* such as hemolysis (destruction of the red blood cells) and hypersplenism (destruction of red blood cells by the spleen).
► *Liver disorders* that prevent the organ from transforming bilirubin. Jaundice can be caused by diseases such as hepatitis (an inflammatory liver disease, frequently viral in origin), alcoholic hepatitis, cirrhosis of the liver due to alcoholism or a virus, as well as certain rare genetic diseases including Gilbert's disease (affecting 2% to 10% of the population).
► *Certain medications.* Toxic reactions to isoniazid (for tuberculosis), sulfonamides, halothane (anesthetic) and erythromycin (antibiotic) can all provoke jaundice.

► *Bile duct obstruction,* such as that caused by gallstones. A tumour of the pancreas can also obstruct or compress the bile ducts, leading to jaundice.

PRACTICAL ADVICE

Beware of false cases. A change in skin coloration may also result from excessive ingestion of carotene (a pigment found in carrots and tomato juice, for example). This is benign and will resolve without treatment over time.

Listen to those around you. Jaundice can appear gradually and subtly. People close to the sufferer are usually the first to notice.

Physiologic neonatal jaundice

In the womb, the fetus is nourished by fetal hemoglobin (or fetal blood), which is progressively replaced by "adult" hemoglobin as the fetus matures. At birth, when the leftover fetal hemoglobin becomes inessential, the body begins to destroy it, causing an increase in bilirubin levels. In most cases, this process goes unnoticed.

Premature babies have a greater amount of fetal hemoglobin to destroy, causing a rise in bilirubin levels that often results in jaundice. Some full-term newborns are also susceptible to developing jaundice if they experience a brief dip in the levels of the enzyme necessary for transforming bilirubin, which prevents the liver from properly metabolizing the pigment.

Jaundice generally appears on the third to fifth day after birth and resolves on its own within no more than two weeks. In most cases of newborn jaundice, the babies are kept at the hospital for a few days and exposed to sun lamps. The rays stimulate the excretion of bilirubin by the gallbladder and intestine, facilitating the pigment's elimination. The baby's eyes are, of course, protected from the rays of the lamp.

WHEN TO CONSULT?

► Your skin and the whites of your eyes have an abnormal, yellowish tinge.

► You have developed jaundice in association with one or more of the following symptoms: fever, chills, nausea, vomiting, loss of appetite, weight loss, liver pain, pale stools and dark urine (coffee or tea coloured).

WHAT HAPPENS DURING THE EXAM?

The physician takes a detailed history and performs a complete physical examination including an abdominal exam. Further investigation is determined by the particular case and the results of the physical examination. Blood and urine tests are required.

The doctor may order imaging tests such as an ultrasound, tomodensitometry (CT scan), endoscopy, or liver biopsy. If necessary, the patient is referred to the specialist appropriate to the underlying cause: a hematologist (for a blood disorder), gastroenterologist (for an intestinal problem), internist, surgeon, or other.

WHAT IS THE TREATMENT?

Disorder causing an excess of bilirubin
The underlying cause determines the treatment.

Liver disorders or certain medications
If the condition is caused by medication, alcohol, or drugs, the patient must refrain from consuming the substance. Antiviral agents may be used to treat viral hepatitis.

Obstruction of the bile duct
Kidney stones may require minor surgery to remove the gallbladder. If the obstruction is in the pancreas or intestine, major surgery is necessary.

Jaw Disorders

The temporomandibular joint, commonly known as the jaw, is located just in front of the ear and composed of two main structures: the mandibular condyle (the lower jaw) and the glenoid fossa (part of the skull). The meniscus is a small fibrocartilage cushion located between the two parts that moves with the jaw.

Jaw disorders are fairly common. Although the exact causes remain unknown, bruxism (teeth grinding) is a significant risk factor, along with certain other bad habits (chewing on the end of a pen or pencil, biting your nails), stress, malocclusion (misalignment of the teeth or jaws), trauma (blows or fractures), osteoarthritis, and rheumatoid arthritis.

Jaw disorders take a number of forms:

► Clicking jaw, with or without pain.
► Misaligned jaw, with mouth open.
► Locked jaw, with mouth half-open (half-open lock).
► Locked jaw, with mouth open (open lock).
► Pain in the jaw, ear, and temple.

WHAT ARE THE CAUSES?

Jaw pain

► *Inflammation.* Pain is felt in the jaw (in front of the ear) and may be accompanied by clicking. There are a number of causes for inflammation, including trauma, malocclusion, and bruxism (teeth grinding).

Muscle pain

► *Bruxism (teeth grinding).* The muscle pain is not due to a jaw problem in this case, but to inflammation, tension, or spasms in the muscles resulting from grinding. Bruxism may be accompanied by shooting pain in the temples and jaw.

Radiating pain

► *Sinusitis, toothaches or earaches* can cause pain that radiates to the jaw. There is no jaw problem in these cases.

Clicking jaw

► *Meniscus displacement.* As it moves, the meniscus may become displaced. When it spontaneously returns to its original position, a painful click may result. This problem does not usually require medical treatment unless it causes intense or persistent pain.

Half-open lock

► *Meniscus displacement without reduction.* In some cases, the meniscus does not return to its original position, causing the mouth to lock half-open. Sufferers then run the risk of developing a deviation (misalignment) of the mouth when open or being unable to open it completely, which may be accompanied by pain.

Open lock

► *Dislocation of the lower jaw (mandibular condyle).* For unknown reasons, some people have a loose and distended jaw. The condyle may become displaced, causing the jaw to deviate or lock in an open position, possibly resulting in pain.

PRACTICAL ADVICE

Pain

Take medication. Non-prescription aspirin, acetaminophen or ibuprofen can help ease the pain. Follow the recommended dosage.

Modify your diet. Avoid food that is hard to chew (candy, steak, French bread, etc.), at least while your jaw hurts. Chewing gum or opening the mouth very wide (to take a bite of an oversized sandwich, for example) is not recommended either, as it can cause microtrauma to the joint. Eat fish, poultry, well-cooked vegetables, soup, dairy products, purees, or other soft foods. Cut raw vegetables and hard fruit into small pieces.

Limit jaw movement. If you need to yawn, put your fist under your jaw to keep it in place and hold your tongue against the palate to stop your mouth from opening too widely.

Do not clench your teeth. Your teeth should touch only when you swallow or chew, even when your mouth is closed.

Relax. Stress is one of the most common causes of jaw pain. Put aside time to relax every day: listen to music, take a hot bath, do some yoga or reading, get a massage. There are a number of techniques to choose from.

Apply heat with. You can use a reusable compress, hot water bottle, or hot towel to relax muscles affected by bruxism or clenched teeth.

Avoid bad posture. Sleeping on your stomach with your head turned to the side or resting your chin on your hand exerts pressure on the jaw or chin, causing or aggravating jaw pain.

Clicking Jaw

Don't worry. Clicking does not necessarily indicate a serious problem or lead to half-open or open locking. If you have no pain and your jaw still moves freely, there is no need to consult a physician. In many cases, particularly in children, the condition is temporary.

Half-open lock

See a doctor or dentist. This type of lock requires consultation and treatment.

Open lock

Put your jaw back in place. Place both your index fingers in your mouth on either side of the jaw as deeply as possible and apply gentle pressure downward. If this does not work, see a doctor or dentist.

WHEN TO CONSULT?

- ► You have received a blow to the jaw.
- ► The pain is persistent.
- ► Your jaw is misaligned when your mouth is open.
- ► Your jaw is locked in a half-open or open position.
- ► Your jaw locks frequently.

► The clicking in your jaw has become painful or very bothersome.
► You experience misalignment of the teeth or jaw.

WHAT HAPPENS DURING THE EXAM?

If necessary, your doctor or dentist will refer you to an oral and max-illofacial surgeon, who will perform a complete examination of the mouth and jaw. This involves measuring the jaw to see how wide it opens and check the range of movement. X-rays of the jaw or mag-netic resonance imaging (MRI) tests of the meniscus are also some-times necessary. If there is a malocclusion, the doctor may take an impression of your teeth to study the misalignment.

WHAT IS THE TREATMENT?

Pain

For intense pain, the doctor will prescribe anti-inflammatories and, in some cases, cortisone injections in the joint. If the pain is radiating from elsewhere, he or she will treat the underlying ailment.

If the pain is caused by teeth clenching, the dentist may create a personalized, nearly-invisible retainer to control the problem during the night. In some cases, the dentist will recommend the patient wear the retainer during the day as well.

Half-open lock

The specialist may prescribe physiotherapy exercises for the patient to do at home. In some cases, one or more joint infiltrations are nec-essary. This involves injecting a solution into the jaw to swell the joint capsule, which creates space for the meniscus to return to its original place. The procedure is performed under local anesthesia. In serious cases, the doctor may choose to surgically stabilize the jaw.

Open lock

The doctor or dentist may be able to manually return an open-locked jaw to its original position. If the patient's jaw locks repeated-ly, surgery may be the only way to permanently treat the problem.

Jet Lag

Jet lag is the term used to describe the unpleasant physical symptoms that result from rapid travel across several time zones. It is the body's normal reaction to being "out of sync" with its new environment. The most pronounced symptom is the disturbance of the body's internal clock, which has a marked effect on sleep patterns.

Jet lag is neither a myth nor an exaggeration, but a scientifically proven phenomenon to which everyone is susceptible. While some are fairly resistant and present only mild symptoms, more fragile travellers can feel the effects for several days.

Jet lag can manifest in a variety of ways:
- Sleep disturbance (difficulty falling or staying asleep).
- Diminished physical or mental performance.
- Increased fatigue.
- Gastrointestinal problems.
- General malaise.

WHAT ARE THE CAUSES?

Frequent travel across time zones.
- Airline pilots, flight attendants and business people are affected by jet lag regularly, since their work often requires them to cross a number of time zones.

Rotating shift work
- Employees who alternate day and night shifts experience symptoms similar to jet lag.

Aging
- The older you are, the more jet lag you will suffer when you travel.

Sensitivity to routine changes
- For those who have trouble with routine changes (cannot sleep anywhere but their own bed, for example), recovering from jet lag will be more difficult.

Travelling east
► The body seems to adapt better to an extended day rather than a contracted one, making east-bound travelers (who lose rather than gain time), more susceptible to jet lag.

PRATICAL ADVICE

Adapt to local time as quickly as possible. Do not hang on to the rhythm of the place you are coming from. Go out into the day, eat at mealtimes and adjust your watch to the new time zone. This will help regulate your body's clock.

Take a nap if you need to. You should sleep for either 30 minutes or two full hours. During the first half hour, sleep remains light, making it relatively easy to wake up while still feeling somewhat refreshed. The deep sleep cycle begins after 30 minutes, at which point it is best to sleep through for an hour and a half to two hours until this phase is over and you move back into light sleep before waking.

Sleep in a quiet place. If possible, find a cool, silent, dark room to sleep.

Eat lightly and drink plenty of liquid. Avoid heavy or greasy meals and drink a lot of water to avoid unpleasant symptoms. Remember, however, that your internal clock is influenced more by the time of day you eat, than by what you eat.

Before leaving
Get plenty of rest. If you are tired when you leave, you will be even more so when you arrive. The night before your departure, go to bed early. If you are travelling at night, try to take a nap in the afternoon to store up sleep for the hours you will miss.

Plan some time to rest during your trip. Jet lag gets worse as people get older, so elderly travellers should set aside some time to rest on their trip. Visiting ten cities in ten days, for example, may prove to be more taxing than fun.

During the flight

Eat lightly. It is recommended that travelers eat lightly during flights. Movement is limited and overeating will only make you uncomfortable.

Drink plenty of liquid. Air is particularly dry on airplanes. Drink water or fruit juice to keep the body well-hydrated.

Avoid alcohol or coffee. Unlike water or fruit juice, alcohol and coffee actually dehydrate the body. Drink as little as possible.

Sleep as much as you can. While it neither modifies your body's internal rhythms nor prevents jet lag, sleeping during the flight will leave you better rested when you arrive.

Sleeping pills? Some travelers are tempted to take sleeping pills during a long flight, although it is generally not recommended. Consult your doctor, who will consider your eating and alcohol habits before advising you. Taking a prescription sleeping pill on a full stomach and after drinking alcohol will certainly not help you feel better when you land. If you are nervous on planes, generally anxious, or suffer from insomnia, the doctor may prescribe a mild sedative to help you rest on the flight.

WHEN TO CONSULT?

► You are worried about your health and must travel in the near future.
► You have trouble sleeping, feel anxious and must travel in the near future.

WHAT HAPPENS DURING THE EXAM?

Anyone with heart or respiratory disease should consult a doctor before travelling on an airplane to ensure there is no risk. If the patient's condition is well controlled by medication, the doctor will authorize the trip.

WHAT IS THE TREATMENT?

In general, full recovery from jet lag (synchronizing the body's internal clock to the new environment) requires one day for every time zone crossed.

Of course, this does not mean you have to sit idly by waiting to feel better!

Travelers should beware of products that claim to ease or prevent jet lag. There is currently no effective treatment on the market.

What about melatonin?

Some natural food stores sell melatonin, a hormone naturally produced by the body. Secreted by the pineal gland, melatonin transmits messages to the brain about the hours of daylight and darkness, helping to regulate the body's circadian clock (natural biological rhythms, including sleep).

In the mid-1990s, melatonin was all the rage. Popular magazines devoted full-length articles to this miracle hormone that could, it was claimed, buttress the immune system, fight the effects of free radicals, prevent a number of diseases, and combat aging and the accompanying decrease in sexual activity. Today, the tone is more moderate, although many researchers still believe that melatonin possesses a number of therapeutic properties, even as a treatment for cancer.

Some believe that melatonin helps the body's clock resynchronize itself, enabling travelers to get over jet lag more quickly. Although there is some scientific proof to back up these claims, there is still not enough evidence to be sure. Moreover, since melatonin is not a regulated substance, it is impossible for consumers to know exactly what the pills contain. Melatonin that is marketed as "natural" is in fact extracted from animal pineal glands and many consider the use of this product to be quite controversial, particularly with respect to the risk of contamination it may present ("mad cow" disease, for example). For the moment, melatonin is generally not recommended.

Joint Pain (Polyarthralgia)

Joint pain is without a doubt one of the most widespread health problems. As we age, we all run the risk of developing chronic pain in the shoulders, elbows, wrists, hands, hips, knees, and feet. The back is also vulnerable, since the spinal column is made up of vertebrae held together by small joints.

This problem most commonly results from the various forms of arthritic disease, which cause mechanical problems or inflammation that irritates the nerve endings in the joints. Unfortunately, arthritis cannot be prevented.

Joint pain is easily confused with other types of problems. Rheumatic pain affects the soft tissue near the joints (muscles, tendons, ligaments) and can be very similar to pain in the joint itself. Tendinitis and bursitis are common causes, as is fibromyalgia, a form of generalized rheumatism (*see inset box for more details*). Many people with osteoporosis also experience joint pain, either as a side effect to their medication or because they also have arthritis. Furthermore, certain lipid-controlling drugs can cause muscle pain that resembles joint pain.

Sufferers can have pain in one or more joints at the same time. Over a few months, the pain may gradually spread to the entire joint system. Joint pain usually manifests in the following:

► Pain of varying intensity, appearing suddenly or gradually, with no apparent cause.
► Short-term (lasting a few days/weeks) or persistent (several weeks/months) pain.
► Joint stiffness after a period of inactivity, particularly in the morning.
► Lack of flexibility.
► Loss of mobility (difficulty moving and using limbs).
► Pain in the joints with movement.
► When caused by inflammatory ailments, sufferers experience swelling, redness and a sensation of heat in the joints, along with general fatigue and prolonged periods of stiffness (one hour or more).

WHAT ARE THE CAUSES?

Non-inflammatory arthritis

► *Osteoarthritis,* also known as degenerative arthritis, is the most common form of arthritic disease. Normally, joint cartilage acts as a shock absorber between the bones, allowing them to slide against one another. When a patient is afflicted with osteoarthritis, this cartilage gradually and inevitably disintegrates, causing the bones to grate against each other, leading to pain and reduced mobility. In advanced stages, growths or bumps appear on the bones particularly at the tips of the fingers. Osteoarthritis can affect all joints in the body, but those that support body weight (hips and knees), the spinal column, and the small joints in the fingers are most vulnerable. It is a chronic disease, usually beginning around age 40. It is a common affliction brought about by aging; 85% of people over the age of 70 are affected. Some patients develop the disease in their twenties because of a familial and genetic predisposition. Although it is considered non-inflammatory arthritis, sufferers generally do experience mild inflammation, although it never develops into another form of inflammatory arthritis.

Inflammatory arthritis (the most common forms are listed below)

► *Rheumatoid arthritis* is the most common form of inflammatory arthritis, affecting one in a hundred Canadians (particularly women) between the ages of 30 and 50. This disorder, which causes the synovial membrane around the joint to become inflamed, results from an immune system malfunction and can affect several joints simultaneously (particularly the hands and feet). This disease is chronic (causing persistent pain) and characterized by swelling, long periods of morning stiffness and fatigue.

► *Gout* is a type of recurrent inflammatory arthritis caused by high levels of uric acid leading to the formation of crystals in the joint tissues. Attacks of gout are very painful and followed by periods of remission. During an attack, the area around the joint swells and the skin becomes shiny, red or purplish in colour, and sensitive to the touch. Each attack lasts about three or four days. This is the only form of arthritis that can be controlled by changing diet.

▶ *Pseudogout* is a form of acute arthritis that closely resembles gout but has a different cause: while gout attacks are caused by uric acid deposits, pseudogout results from calcium pyrophosphate crystals forming in the joint tissue. The knee is particularly vulnerable to this form of arthritis, although on rare occasions, several joints are affected at the same time (frequently leading to diagnostic confusion between pseudogout and rheumatoid arthritis). Like gout, pseudogout manifests as recurrent attacks lasting three to four days. The condition affects primarily women between the ages of 50 and 60.

▶ *Psoriatic arthritis.* Some people are born with a genetic disposition to develop two chronic inflammatory diseases, psoriasis and arthritis, at the same time (5% to 10% of psoriasis sufferers). In 70% of cases, the psoriasis appears slightly before the arthritis. Generally, only a few joints are affected, possibly including the spinal column.

▶ *Ankylosing spondylitis* is another form of chronic inflammatory arthritis caused by a malfunctioning immune system. It affects both men and women between the ages of 20 and 30, although the symptoms are more pronounced in men. It causes prolonged periods of stiffness in the spinal column and may also affect the hips, knees, and shoulders. In advanced stages, the disease causes intense pain and severe loss of spinal mobility, making it very difficult for the person to move around.

Yes, you're right! Joints do react to the temperature!

Many people claim their joints hurt more when it rains, snows or the weather is humid. Some even swear they can predict the weather by how their joints feel. Well, they are probably right! It seems that the weather, or more specifically changes in barometric pressure, do have an influence on arthritic pain, although the precise mechanism is not yet understood.

► *Polymyalgia rheumatica* is an inflammatory arthritic disease caused by a malfunction of the immune system. The condition appears suddenly in elderly people, causing pain in the shoulders and hips. It is one of the only forms of inflammatory arthritis with a quick reaction time to treatment; it generally lasts less than a year.

► *Systemic lupus erythematosus.* This chronic and inflammatory arthritic disease is caused by a malfunctioning immune system and is most common in young women. It is accompanied by fatigue, rash (commonly butterfly-shaped red blotches on the cheeks) and may cause pain in a number of joints.

Other causes

► *Viral infections.* Influenza (the flu) and the parvovirus (responsible for "fifth disease" or erythema infectiosum in children) can cause temporary joint pain and in the latter case, swelling.

► *Bacterial infections.* A bacterial arthritic disease usually affects only one joint and causes intense pain accompanied by swelling, fever, and shivering. The most common type of infection is staphylococcus, a type of bacteria found on the skin surface that can cause pain if it enters the blood stream through a cut or lesion. Streptococcal pharyngitis (strep throat) is one of the few bacterial infections that affects more than one joint simultaneously.

► *Cancer* can result in joint pain without swelling, due to a general deregulation of the immune system. This is a fairly rare occurrence, though possible in all types of cancer.

PRACTICAL ADVICE

Osteoarthritis

Don't be too fatalistic. Remember that it is generally possible to ease the pain caused by osteoarthritis and live a normal life. Even the most serious cases can be controlled with medication.

Deal with the pain. When you feel pain, avoid using the joint unnecessarily and apply a heat compress to stimulate blood circulation, encouraging the muscles and tendons to more effectively support the affected joints. Place a hot water bottle, a re-usable hot compress, or a heating pad on the sore area for 10 to 15 minutes, three or four times a day.

Take acetaminophen or anti-inflammatories. To ease the pain, take one or two tablets of acetaminophen (235 mg to 500 mg) every six hours, never exceeding 4 grams daily. In people over age 65, the maximum daily dose is 3 grams, since acetaminophen can be toxic to the liver. Anti-inflammatories can also help soothe the pain, although be sure not to exceed the manufacturer's recommended dosage, since osteoarthritis

---

Fibromyalgia—a controversial syndrome

The scientific community is divided when it comes to fibromyalgia. While some researchers believe it is a problem with the locomotive apparatus, others think infections may be responsible. Some even suspect it of being a physical manifestation of an emotional disorder, such as depression, stress, or professional burnout. While there are doubts about the cause, however, no one refutes the fact that patients are indeed suffering.

The term fibromyalgia is fairly new, although the syndrome itself has been recognized for years by other names, including soft tissue rheumatism, fibrositis, and nonarticular rheumatism. Studies show that it affects three out of a hundred Canadians and is much more prevalent in women (representing 90% of cases).

Fibromyalgia is characterized by generalized muscle pain with focal points on both sides of the body. Other symptoms include limb stiffness, insomnia or non-restful sleep, headache, intense fatigue, intestinal problems, lapses in memory and concentration, stress, and anxiety.

There is still no cure for fibromyalgia. A specially-adapted aerobic exercise programme may provide partial relief and drugs such as amitriptyline or cyclobenzaprine can be used to control the symptoms, although success rates are fairly low. In some cases, a multidisciplinary approach involving a doctor, physiotherapist, psychologist, and even social worker is the best means of treatment.

causes only minimal inflammation and extra amounts of this type of medication will not help. Take acetaminophen or anti-inflammatories as preventive measures when you know you will be using a sensitive joint (before running your errands or playing golf, for example).

Use rub-on analgesic creams. To ease the pain, apply methyl salicylate-based creams (such as Rub A535) or creams with a capsaicin (red pepper extract) base, on sale over the counter in pharmacies. To prevent morning stiffness, apply the cream on sore areas at bedtime. This treatment can be effective for mild forms of osteoarthritis.

What about glucosamine? Glucosamine sulphate is an increasingly popular dietary supplement that many believe can prevent joint erosion and soothe joint pain. However, rigorous scientific studies have not been able to prove this claim. Furthermore, because there is no governmental regulation of so-called "natural" products, the concentration of glucosamine in the supplements can vary from bottle to bottle. Should you take it? If non-prescription acetaminophen and anti-inflammatories provide no relief, try glucosamine for a few months and stop if the pain dissipates (apparently its effects last for a while). Buy the brand with the highest concentration. But be careful: people over the age of 65 should avoid this substance, as they can be more sensitive to the potassium and magnesium it contains. Glucosamine is also contra-indicated for diabetics, as it can increase blood sugar levels. It should also be noted that this product is not beneficial in cases of inflammatory arthritis.

Exercise. Specific exercises to reinforce your muscles will protect your joints, while range of movement exercises help prevent ankylosis. Ask your doctor for information, or consult an occupational therapist or physiotherapist. Remember that while physical activity can be generally beneficial, not all forms will help your joints. For example, biking will not make your knee feel better, and might even aggravate the condition.

Do aquatic exercises. All the specialists agree: activities performed in water take the pressure off the joints and can greatly help relieve arthritic pain. Find an aquatic activity you like (swimming, water aerobics) and do it regularly, once or twice a week, in a heated pool.

Maintain a healthy weight. Keep off excess weight so as not to over-load your hip and knee joints.

Get a massage. The pain of osteoarthritis increases muscle tension. Massage helps you relax and provides temporary pain relief by free-ing up endorphins, a natural analgesic produced by the body.

Inflammatory arthritis
Get some rest. If you are in pain, the wisest thing to do is to avoid or at least limit movement of the joint. Because arthritic diseases are usually accompanied by general fatigue, it is important to take good care of yourself. Do not try to do too much as this will only aggra-vate your symptoms and make you more tired.

Apply hot or cold compresses. If you have recently developed intense pain concentrated in the joint area that is accompanied by swelling, apply a bag of ice to the joint for ten minutes, a few times each day. Consult a doctor. If you know you have a chronic arthritic disease, on the other hand, apply heat (inflammatory mechanisms vary according to whether the disease is acute or chronic). Use a hot water bottle, heating pad, or re-usable hot compress.

Take anti-inflammatories. Acetaminophen can provide only minor relief for inflammatory arthritic pain. Anti-inflammatories (such as ibuprofen) are a better bet. Follow the manufacturer's recommendations. Be careful: people with digestive tract ulcers or kidney disease should avoid anti-inflammatories, as they can aggravate their disease. Elderly people should also be careful, as they can increase (or even trigger) high blood pressure.

Changing your diet will not help. Eating less acidic food and using dietary supplements (such as amino acids or vitamin A or E) will not change a thing. Just be sure to keep eating well and maintain a healthy weight. Gout is the only form of inflammatory arthritis that can be improved by diet. Sufferers of the latter should avoid seafood, game and cold cuts, which encourage uric acid build-up in the blood. It is important to note that pseudogout cannot be controlled by diet.

Stay active. Keep moving even though you have arthritis, being sure to respect your own limits. Go about your daily activities and do mild exercises that avoid putting pressure on the sore joint as much as possible. Ask your doctor for advice about which activities suit you best, or see an occupational therapist or physiotherapist.

Stay in contact with people. Some people with inflammatory arthritis withdraw from social contact, letting the disease negatively affect their quality of life. This is a mistake. Keep going out and doing your favourite things. See your friends and talk about your pain with those closest to you. If the disease is in an advanced stage, an occupational therapist can give you advice about adapting your environment to your physical capacities (moving doorknobs, using special utensils and tools, getting dressed, etc.)

WHEN TO CONSULT?

► There is pain, swelling and redness around the joint, accompanied by fever or shivering. This is a medical emergency.
► There is swelling, pain, possible redness and a sensation of heat. Consult a doctor as soon as you can.
► You have an attack of gout that lasts more than five days.
► Pain cannot be controlled by non-prescription medication and regularly disrupts your sleep and daily activities.

WHAT HAPPENS DURING THE EXAM?

The doctor will take a complete history and proceed with a physical examination of the locomotive apparatus (joints, bones and muscles). A complete exam (of the abdomen, lungs and the cardiovascular system) is particularly necessary in cases of inflammatory arthritis to understand how far the condition has spread and whether there is an underlying disease. The doctor may also request blood tests, X-rays, and a bone scan. It may also be necessary to aspirate some synovial liquid from the joints to determine whether there is a bacterial infection and if so, which antibiotic to prescribe.

WHAT IS THE TREATMENT?

Osteoarthritis

This is an incurable, chronic disease. Treatment is aimed at easing the pain and improving joint function.

An exercise programme adapted to the patient's needs will strengthen the muscles and tendons for better support of the affected joints.

Painkillers (such as acetaminophen) or non-steroidal anti-inflammatories (such as ibuprofen) are also generally prescribed. A new family of anti-inflammatories known as anti-COX-2 can also provide relief. The latter may be better tolerated by the digestive system and reduce the risk of side effects such as stomach and intestinal ulcers. It should be kept in mind, however, that they may also aggravate high blood pressure or kidney disease. If the disease affects only a few joints, the doctor may perform an infiltration, injecting cortisone-derived substances into the joints. New, hyaluronic acid-based injectable products may be used for mild cases of osteoarthritis of the knee. As a last resort, the doctor may recommend hip or knee replacement surgery.

A topical anti-inflammatory known as Pennsaid has recently been approved in Canada for osteoarthritis of the knee. It is very important to follow the doctor's or pharmacist's instructions, as overuse can lead to side effects similar to those of other anti-inflammatories. Patients must also be sure to wash their hands after each application.

Orthotics (orthopaedic soles, braces, or canes, for example) can also be helpful.

Inflammatory arthritis

For all forms

All forms of inflammatory arthritis can be treated with the same types of anti-inflammatories used for osteoarthritis. Patients with inflammatory arthritis simply have to take larger doses.

In most cases of chronic arthritis (rheumatoid arthritis, for example), the doctor will also prescribe a slow-acting anti-rheumatic agent (such as Plaquenil or Methotrexate). This modifies the immune system's response, slowing down and sometimes even halting the progression of the disease. This is a long-term prescription.

New treatments (such as Remicade and Enbrel) have also recently become available. Known as biologic agents, they are laboratory-synthesized products that mimic substances produced by the immune system, thereby creating a more focused immune response. Since these drugs have only been developed recently, however, and have not been used extensively because of their high cost, long-term side effects are not well understood.

Gout and pseudogout

Acute gout attacks may be relieved with non-steroidal anti-inflammatories and colchicine. As a preventive measure, the doctor may also prescribe an agent to inhibit the synthesis of uric acid that leads to the formation of crystals. Regular follow up is necessary to verify uric acid levels and prevent the recurrence of attacks. Pseudogout is treated with anti-inflammatories and cholchicine.

Polymyalgia rheumatica

This is one of the only forms of arthritis that can be cured. Treatment involves low doses of cortisone taken orally.

Infection

Joint pain due to infection disappears with treatment of the underlying ailment.

In all cases of joint pain, rest and healthy moderate habits will help patients control the disease.

Locked Knee

Moving from place to place, everyday chores, sports, recreational activities—all these daily activities put the knee under constant pressure. Of all the joints in the human body, it is the most vulnerable to mechanical problems affecting locomotion.

The most frequent problem is locked knee, which prevents sufferers from fully extending their legs and causes pain with attempts to do so. The intensity of the pain will vary according to the origin of the problem and there may be swelling. The sufferer might also have trouble walking.

A locked knee can manifest in two ways:

Acute form (due to trauma or a false move)

- Mechanical lock, characterized by swelling, pain and inability to fully extend the leg.
- Torn ligament, characterized by intense pain, inability to fully extend the leg and, in some cases, swelling. The body's reflexes lock the knee to prevent painful movement.
- Antalgic lock, characterized by decreased mobility of the knee due to intense pain, sometimes accompanied by swelling. The body's reflexes lock the knee to prevent movements that cause pain.

Chronic form

- Progressive loss of capacity for movement (arthritis)

WHAT ARE THE CAUSES?

Acute form
Mechanical lock

- ***Detached cartilage.*** A piece of cartilage can detach and block the free movement of the knee joint.
- ***Torn meniscus.*** A tear in the meniscus (the cartilage protecting certain joints, including the knee) prevents the free movement of the knee joint.

Torn ligament

► **Torn ligament.** The internal lateral ligament or cruciate anterior ligament can tear at the point it attaches to the knee, preventing extension.

Antalgic lock

► **Sprain or serious injury** causes swelling or pain, preventing full extension.

► **Mechanical lock, torn ligament or capsule.** An antalgic locked knee may also be related to these problems.

Chronic form

► **Degenerative problems** causing the disintegration of the joints or bones, such as arthritis, aging, or badly treated sports injuries.

PRACTICAL ADVICE

Acute form

See a doctor immediately. An acute locked knee requires medical attention.

Do not wear a splint. To immobilize the knee, put your leg up on a chair.

Avoid putting weight on an injured leg. Use crutches to move around.

Combat inflammation. To prevent inflammation during the first three days, apply ice or cold water compresses for fifteen minutes at a time, four to six times a day. Note that the cold also has an analgesic effect, freezing the nerve endings. After three days, apply heat to encourage blood circulation, which will also help fight inflammation. Take hot baths, and use compresses or heating pads (be very careful not to fall asleep while using a heating pad, as it can burn the knee).

Take a painkiller. Ease the pain with one or two acetaminophen tablets (325 mg to 500 mg), four times a day, not exceeding 4 grams daily. Anti-inflammatories are also helpful. Follow the manufacturer's dosage recommendations. Take both medications at once if the pain is difficult to control.

Respect your limits. Forcing your knee to straighten can damage the cartilage.

Chronic form
Do more gentle sports. Avoid sports (such as running) that cause repeated microtraumas. Go biking or swimming instead.

Do not gain weight. Try to maintain a healthy body weight to avoid putting any excess pressure on your knees.

Take hot baths. Heat helps you relax and get rid of muscle stiffness.

Apply a hot compress. Reusable compresses (Magic Bags) are available in drugstores over-the-counter. Heat in a microwave and apply to the painful area.

Take glucosamine with an anti-inflammatory. Available in pill form over-the-counter in drugstores, glucosamine is a natural product used in combination with anti-inflammatories to treat arthritis pain. Take three times a day. Be careful: glucosamine is contra-indicated for diabetics, as it increases blood sugar levels.

Wear shock-absorbing arch supports. Especially if you are young and suffering from arthritis. This will help slow progressive degeneration.

Use an elastic bandage for support and to keep the knee warm. Be careful not to wrap it too tightly and remove it before going to bed. It is also important to take it off when sitting, since a bent leg makes circulation more difficult and may cause phlebitis or other complications.

WHEN TO CONSULT?

► A locked knee always requires medical attention. In acute cases, consult a doctor as quickly as possible.

WHAT HAPPENS DURING THE EXAM?

Acute form

The doctor will ask questions about how the injury happened, what position the patient was in when it occurred, what side of the knee took the impact, and when the swelling appeared (immediately after the injury or two or three days later). He or she will perform a physical examination to determine the state of the ligaments and whether there is inflammation. X-rays may be necessary to ensure the meniscus has not been damaged.

Chronic form

The doctor will take a medical history, with a particular focus on previous injuries (how they were treated, how the problem developed, which treatments were successful, etc.). He or she will palpate the knee to determine the location of the pain and look for any leg deformities (such as bow legs). X-rays are usually required.

WHAT IS THE TREATMENT?

A locked knee will generally heal with traditional standard treatment (anti-inflammatories, crutches, physiotherapy), although special measures are required if it is caused by a problem with the anterior cruciate ligament (at the front of the knee), which is responsible for the knee's pivot movement. This is the ligament commonly injured in skating, hockey and ski accidents. Surgery is often necessary in these cases.

Acute form

Mechanical lock

Minor arthroscopic surgery is required, involving an internal examination of the joint and the removal of the meniscus or the piece of cartilage blocking movement.

Torn ligament

The patient may undergo either standard treatment or surgery, depending on his or her needs. If the patient is seriously involved in athletic activities and wishes to resume them, surgery is necessary. Everyday activities can be resumed without surgical treatment.

Antalgic lock

The doctor will attempt to fix the problem causing the locked knee.

Chronic form

To slow the progress of the disease, the patient may be required to adapt his or her diet to reach an ideal weight. It may also be necessary to modify the patient's athletic regimen and reduce activities that cause repeated trauma.

The physician will prescribe analgesics, anti-inflammatories, and physiotherapy to help control the pain.

The doctor may also recommend orthotics to secure the knee in its axis and avoid deterioration. In certain cases, a lubricant (Synvisc) may be injected into the joint to improve the quality of the joint fluid and increase shock absorption. Advanced cases of arthritis may require surgery.

Loss of Balance

For humans, balance is defined as stability while standing and depends on two opposing forces: body weight (which pulls us towards the ground) and muscle contractions (which keep the body vertical). Loss of balance describes difficulty remaining in a standing position.

The balancing mechanism is a remarkable data processing system. When a person gets up, messages are sent from the soles of the feet, muscles, joints, head, neck, inner ear (controlling balance), eyes, cerebellum (controlling and refining movement), and the deep structures of the brain (where information is transferred). Once the data is recorded, the cerebral cortex commands the muscles to hold the body upright.

A problem with any one of these body parts can lead to loss of balance, which in itself is not a disease, but a symptom.

Loss of balance may be accompanied by:

► Vertigo.
► Dizziness.
► Loss of hearing.
► Tinnitus (noise in the ear).
► Visual instability (static objects seem to move around).
► Nausea.
► Falling.
► Other symptoms, according to the cause of the problem.

WHAT ARE THE CAUSES?

► *Vision problems.* Good balance requires adequate vision. Any loss of vision—for example, due to cataracts, glaucoma, or, in some cases, dim lighting—can disturb balance. Strabismus, thyroid problems, or trauma (blow to the head, accident) can weaken the eye muscles, leading to double vision or involuntary shaking of the eyes (nystagmus) causing visual instability.

► *Inner ear disorders.* A number of problems can affect the inner ear and the balancing mechanism: benign positional vertigo (caused either by changing your position rapidly or holding the same one for a prolonged period), labyrinthitis (inflammation of the inner ear), Ménière's disease (inner ear congestion and water retention), skull trauma (disturbing the inner ear and fracturing the petrous part of the temporal bone), acoustic neuroma (benign tumour affecting the auditory nerves), or a thrombosis of the auditory arteries.

► *Postural problems* can disturb the centre of gravity (normally located in the pelvis) and cause loss of balance. Postural problems can be caused by:

▷ Motor disorders: hemiplegia (paralysis of half of the body), hemiparesis (weakness in half of the body), and Parkinson's disease.

▷ Osteoarticular (bone and joint) problems: femur fracture, osteoarthritis of the knees, osteoporosis.

▷ Muscular problems: myopathy (general term to describe muscle diseases like muscular dystrophy and Duchenne's disease, for example).

▷ Nerve disorders: sensitive polyneuritis (infection, inflammation, or vitamin deficiency affecting the nerves).

Vertigo or Dizziness?

Although frequently confused, vertigo and dizziness are distinct phenomena.

Vertigo is characterized by the sensation of movement, giving the sufferer the feeling that the room is spinning, or that he or she is being spun around, pitched back and forth, or rocked side to side, as during an amusement ride. The length of time vertigo lasts varies considerably.

Dizziness gives the sufferer the impression that his or her head is "floating". Images and ideas are blurry, the floor may feel unstable, and the sufferer may fear falling. This sensation is usually brief.

► *Damage to the brain or cerebellum.* The following diseases affect posture and balance: multiple sclerosis, cardiovascular accident (cortex or cerebral infarction), hydrocephaly, infections (such as encephalitis or meningitis), tumours, and trauma.

► *Metabolic and vascular disorders.* Cholesterol, diabetes, and high blood pressure encourage atheriosclerosis, which can block the blood vessels and impede the flow of oxygen to the brain.

► *Anxiety.* Extreme anxiety can inhibit the nervous system, triggering nausea, dizziness, and loss of balance (among other symptoms). This can occur when a person suffers a sudden shock or is going through a particularly trying time.

► *Drug toxicity and certain medications.* Medications (certain antidepressants, anxiolytics, or antibiotics), alcohol, and illicit drugs dull the brain.

► *Aging.* In the elderly, the reasons for loss of balance are often unclear. Loss of vision and polyneuritis (aggravated by medication), are possible causes.

PRACTICAL ADVICE

Don't worry. Loss of balance can be normal. If you lose your balance when you get up to go to the bathroom in the middle of the night, there is no cause for concern. Your brain is probably still half asleep and unable to properly decode the messages it is receiving, or your eyes have not fully adjusted to the dark.

Go for a check-up. Adult women and men over the age of 50 should have a complete check-up once a year. Men between the ages of 14 and 50 should have a check up every five years.

Adopt a healthy lifestyle. The way you live affects your health. A healthy and varied diet, regular physical exercise, and a good balance between your work and personal life will help you maintain physical and mental health. Also be sure to listen to your body and respect your own limits, particularly as your body goes through normal biological changes as it ages (remember, aging is not a disease). Develop some hobbies.

Avoid anxiety. Try to be more philosophical about the big issues, such as birth, health, disease, and death. Exaggerating your fear can cause psychological problems that may lead to dizziness and loss of balance. In other words, mental balance is essential to physical balance.

Adapt your environment. If you frequently lose your balance, take a few precautions at home to avoid falling: install handrails in hallways and stairwells, and non-slip mats on slippery floors and in bathtubs. Putting a nightlight in the bedroom and the hallway is also recommended.

Avoid stimulants. Caffeine, sugar, and alcohol can cause balance problems if consumed in excess. After the initial boosting effects subside, energy to the brain drops off quickly, possibly causing dizziness and loss of balance.

Control your medication intake. Many people tend to over-consume certain types of medication (particularly tranquilizers), impeding the reactions of the brain.

WHEN TO CONSULT?
► You have lost your balance (even if this has occurred only once).

WHAT HAPPENS DURING THE EXAM?
The doctor takes a history and performs a complete physical examination. Diagnostic tests and treatments are adapted to the individual patient.

WHAT IS THE TREATMENT?
Vision problems
Cataracts require a surgical procedure known as phacoemulsification, which involves making an incision in the eye, breaking the defective crystalline lens into small pieces, suctioning out these pieces, and replacing the cataract with an artificial crystalline lens. This day-surgery procedure has a short recovery period after which the patient can resume regular activities.

Acute glaucoma is treated with laser surgery, while chronic glaucoma is controlled with hypotensives or beta-blockers in eye drop form.

Vision loss in dim lighting is usually caused by vitamin deficiency. This is easily treated with diet modification and vitamin supplements.

Strabismus is controlled with special lenses.

Thyroid problems are treated with specific medications.

Inner ear problems

Benign positional vertigo requires no medical treatment, although the doctor may prescribe anti-nausea medication, if necessary.

Labyrinthitis usually resolves on its own and requires no medication or treatment beyond acetaminophen and rest. Products such as Serc, Antivert and Gravol may ease the symptoms. Certain cases require ear-reconditioning exercises, which are simple to perform at home.

For Ménière's disease, the doctor prescribes specific medication, explaining its mechanism of action and side effects. This disease requires regular medical follow-ups.

In cases of acoustic neuroma, the removal of the benign tumour leads to complete recovery.

Postural problems

In cases of hemiplegia and hemiparesis, a physiotherapist will help the patient recover lost capacity, while occupational therapy will teach him or her how to function within new limitations (find another way to get out of bed, for example). If the underlying problem is vascular (blood clot), medication is also prescribed to prevent the formation of new clots. If a hemorrhage is responsible, physiotherapy is indicated.

Parkinson's disease is chronic and can be controlled with antiparkinsonian drugs.

A fractured femur requires surgery and physiotherapy.

Osteoarthritis in the knee is treated with analgesics and anti-inflammatories, or by injecting substances that facilitate the sliding of the joints (to avoid friction and premature erosion).

In cases of osteoporosis, the doctor prescribes medication to help the bones absorb calcium and stimulate bone tissue regeneration.

The underlying cause for myopathic problems must be treated. In most cases, physiotherapy is used to rebuild muscle mass.

If the patient is suffering from sensitive polyneuritis, the underlying condition must be treated. The patient's recovery depends upon the degree of nerve damage.

Damage to the brain or cerebellum
Multiple sclerosis is a chronic and degenerative disease that can be controlled with various medications.

Cerebrovascular accidents require hospitalization.

Infections such as encephalitis or meningitis usually respond well to antibiotics.

In cases of tumour or skull trauma, the appropriate treatment is immediately undertaken.

Metabolic and vascular disorders
The patient must control his or her cholesterol levels, diabetes, or hypertension to stimulate blood circulation and help correct balance problems.

Anxiety
If necessary, anxiolytics or antidepressants are prescribed.

Drug toxicity and certain medication
If medication is causing the loss of balance, the prescription may be modified. If the patient has a drug or alcohol problem, the doctor may recommend a detoxification program.

Loss of the Sense of Taste or Smell

The senses of taste and smell are intimately linked. Taste buds perceive sweet, salty and acidic flavours, while the sense of smell determines the nature of the substance. For example, the tongue detects sugar, but the nose identifies the food as chocolate or caramel.

In 85% of cases, total loss of the sense of smell (anosmia) is accompanied by a loss of the sense of taste, although it is possible for patients to lose only their sense of smell. Sufferers might also perceive a real or hallucinatory bad odour (objective or subjective cacosmia), or nonexistent odours (phantosmia). It is also possible to lose only one's sense of taste, or for this sense to become altered (metallic or unpleasant).

Problems with taste and smell have a negative effect on both quality of life and safety. Not only are sufferers unable to enjoy food and cooking, they cannot recognize the smell of burning, gas, or spoiled food. It may also result in a decreased libido and, in some cases, depression.

WHAT ARE THE CAUSES?

Anosmia (total loss of the sense of smell) and hyposmia (diminished sense of smell)

- ► *Infections* such as colds, flu, or sinusitis, are the most common cause.
- ► *Inflammation of the nasal passages* such as a respiratory allergy, acute or chronic rhinitis, or naso-sinus polyposis (formation of polyps or tissue masses in the nasal passages).
- ► *Head trauma* may shear the olfactory nerve linking the nose to the brain.
- ► *Brain surgery.*
- ► *Certain medications,* including codeine, morphine, tetracycline, methotrexate, clofibrate, and others. Certain medical treatments such as cervical spine radiation therapy, chemotherapy, and hemodialysis may also have this effect.

► *Neurological disorders,* including Alzheimer's disease, tumours in the olfactory passages and centres, multiple sclerosis, Parkinson's disease, and amyotrophic lateral sclerosis.

► *Diabetes and pregnancy.* Diabetes can damage the olfactory nerves. Pregnancy can cause nasal congestion, temporarily impeding the sense of smell, but things should return to normal when the pregnancy ends.

► *Inhalation of toxic substances* such as tobacco, natural gas, cement dust, tar, gasoline, lead, zinc, sulfur dioxide, and chromium. *Aging,* particularly after the age of 80.

Objective cacosmia (perception of an existing unpleasant odour)

► *Foreign object in the nasal passages.*

► *Bacterial infection.*

► *Necrotic nasal tumours* (benign or malignant) cause a lack of oxygen, possibly leading to a secondary infection, destroying the tissues.

► *Chronic atrophy of the nasal mucous membranes* (ozena) is accompanied by brown, crusty scabs lining the nasal passages.

Subjective cacosmia (hallucinatory perception of unpleasant odour) and phantosmia (hallucinatory perception of any type of odour)

► *Mental disturbance* such as hysteria, psychosis, schizophrenia, hypochondria, and anxiety.

► *Brain injury or tumour.*

► *Epilepsy.*

Loss or alteration of sense of taste only

► *Dental problems,* such as cavities, gingivitis, or periodontitis, as well as dentures, fillings, and bad dental hygiene.

► *Infections or diseases,* such as otitis media, diabetes, fungal infection of the taste buds, respiratory tract infections, anemia, and tumours on the nerves controlling the sense of taste.

► *Certain medications and medical treatments,* such as antibiotics, radiation therapy, and chemotherapy.

► *Smoking and alcohol* can damage the taste buds.

PRACTICAL ADVICE

Be patient. If you have a cold, flu, or sinusitis, things should return to normal within ten days.

Treat nasal congestion. Fast-acting oral decongestants can help clear your sinuses. Nasal spray saline solutions are also effective, but should be avoided if you have high blood pressure as it can aggravate the condition. While a dry environment dehydrates nasal secretions, humidity levels between 40% and 50% can help ease nasal congestion. Be careful the air is not too humid, however, as this will encourage the proliferation of dust mites. Hot showers also help decongest the sinuses.

Do not use nasal spray decongestants for more than five days in a row. Regular use of decongestants creates a dependency, causing the nose to block after a few hours or even minutes (rebound congestion). Because of their side effects, decongestants are also contra-indicated for people with high blood pressure, diabetes, or heart disease.

Treat respiratory allergies. Liquid or pill-form antihistamines reduce inflammation of the nasal passages.

Wear a mask. Working with chemical products can damage the olfactory nerves. Wear a mask to protect yourself.

Install smoke detectors. Smoke detectors become even more crucial to your safety if you cannot rely on your sense of smell. Install one or a number in your home (particularly in the kitchen, hallway, and basement) and be sure to check the batteries regularly.

Pay special attention to your personal hygiene. If your sense of smell is unreliable, be extra-careful with your personal hygiene to avoid embarrassment. It is also a good idea to visit your dentist to ensure proper oral hygiene.

Ask for help. Losing your sense of smell or taste affects the details of your daily life. Ask your partner or a friend to tell you if you are wearing too much perfume, add spices to cooking, or check the freshness of food (also be sure to check the expiry date).

Add extra spices to your own meals. If food has lost its flavour, try adding pepper, herbs, spices, condiments or lemon juice (do so cautiously, if you suffer from high blood pressure).

Do not smoke. Tobacco can cause irreversible damage to the nerves responsible for taste and smell.

WHEN TO CONSULT?

► Nasal congestion lasts for more than ten days.
► Your nose is not congested, but your sense of smell has diminished.
► You frequently or continuously perceive unpleasant odours.
► You are experiencing olfactory hallucinations (i.e., smell things that are not there).
► Food has lost all its flavour.

WHAT HAPPENS DURING THE EXAM?

The doctor will try to determine the degree to which the patient has lost his or her sense of smell or taste and identify the cause. He or she will examine the nasal passages for mechanical or physiological problems, as well as the mouth and throat to verify the state of the tonsils (in some cases, food debris can accumulate in the grooves of the tonsils, resulting in a bad taste in the mouth). A neurological exam is undertaken to rule out any damage to the cranial nerves. The doctor will also check for digestive problems (regurgitation leaves a bad taste in the mouth).

Allergy and blood tests as well as a sinus CT scan are standard diagnostic tests. An olfactometry test (to determine whether the patient can detect certain odours) may be necessary for a precise diagnosis.

WHAT IS THE TREATMENT?

Anosmia and hyposmia

Infections or inflammations are treated with antibiotics or cortisone drugs (often in nasal spray) and generally heal quickly.

If patients suffering from naso-sinusal polyposis receive oral cortisone treatment, they should recover their sense of smell within 72 hours. If this is not successful, surgical removal of the polyps (with or without cortisone therapy) may be effective. It should be noted that naso-sinusal polyposis is a chronic disorder that requires regular follow up to control any recurrences.

The cranial nerves controlling the sense of smell do not regenerate. If the patient has not, therefore, regained his or her sense of smell within six months of a head trauma or neurosurgery, full recovery is unlikely.

If the condition is caused by medication or medical treatment, the sense of taste or smell is generally regained after the treatment comes to an end.

In cases of diabetes or neurological disease, the loss is usually severe and permanent.

The degree of damage caused by inhaling toxic substances determines whether recovery is possible; in severe cases, it is not. Industrial environments where dangerous products are used (natural gas, for example) must have special equipment to detect toxic fumes and protect workers who have lost their sense of smell.

If hyposmia is not caused by an underlying medical condition, recovery may occur after one or two years. Cortisone may improve the condition somewhat.

Objective cacosmia

In most cases, bacterial infections respond well to antibiotics.

Surgery is recommended to remove necrotic nasal tumours.

In cases of chronic atrophy of the nasal mucous membrane, hormone-based ointments can control the formation of purulent scabs.

Subjective cacosmia and phantosmia

Medication can control the symptoms of epilepsy.

In cases of brain damage or tumour, the appropriate treatment is undertaken. The degree of recovery depends on the severity of the loss.

Loss of the sense of taste

Treatment of the underlying dental problem, infection, or disease, proper management of the patient's diabetes, or the end of cancer treatments or drug therapy will usually allow patients to recover their sense of taste. If caused by smoking or excessive alcohol consumption, the degree of recovery depends on how severely the taste buds are damaged.

Low Blood Pressure (Hypotension)

Low blood pressure, or hypotension, occurs when the circulating blood volume in the body is below normal, causing an inadequate blood supply to the brain. Blood pressure depends on three factors: the heart's pumping ability; circulating blood volume throughout the tubes, or vessels; and the quality of the vessels. Blood pressure (BP) is expressed as a fraction, with a reading of 120/80 designating what is normal. A reading of 140/90 indicates slightly elevated pressure; if it drops to below 100, regardless of the denominator (i.e., lower number) low blood pressure is indicated.

Hypotension is under-diagnosed for several reasons. Most often, for example, it is measured while the patient is sitting whereas hypotension usually becomes apparent while standing. There are also psychological factors. Some people experience "white coat syndrome", a fear of going to the doctor that causes blood pressure to rise during an examination. Moreover, the symptoms of hypotension may mimic those of chronic fatigue, anxiety or hypoglycemia. Hypotension manifests in the following symptoms:

► Nausea and vomiting.
► Vertigo.
► Sweating.
► Vision disturbance.
► Headache.
► Drowsiness.
► Anxiety and confusion.
► Fainting (in extreme cases).
► Rapid heart rate (also known as tachycardia), caused by the adrenal glands working harder to raise blood pressure and maintain adequate blood flow to the organs.

WHAT ARE THE CAUSES?

▶ **Blood loss** as a result of acute or chronic bleeding. This is the most common cause of hypotension and the reason people with anemia often faint.

▶ **Dehydration** from vomiting, diarrhea, excessive heat or rigorous exercise with inadequate hydration (typical of marathon events).

▶ **Varicose veins** (generally found in the lower body) are another relatively common cause, as they reduce blood volume. Because the walls of the vessels are distended (stretched or enlarged) and of poor quality, varicose veins accumulate blood that would normally circulate (up to one litre after only half an hour of standing).

▶ **Drugs,** notably those that cause a drop in blood pressure to manage hypertension (high blood pressure) such as diuretics and vasodilators.

▶ **Aging.** When the vessels become hard and stiff, as they often do in the elderly, the stomach requires a large amount of blood for digestion, resulting in a reduction of circulating blood volume and lower blood pressure after meals.

▶ **Likely hereditary factors.**

▶ **Long-standing diabetes** damages the nerves that control blood vessel tonicity, disturbing blood circulation throughout the body.

▶ **Certain diseases of the nervous system,** such as Parkinson's disease and Guillain-Barré syndrome.

PRACTICAL ADVICE

Consume salt. While salt is not good for persons with hypertension, a sufficient amount is essential for hypotensive individuals, as it retains water in the arteries, helping increase blood pressure. Drinking mineral water is beneficial, especially if it has a high sodium content.

Drink lots of fluids. They increase blood volume.

Avoid alcohol. Alcohol dilates the blood vessels, reducing blood pressure. Alcohol is also a diuretic, causing the body to produce more urine than the amount of liquid consumed. Loss of fluid aggravates hypotension.

Do not get up suddenly. If you are hypotensive, getting up suddenly can cause an extreme drop in blood pressure (known as orthostatic hypotension) that may make you fall and lose consciousness.

Stretch before getting up. When you get up in the morning, for example, sit on the edge of the bed for a few seconds before standing. Stretching and contracting the muscles will raise your pressure and adapting the body to the upright position gradually will prevent dizziness.

Wear support hose for varicose veins. Remember to slip them on when you know you will be standing for prolonged periods of time.

Take a nap after eating if you are over 60. Since digestion consumes a tremendous amount of energy in terms of blood flow, physical activity after meals can impede sufficient blood flow to the brain and cause hypotension.

Wriggle your toes and contract your calf muscles. This will help if you have to remain standing in one place for a certain length of time.

Take preventive measures. If you are prone to low blood pressure, even without being sick, make sure to replenish fluids and consume enough salt in hot weather, especially when exercising. Although

Women and Hypotension

While statistics on hypotension are not available, one in 20 people are believed to suffer from it, and particularly women: for every 60 women, only 2 men have low blood pressure. Menstrual blood loss appears to be a risk factor. It should also be pointed out that low blood pressure is normal in children, because their arteries are smaller, the tissues of their veins are more flexible, and their blood vessels are not obstructed.

regular physical activity is generally recommended (especially in cases of hypertension), there is no evidence that it is particularly beneficial for hypotension.

Know what to do during a fainting spell. Most people react by raising the victim's head, but this is a serious mistake. In fact, it is the feet that should be raised so the blood can flow back to the brain. If the person does not regain consciousness immediately, hypotension is not the problem and you should call an ambulance.

WHEN TO CONSULT?

► You feel dizzy or weak when upright, or experience these symptoms when standing up after lying down or sitting.
► You experience dizziness or weakness after a meal.
► You lose consciousness after remaining upright or stationary for a certain length of time.

WHAT HAPPENS DURING THE EXAM?

The doctor will take a blood pressure reading while the patient is standing. He or she will then select one of the many exams available to make a diagnosis. The patient may be outfitted with a monitoring device (to be worn for several days) in order to measure blood pressure 24 hours a day. The doctor will check the heart's pumping ability, the blood volume, and blood level of certain hormones. He or she may then perform the tilt-table test, which involves securing the patient to the table, then tilting it upright so the head is up and the feet are down. People with hypotension will faint after 5 minutes.

WHAT IS THE TREATMENT?

Unlike hypertension, hypotension does not shorten life expectancy. It can, however, affect quality of life considerably. If necessary, the doctor can prescribe drugs that increase blood volume (by maintaining salt levels), contract the vessels, or prevent them from dilating. Complex cases will require several drugs.

Lump in the Groin Area

A lump in the groin may be caused by any number of problems, most of which are entirely benign. There is usually no cause for concern.

A lump in the groin presents in the following manner:
- One or two lumps in the groin area.
- May be painful.
- Lumps may be either soft or hard.
- Lumps may be the size of a chestnut, egg, lemon, or even larger.
- May be accompanied by fever and redness in the area.

WHAT ARE THE CAUSES?
- ***Hernia.*** A hernia occurs when an organ (or part of one) protrudes from the abdominal cavity. Two types of hernias can cause lumps in the groin area: inguinal (the most common) and crural (or femoral). In both cases, the lump varies in size, can be either hard or soft, and may or may not be painful. In adults, groin hernias occur during extreme physical exertion and are caused by a weakness in the abdominal wall. Prostate hypertrophy, which requires men to force urination, also increases the risk of the peritoneum (membrane lining the abdominal cavity) protruding into the inguinal canal (the area just above the groin). In male infants, inguinal hernias are relatively common, occurring when the inguinal canal fails to close after one or both testicles descend into the scrotum just before birth.
- ***Inflammation of the lymph nodes.*** The body's defense system is regulated by the lymph nodes in the neck, armpits and groin. One or all of the nodes can swell as they fight an infection, causing pain and in some cases, fever and redness. Pain can radiate as far down as the thigh or leg, if a swollen node in the groin presses on a nerve. Sexually transmitted infections, wounds, viruses, and certain bacteria can also trigger swelling.
- ***Cancer.*** In very rare cases, lymph nodes swell as they try to fight off the cancer. In lymphatic cancer, the lumps in the groin are highly perceptible. Cancer of the prostate, liver, colon, rectum,

or anus may metastasize to the groin, creating hard, irregular (ill-defined) lumps, sometimes grouped together and rarely painful.

PRACTICAL ADVICE

Consult a doctor. Even if the lump is very small or painless.

Is it a hernia? You can perform a very simple test to determine whether you have an inguinal or femoral hernia by lying on your back. If the lump withdraws into the groin, you have a hernia; if it is painful and does not recede, you may have an irreducible hernia.

Stay in shape. Good muscle tone solidifies the tissues of the body and protects against hernias. Exercise regularly. If you have a sedentary lifestyle, start slowly and build up your exercise routine gradually. Avoid high-impact sports at the beginning, as excessive exertion can cause a hernia.

Watch out for animals' claws. A virus can enter your system through a dog or cat scratch. Even if the scratch is disinfected, the lymphatic system will react, possibly causing the lymph nodes in the groin to swell. File down the claws on your dog. Have your pets vaccinated regularly.

Practice safe sex. This will prevent contracting a sexually transmitted infection that might cause a lymph node reaction in the groin.

WHEN TO CONSULT?

► You have a lump in the groin.
► The lump is painful. Consult immediately.

WHAT HAPPENS DURING THE EXAM?

The doctor performs a physical exam to diagnose a hernia. If necessary, he or she will order blood tests or a biopsy to assess the cells in the lump and narrow down the cause of the swelling. An abdominal and groin ultrasound or tomodensitometry scan are useful tools for precise diagnosis.

WHAT IS THE TREATMENT?

Hernia

Inguinal, femoral, and strangulated hernias are corrected through surgery to replace the organ in its cavity and repair the abdominal wall. The patient must take analgesics, rest for a few days after the operation, and avoid excessive physical effort and high-impact sports for the next two or three months.

In the case of infant hernia, surgery is required to move the testicle to the scrotum. If the testicle remains in the inguinal canal for a long period of time (a condition known as cryptorchidism), there is a risk of infertility. If it is moved down before the age of five, there will be no negative effects. An undescended testicle in a pre-adolescent child must be removed to eliminate the risk of cancer, but this does not generally affect fertility, as one functioning testicle is usually enough.

Inflammation of the lymph nodes

The lymph node infection is treated with antibiotics.

Cancer

The appropriate treatment is undertaken without delay.

Memory Loss

It is completely normal to suffer the occasional memory lapse. If you sometimes forget where you put your keys, when that meeting is, or what you had to pick up at the store, there is no cause for concern. Little slips like these tend to occur when we are preoccupied and become more common with age.

After the age of 65, the brain loses its ability to store new information. This is why the elderly may forget the names of people they have just met, while still being able to perfectly recollect events of long ago.

Even though some types of memory loss are normal, others are not and can seriously impede the daily life of the sufferer. In most cases, language, basic skills, and functional skills (capacity for organization, planning, and self-correction), are also affected. For example:

- Sufferers cannot remember appropriate vocabulary and shorten or simplify their sentences.
- They may forget simple skills like how to use the microwave or remote control.
- They may forget the order of ingredients in a favourite recipe.
- They may not be able to draw up a grocery list.
- They are often unaware of these impairments.

Individuals whose functional capacity is only moderately disturbed are said to be suffering from mild cognitive impairment or isolated memory loss. The term "dementia" is reserved for more serious cases (where the sufferer forgets how to get dressed or wash, for example).

WHAT ARE THE CAUSES?

Mild cognitive impairment (isolated memory loss)

- *Medications.* Certain sleeping pills or tranquilizers have a dulling effect on the brain, which can disrupt proper transmission and reception of information.

► *Nervous breakdown or mental anguish* can disturb normal daily functions. Being preoccupied or unmotivated impedes our ability to retain information.

► *Hypothyroidism.* The inadequate production of hormones by the thyroid gland can slow down intellectual function and cause memory lapses. Other symptoms include lack of appetite, chronic fatigue, muscle weakness, constipation, sensitivity to the cold, dry, rough skin, hoarseness, and brittle hair.

► *Brain damage.* Cerebrovascular accidents and brain tumours can damage the neurons responsible for intellectual function.

Dementia

► *Alzheimer's disease.* Of unknown origin, this degenerative disease primarily affects the elderly (5% of those over the age of 65; 25% of those over 85), causing dementia and personality changes. There seems to be a hereditary factor, as the risk of developing Alzheimer's is four times higher for those with an immediate family member (parent, brother, sister) suffering from the disease.

► *Multiple infarct dementia (cerebral arteriosclerosis)* is a degenerative disease characterized by tiny hemorrhages or blood clots causing brain damage. This type of dementia is most common in elderly people suffering from high blood pressure, diabetes, or heart disease. Symptoms may also include speech difficulties or loss of sensitivity in an arm or leg, depending on the location of the lesion.

PRACTICAL ADVICE

Develop habits to help you remember. If you frequently forget things, teach yourself a few tricks: always put your keys in the same place, write down things you don't want to forget, look for landmarks (to help find your car, for example), and remind yourself out loud ("I will remember to turn out the lights when I leave the house.").

Learn to relax. Stress and daily worries can take up too much room in your brain and make you forget things. Set aside some time for relaxation every day.

Exercise your brain. Recent discoveries have proven that remaining intellectually active throughout your lifetime will help protect you from Alzheimer's disease. Read a lot, do crossword puzzles, play scrabble—keep your brain in shape!

Exercise your body. Certain studies have shown that physical exercise is also good for memory. Choose an activity (bicycling, swimming, walking, etc.) and do it for at least 20 minutes three times a week.

Prevention is better than a cure. Early detection and treatment of high blood pressure or diabetes is an important step in the prevention of multiple infarct dementia (cerebral arteriosclerosis).

Get regular check-ups. People suffering from mild cognitive impairment (isolated memory loss) are at risk of developing Alzheimer's disease. To be safe, get a medical check-up.

Take note of an elderly person's behaviour. When elderly people begin to lose their memory, they are usually unaware of the problem. Take them to see a doctor and accompany them when they go out or take part in various activities.

Be legally prepared. Everyone should take legal steps to protect themselves and their loved ones in case of future incapacity. Prepare a living will and set up a power of attorney, appointing another person to make medical decisions on your behalf and manage your property and finances if you become unable to do so yourself. Various forms are available. Speak to a lawyer.

Contact the Public Trustee. If a loved one has Alzheimer's disease or another form of dementia, legal steps must be taken to manage his or her property and finances. If a document exists appointing someone with power of attorney, it may need to be validated. If the sufferer has not made any legal provisions, the Public Trustee (a government agency responsible for managing the affairs of those who are unable to do so themselves) will administer the sufferer's property.

Ask for help. Contact a branch of the Alzheimer's Society of Canada in your area. They can provide advice and support.

WHEN TO CONSULT?

- ► Memory loss is disturbing your daily activities.
- ► Other intellectual capacities are also affected (language, basic skills, etc.).
- ► Isolated memory lapses are happening with increasing frequency.

WHAT HAPPENS DURING THE EXAM?

The doctors' first step is to rule out any curable physical or mental problem that may be impairing the patient's intellectual capacities.

If no such condition is detected, the doctor performs a medical examination and administers specialized tests to determine whether the patient is suffering from a degenerative disease. Blood tests, X-rays, and, in some cases, an in-depth neuropsychological exam are required.

WHAT IS THE TREATMENT?

Mild cognitive impairment (isolated memory loss)

In all cases, regular intellectual and physical exercise can be beneficial.

Medications

The doctor will review the patient's prescriptions, making the modifications necessary to improve the patient's cognitive function.

Nervous breakdown or mental anguish

The doctor may prescribe antidepressants and advise the patient to rest. In most cases, memory and other impaired intellectual skills will be recovered.

Hypothyroidism

Treatment involves thyroid hormone replacement therapy. The level of recovery depends on when the treatment is begun and the degree of damage.

Brain damage

Cerebrovascular accidents and brain tumours require specific treatment. While some patients will continue to suffer memory loss, those with less severe damage may partially or completely recover their capacity for memory through rehabilitation therapy (speech and occupational therapy, for example).

Dementia
Alzheimer's disease

Three medications currently on the market slow down the progression of the disease in its mild or moderate stages. The doctor will prescribe donezepil (Aricept), rivastigmine (Exelon) or glantamine (Reminyl), depending on the patient's response to the drug and tolerance for the side effects. As these are new medications, it is still too early to observe their effectiveness in the long term or advanced cases. Other promising medications are currently in the experimental stage.

Multiple infarct dementia (cerebral arteriosclerosis)

The patient's high blood pressure or diabetes must be treated first, after which the doctor may prescribe medications for Alzheimer's disease that have also shown some success as treatment for multiple infarct dementia.

Mild Depression

Occasional feelings of sadness or mild depression is a part of life. Everyone has felt this way at one time or other; it is a universal human response to failure, disappointment, and other situations of adversity.

While major depression lasts for an extended period, the symptoms of mild depression are temporary and most sufferers regain their sense of optimism fairly quickly. Symptoms of mild depression may last several hours, days or weeks and include: loss of interest in work or daily tasks, insomnia, loss of appetite, inability to concentrate, and irritability. People with mild depression can still enjoy certain pleasurable activities, unlike those suffering from a major depressive disorder.

WHAT ARE THE CAUSES?

- *A sad or traumatizing event,* such as separation, bereavement, job loss, or even something as apparently minor as an argument.
- *A difficult financial situation* (job loss, increased cost of living, etc.) contributes to a general feeling of gloom.
- *Pessimism in the face of adversity.* Pessimists frequently suffer recurrent bouts of mild depression because of their bleak perspective on the world. They are often convinced they have been singled out to suffer all manner of troubles and tend to find the negative in any given situation.

PRACTICAL ADVICE

Try to see events as opportunities for growth. Using our troubles as opportunities for learning and personal growth can help us emerge from our ordeals with an even greater sense of equilibrium than before. Failure and mistakes can teach us how to avoid the same problems in the future.

Re-evaluate pessimistic attitudes. Be realistic, but try not to see only the negative in every situation. Do not use your limitations as an excuse for your problems. Remember your good points: your successes, good deeds, strengths, and positive qualities. Do not feel responsible for things you cannot control.

Talk. Keeping everything inside is the worst thing you can do. Long term isolation can only make you sink deeper into despondency. Talk to reliable confidants. Simply sharing your emotions and feeling like someone is listening to you will probably make you feel better.

Plan pleasurable activities. Enjoyable activities help remind us that pleasure is available if we make even a small effort to find it.

Avoid isolation. Difficult events in your life will have less of an impact if you maintain contact with your friends and family. Tell them what you need and how you would like them to help you.

Avoid people or situations that make you feel bad. People who cause you anxiety and make you feel powerless and dependent should be avoided at all cost.

Deal with money and stress. If your emotional state is due to finances, the first thing to do is contact your creditors and explain your temporary problems. They will help you find solutions. If you have just lost your job, look at it as an opportunity to find a better position. You have professional qualities no one else has; you just have to find a way to present and draw them out.

Do exercise. Physical activity is one of the best ways to deal with mild depression. Walk, cycle, go rollerblading, play golf—any of these activities will give you the physical and mental energy to see things from a better perspective.

Go to bed early. If you feel depressed or pessimistic, you might be suffering from a lack of sleep. Give up late-night television and go to bed. You will wake up fresher and more dynamic in the morning. If you have nightmares or wake up frequently during the night, talk to a doctor.

Beware of stimulants. Limit your consumption of coffee and sweets. Too much of these stimulants can lead to irritability and aggravate your depression.

Use your sense of humour. The ability to laugh and enjoy ourselves gives us the energy we need to face life and get through tough times.

It's healthy to mourn. Our overwhelming feelings of sadness after the death of a loved one can help us accept our new reality. Take the time to cry and really experience the pain caused by your bereavement. If you are having trouble believing that your loved one is really gone, or if you find it impossible to think of anything else, you are perfectly normal and these feelings will dissipate in time. How much time this takes is unique to each person.

WHEN TO CONSULT?
- Your feelings of depression last for more than a few weeks.
- You have trouble sleeping.
- You have suicidal thoughts.

WHAT HAPPENS DURING THE EXAM?
The doctor will interview the patient and perform a physical examination. If you are suffering from major depression, he or she will prescribe the appropriate treatment.

WHAT IS THE TREATMENT?
Doctors do not prescribe medication for mild depression. For serious sleeping problems, short-term help is available in the form of benzodiazepines. However, these tranquilizers are addictive if taken over a long period of time and can hide symptoms. Doctors therefore encourage natural sleep aids: exercise, refraining from eating before bedtime, taking hot baths, reading, and establishing a regular bedtime.

Muscle Cramps and Spasms

The pain of muscle cramps and spasms is caused by involuntary contractions of the fibres, that impede blood circulation in the muscle.

Muscle cramps and muscle spasms are defined differently:

Cramp
► Short, involuntary, painful contraction.

Spasm
► Prolonged cramp. As they contract, the fibres expel blood, leading to a lack of oxygen, irritation and pain in the muscles that intensifies the contractions and stiffens the muscles even more.

WHAT ARE THE CAUSES?
► *Muscle fatigue due to prolonged inactivity* (more than a few days).
► *Reckless workouts.* Cramps and spasms can result if the patient neglects to warm up before exercising, or pushes his or her muscles too hard. During exertion, muscles produce waste products (particularly lactic acid), which cramps and spasms trap in the muscles, causing irritation and pain.
► *Bad posture.*
► *Viral infections.* A virus causes an immune system response in the body that sometimes includes muscle cramps, as in the case of the flu.
► *Trauma.* Pain can result from any number of injuries, including wounds, contusions, muscle tears and sprains. The type of discomfort varies according to the source, from sensitivity, to shooting pain, to burning sensations and cramps. In a lumbar sprain, for example, the pain is caused by the reflexive contraction of muscle fibres (in a cramp or spasm), which protects the lesion by stopping the muscle from extending.
► *Dehydration.* If not replaced, excessive loss of liquid (caused by sweating due to physical exertion, unusual weather conditions, or severe diarrhea or vomiting) will lead to decreased blood circula-

tion. This prevents the muscles from purging their waste products, causing painful irritation. Dehydration also causes depletion of the mineral salts (particularly calcium, sodium and potassium) necessary for muscle function.

► *Pregnancy.* Pregnancy significantly increases the body's calcium requirements. Insufficient calcium can cause muscle cramps, particularly during the third trimester, when the weight of the foetus compresses the nerves in the lower limbs.

How to get rid of a cramp

► Massage the cramped area, gently extending the muscle with one hand, while alternately tightening and releasing your grip on the same muscle with the other. This will stimulate a fresh supply of blood, and should ease the cramp in a few seconds.

► If this does not work and the cramp is developing into a spasm, rub an ice cube over the muscle for three to five minutes. Avoid burning the skin by not rubbing too quickly.

► For a cramp in the calf, point your toes upward, hold your calf in one hand, and gently tighten your grip for 15 seconds. Let go and repeat if necessary. You can also place your feet flat on the floor, about 60 cm from a wall. Press your hands against the wall and lean in, maintaining the stretch for at least 30 seconds. Bring your weight back, resting it all on one leg, and shake the other foot for 15 seconds. Repeat on the other side.

► For a cramp in the thigh, bring your heel up to your buttocks.

► For a cramp in your back, lie on the floor and slowly bring your knees up to your chin. Stay in this position for one minute then let go, resting your legs on a chair, with your knees bent at a 90-degree angle.

► For a cramp in the neck, rub the area with an ice cube and slowly twist your neck from side to side (as though you were shaking your head to say "no").

► *Electrolyte imbalance* (lack or excess of mineral salts such as sodium, potassium, calcium, phosphorus, and magnesium) is rare and often linked to a tumour in the parathyroid or adrenal gland. The condition disturbs muscle function and causes pain because electrolytes are responsible for transmitting the contract-relax message to the muscle fibres.

► *Ossifying myositis.* This condition involves the progressive hardening of muscle fibre. Bony nodules reduce elasticity and impede the muscles' response to the contract-relax message.

► *Tetanus.* This infection has become increasingly rare since the vaccine and booster shots were developed. Tetanus invades the body through an open wound, causing violent and generalized muscle contractions. It can also cause contraction of the respiratory muscles and is fatal in 80% of cases.

PRACTICAL ADVICE

Follow these golden rules:

► Do not remain inactive or immobile for long periods of time.

► Avoid vigorous physical activity less than 2 hours before bedtime. If the muscles are fatigued, any normal movements you make during the night can cause pain, sending a signal to the spinal column. It may then be translated into muscle spasms, which disrupt sleep.

► Avoid sudden movements.

► Avoid walking if you have suffered an injury to a lower limb, particularly if you have not yet seen the doctor.

► In cases of injury, painkillers can deceive the sufferer into thinking they are capable of more movement than they actually are. Be careful not to aggravate the injury with prematurely vigorous activity.

► Avoid intense or prolonged exercise during hot weather.

► Avoid excess consumption of salt, alcohol and caffeine. The salt in soft drinks, for example, drains water from the muscles, as do coffee and tea.

Take precautions before and after physical exertion. Know your limits. Do warm-up exercises before your workout and cool-down exercises afterwards.

Cold and hot shower. If your muscles have been overworked and you want to eliminate lactic acid build-up, step into a hot shower for 2 minutes, then switch to cold water for 30 seconds. Repeat this five to ten times. If you are sore the next day, take a hot bath with Epsom salts to refresh the body and relax the muscles.

Massage the affected limb. Light manual massage will stimulate circulation and eliminate waste products. Always massage towards the heart.

Use warming or cooling ointments. Never use them in combination with a hot bath or a cold compress, as this can burn the skin.

Maintain good posture. Keep your back straight, your arms to your sides and your legs uncrossed. If you must lift something heavy, be sure to keep your back straight, knees bent and arms close to the body.

Treat cramps and muscle tears. Apply a cold compress, bag of ice, or ice pack to the area for the first 72 hours, then use a heating pad, hot compress, or hot bath to increase blood circulation. When at rest, keep the injured area above heart level with a scarf or elastic bandage sling. Take painkillers. If it is a large muscle tear, consult a doctor to prevent the risk of developing ossifying myositis (*see above in the section on causes*), which occurs if the hematoma calcifies.

If wearing a cast. Lightly massage the area directly around the cast and move the fingers or toes regularly.

Rehydration. Drink bottled water, fruit juice mixed with 50% water, or sports drinks. Take three or four sips at a time. Even if your thirst is quenched, keep drinking until your urine has no colour.

Stay comfortable during pregnancy. Following the *Canada Food Guide* recommendations, consume four to six portions of dairy products a day. If you develop cramps, do the appropriate exercises (*see box*). Stop the compression of your lower limbs by lying on your left side.

Get some rest and take painkillers. If you have a viral infection, rest and take analgesic medications (acetaminophen or anti-inflammatories). Ease the pain with one or two acetaminophen tablets (325 mg to 500 mg) four times a day, not exceeding 4 grams daily. Anti-inflammatories are also effective. Follow the manufacturer's dosage recommendations.

Prevent tetanus. Keep your booster shots up-to-date (once every ten years for adults), and be sure to wash any open sores thoroughly with soap and water.

WHEN TO CONSULT?

- ► You have a muscle spasm in your back or neck, accompanied by numbness, tingling, or weakness in the arm or leg muscles.
- ► You experience repeated cramps or prolonged spasms. They do not disappear when using home remedies.
- ► You notice a change in one of your muscles, in the form of a lump, hernia, or nodule.
- ► Your injury swells rapidly and you can no longer put any weight on your limb.
- ► Your injury is not healing well. There is swelling, redness and the sensation of heat around the injury. You also have a fever.
- ► You are wearing a cast and your cramps last longer than an hour.
- ► You cannot keep anything down and even vomit water, making rehydration impossible.

WHAT HAPPENS DURING THE EXAM?

The doctor performs a clinical examination and takes X-rays to identify the injury. Ossifying myositis is diagnosed with the help of ultrasound, magnetic resonance imaging, or bone scintigraphy. A serious case may be visible by X-ray.

Testing for electrolyte imbalances involves urine and blood tests, as well as X-rays and scanner examinations.

WHAT IS THE TREATMENT?

Pain
Your doctor can prescribe a muscle relaxant or an anti-inflammatory (aspirin, ibuprofen).

Viral infection
The appropriate medication is prescribed.

Dehydration
Cases of severe dehydration that resist home remedies can be treated with an intravenous drip.

Tumours, ossifying myositis and complete muscle tears
Surgery is usually required.

Electrolyte imbalance
Chronic imbalance requires medication and constant medical supervision.

Tetanus
The patient will receive antitetanic serum and be given respiratory assistance in hospital.

Muscle Weakness

Muscle weakness, or the feeling of having no strength, occurs when one or several muscles lose function or the body is exhausted. The sensation may affect a limb, a single muscle, a group of muscles (shoulder, wrist, knee, foot, etc.), or the entire body.

There are three broad categories of muscle weakness: weakness due to fatigue, weakness due to musculoskeletal problems, and weakness due to neuromuscular problems.

When weakness is caused by fatigue, the muscles themselves are not affected. The person is simply too sick or exhausted to function normally.

Weakness due to a musculoskeletal problem is common and almost always accompanied by pain in the affected area.

In these cases, the pain itself is the underlying cause of the weakness. Because the sufferer avoids using the painful limb, the muscles develop ankylosis (become stiff), atrophy (lose mass), and weaken.

Weakness due to neuromuscular problems usually takes the form of paralysis or paresis (partial or mild paralysis). The muscles lose their ability to contract and move. The problem may originate in the brain, nerve roots or nerves, or be caused by diseases and metabolic defects of the muscles.

WHAT ARE THE CAUSES?

Weakness due to fatigue

- ► *Substance abuse or overuse of muscles.* Over-consumption of alcohol or drugs can cause temporary (and generally harmless) muscle weakness. Intense exertion, particularly by those with little physical training, has the same effect.
- ► *General exhaustion.* People suffering from exhaustion very often experience muscle weakness, stress, anxiety and depression, as well as disturbed sleeping patterns, appetite and mood. These symptoms can last anywhere from a few weeks to a few months.
- ► *Diseases.* A very large number of diseases can cause muscle weakness, including the flu, colds, anemia, gastroenteritis, infectious

diseases, metabolic problems (disturbance of the body's biochemical reactions), adrenal gland disorders, hyperthyroidism, diabetes, and organ failure (liver, kidneys, etc.).

► *Malnutrition.* The muscles are energy reservoirs. During prolonged periods of fasting or malnutrition, the available energy (measured in calories) is insufficient to maintain muscle function. Muscles therefore become weak.

Weakness due to musculoskeletal problems

► *Trauma.* Muscle weakness almost always occurs in cases of bone fracture, due to the fracture itself as well as the immobilization of the limb in the cast. Tendinitis, bursitis, sprains and torn ligaments are other causes of weakness.

► *Osteoarthritis,* usually part of the aging process, is the normal but often painful erosion of the joints. Pain in the knee or the hip can cause not only muscle weakness but also limping, slowing of movement, or inability to walk. Lack of physical fitness, excessive effort, and obesity can aggravate the condition. Joint inflammation (arthritis) can occur at any age, and is accompanied by pain, swelling, stiffness and muscle weakness.

Weakness due to neuromuscular problems

► *Pinched nerve or nerve root.* A fracture or a herniated disc, for example, may pinch a nerve root in the spinal cord, leading to paresis of a limb. This problem is usually reversible.

► *Spinal cord injury.* Paralysis or severe paresis can occur if the spinal cord is injured (in a motorcycle or car accident, for example), whether or not there is any damage to the spine itself. The degree of paralysis corresponds to the area of injury to the cord (at the level of the neck, upper back, or lower back). Trauma survivors may suffer from quadriplegia (paralysis of all four limbs) or paraplegia (paralysis of both legs).

► *Brain injury.* Accidental brain injury, with or without skull trauma, can cause paralysis or paresis of half the body (one arm and leg) or the entire body. When the spinal cord or brain is injured, the resulting paralysis is associated with spasticity (involuntary muscle contractions).

▶ *Neurological diseases.* Polyneuritis (nerve inflammation) can cause muscle weakness beginning in the legs. Guillain-Barré syndrome is an infectious disease causing full-body paralysis (including the respiratory muscles) in just a few days. Muscular dystrophy is a chronic and progressive hereditary disease leading to eventual irreversible muscle weakness. Multiple sclerosis is a chronic disease that can progress either slowly or quickly, causing paralysis of different parts of the body. Its origin is unknown. Infections or tumours may compromise the spinal column or the brain, leading to paralysis. Cerebrovascular accident (CVA or stroke) is the most frequent cause of paralysis originating in the brain. In these cases, paralysis usually occurs in half the body (one arm and leg).

PRACTICAL ADVICE

Get some rest. If general weakness is caused by exhaustion or the flu, drink plenty of water and rest for 24 to 48 hours.

Avoid using the weakened muscles. If you have bursitis or tendinitis, or if you have over-exerted yourself physically and only one part of the body is weak (the shoulder or the elbow, for example), rest these muscles for 24 to 48 hours.

Ease the pain. Take one or two acetaminophen tablets (325 mg to 500 mg) four times a day, never exceeding four grams a day. Anti-inflammatories may also be helpful; follow the manufacturer's recommended dosage. Take both medications if the pain is difficult to manage. Wrap some ice in a towel and apply to the sore area as often as possible during the first two days.

Gently resume regular activities. If a muscle remains inactive for more than three days, it will become even weaker. After two days of rest, gently move the weakened muscles and resume your regular activities.

Adopt a healthy lifestyle. A healthy and balanced diet and regular physical activity will maintain muscle mass and control your weight.

Choose a sport you enjoy and do it at least two or three times a week. People who are confined to a bed (particularly the elderly) should get up and walk around at least twice a day. Walking outside for one hour every day prevents osteoporosis and preserves muscle tone.

Avoid certain substances. Abstain from toxic substances, like alcohol, nicotine, and other drugs. Above all, never drink and drive.

WHEN TO CONSULT?

- ► You have suffered a serious injury (in an accident, a fall, etc.).
- ► You are unable to move one of your limbs.
- ► Your muscles suddenly feel weak, for no apparent reasons.
- ► Muscle weakness has lasted for more than one week.
- ► Muscle weakness is spreading to other parts of the body.
- ► Muscle weakness is accompanied by pain.

WHAT HAPPENS DURING THE EXAM?

The doctor will interview the patient and perform a complete physical exam. X-rays and blood tests are usually ordered. In some cases, more detailed tests are required, such as lumbar puncture tests, tomodensitometry, magnetic resonance imaging (MRI), or ultrasounds.

WHAT IS THE TREATMENT?

Weakness due to fatigue

Most of the problems will resolve themselves after a few days' rest. In cases of exhaustion, however, the doctor will prescribe a longer period of rest and perhaps some medication (such as antidepressants, if the problem has a psychological origin).

Diseases like anemia, diabetes, metabolic problems, adrenal gland disorders, and hyperthyroidism each require specific medical treatment.

Weakness due to musculoskeletal problems
Trauma

A cast, sling, or bandage may be required to heal the fracture, tendinitis, or bursitis. Physiotherapy may be required.

Osteoarthritis

Physiotherapy is very effective, as it can help the patient learn ways to diminish the pain while maintaining use of the limb.

Weakness due to neuromuscular problems

Pinched nerve or nerve root, spinal cord injury, brain injury, neurological diseases.

In cases of paralysis and paresis caused by neuromuscular conditions, acute care is almost always followed by rehabilitation, to help the patient regain the use of his or her body and maintain autonomy.

Physiotherapy is necessary if the patient must learn how to walk again. Rehabilitation requires the services of a doctor, a physiotherapist, and, in some cases, an occupational therapist, a psychologist and a social worker, all working with the patient and his or her support group. The patient's physical environment and the way he or she moves around are adapted, often using specific equipment (hallway or bathtub handrails, for example).

Nail Abnormalities

While some people pay no attention to their nails, others spend considerable time and money keeping them healthy and attractive. Whatever your attitude, remember that they are a reflection of a person's general state of health and have a primary function of protecting the fingers and toes.

Nail abnormalities can take several forms:

Deformities
- Ridges (parallel straight lines); this is the most common deformity.
- Bumps (in the form of a staircase).
- Pitting.
- Clubbed nails (arced, like the back of a teaspoon).

Thickening and chalkiness of the nails
- The outer layer of the nail thickens while the deeper layers crumble.
- Light yellow discoloration.
- Frequent, insidious problem, primarily affecting the toenails.
- May be painful, particularly when caused by an infection.
- Elderly people are at greater risk.

Brittleness or splitting
- Nails break easily.

Discoloration
- Bluish colour under the nail, with or without pain; this is the most common discoloration.
- Small red spots under the nail, sometimes accompanied by fatigue.
- Unusual paleness under the nail.

Pain
- Pain around the nail (perhaps throbbing, following the heartbeat); if located in the toes, the pain intensifies with walking.

► Often accompanied by redness, the sensation of heat, swelling, and occasionally a discharge of pus.

Nail-biting (onychophagia)
► Compulsive biting of the fingernails

WHAT ARE THE CAUSES?
Deformities
► *Inflammation of nail root* causes ridges or "staircase" bumps. The inflammation may be the result of frequent immersion of the hands in water, chemical exposure (working with detergents and chemical products) or physical trauma (such as an accidental hammer blow to the finger, for a classic example). Some traumas may go unnoticed (such as when the nail area is pinched).
► *Certain generalized illnesses* such as psoriasis cause the formation of small pits on the nail surface.

Treating ingrown nails and whitlow

Before going to the doctor, there are a few things you can do:
► Prepare the following solution: 1 litre lukewarm boiled water, 1 tablespoon non-concentrated laundry bleach, and 1 teaspoon salt. Soak your foot or hand in this solution for 20 minutes, four to six times a day. This will stimulate circulation, soften the nail and clean out the pus and debris. This can heal an ingrown nail in as little as 48 hours.
► With clean scissors, make a small cut in the shape of a V or triangle at the tip and in the middle of the nail. This will release the pressure.
► Apply a clean bandage over the nail. Keep the nail dry; do not apply antibiotic ointment.
► Place a piece of cotton under the end of the nail until it grows over it.

If these steps do not help, consult a doctor.

► *Immune system disorders or chronic respiratory diseases.* Respiratory failure can lead to hypertrophy of the blood vessels in compensation for the lack of oxygen. In rare cases, this causes clubbed nails. In extremely rare cases, clubbed nails are a symptom of lung cancer.

Thickening and chalkiness of the nails

► *Yeast infection or onychomycosis.* Humidity is a triggering factor. Excessive sweating or walking barefoot poolside or in public baths increases the risk of infection.

► *Predisposing illness,* such as diabetes or poor blood circulation.

► *Trauma.*

► *Immune system deficiency.*

Brittleness or splitting

► *Repeated exposure to humidity.*

► *Excessive exposure to heat,* especially in contrast to cold weather. Nails are 75% water, and like skin, react to extreme temperature and humidity changes. Dryness causes the nails to become brittle.

Discoloration

► *Bluish colour under the nail.* A bluish spot is usually the result of a hematoma caused by trauma. If the shock to the finger was slight, there may be no pain. A diffuse bluish colour is sometimes a symptom of respiratory failure. In very rare cases, a dark spot under the nail, unchanging as the nail grows, is a sign of melanoma.

► *Small red spots.* These can be a sign of endocarditis, an infection of the heart valves. They generally appear in people with heart abnormalities or those who have used contaminated syringes.

► *Unusual paleness under the nail.* This usually reflects a generalized illness such as anemia or a disease of the circulatory system, kidneys or liver. It may also be a sign of vitamin C deficiency, although this condition is extremely rare in developed countries.

Pain
- *Infected ingrown toenail.* If the nail is cut too short, has suffered trauma, is irritated by a foreign object (for example, a grain of sand), or is pressed against the skin in narrow shoes, it can become ingrown and infected. In rare cases, no infection develops.
- *Whitlow.* This infection of the soft tissue around the nail may develop if bacteria or tiny foreign objects are let in through skin abrasions. The nail is not ingrown.

Nail-biting (onycophagia)
- *Stress or anxiety.*
- *Habit.*
- *Poor hygiene.* People frequently bite their nails because they don't like their irregular shape, but this merely aggravates the problem.

PRACTICAL ADVICE
Trim your nails to a reasonable length. If you frequently catch your nails on objects, they are too long.

Cut your nails in a straight line across your finger or toe. If they are cut too short or in a semi-circle, they may become ingrown.

How to stop biting your nails

- Look at yourself in the mirror when you bite your nails.
- Keep a diary and try to identify situations in which you are more likely to bite your nails (watching television, during school, etc.).
- File your nails; people are more likely to bite their nails when they are already in bad shape.
- Cover your nails with a bad-tasting product like lemon juice or a special nail polish made for this purpose (check your local pharmacy).
- As a last resort, wear gloves... and get some help from a psychotherapist!

Be gentle. Do not try to correct a nail deformity (bumps, ridges) by yourself.

Avoid biting your nails. Onychophagia can quickly develop into a habit that is hard to break (*see box*).

Use a clean nail clipper. Disinfect it with rubbing alcohol before use. If you suspect a yeast infection, disinfect the clipper before moving on to the next nail.

Dry your hands well. Every time you wash your hands, be sure to dry your nails as well.

Use moisturizing lotion regularly. This will keep your nails soft. Use good quality products, especially on your hands.

Protect your nails. Shield them from excessive cold, heat, humidity, and irritating chemical products. If your hands are frequently immersed in water or you work with chemical products, wear a good pair of gloves.

Wear proper shoes. Choose shoes that "breathe" well (this will help avoid yeast infections), and be sure they are the proper width. Lower your risk of getting yeast infections, athlete's foot or a plantar wart by never wearing other people's shoes.

Never walk barefoot in public places. Wear bath sandals in public showers or around public pools.

Drink plenty of liquids. Like skin, nails need proper hydration.

WHEN TO CONSULT?

► You notice a deformity in one or more nails. There is no apparent cause (no trauma, for instance).
► You notice a deformity developing. You may feel some pain.

▶ The outer layer of the nail is very thick while the deeper layers are crumbly and chalky in texture. The nails are yellowish. You may feel some pain.

▶ Your nails have an unusual colour (bluish, reddish or very pale).

▶ You feel pain (possibly throbbing) around the nail. If it affects your toenail, the pain increases when you walk. It may be accompanied by a heat sensation and swelling.

▶ You bite your nails compulsively.

WHAT HAPPENS DURING THE EXAM?

The doctor will proceed with a visual examination and order additional tests (X-rays or blood tests) if there is reason to suspect respiratory or generalized illness. If the nail presents signs of fungal infection, the doctor will scrape off a sample. The diagnosis will be confirmed by laboratory analysis.

WHAT IS THE TREATMENT?

Deformities

In those rare cases where generalized illness has caused a nail deformity, the disease itself will be treated. There is no treatment for deformities due to trauma; they will disappear as the nail grows out, which may take six to nine months. If there has been serious trauma (for example, a deep cut), the deformity may become permanent.

Thickening and chalkiness of the nails

Infections are persistent and difficult to treat. Topical lotions are not very effective since they cannot reach the root of the nail, where the infection is usually located. In such cases, the doctor will prescribe oral medications (such as ketoconazole or terbinafine) for four to six months. If the nail is extremely misshapen, it may be removed surgically. The nail that grows in to replace it will be healthy.

Brittleness or splitting

This is not a serious condition and there is no particular treatment.

Discoloration

A bluish spot due to trauma will be left to grow out on its own. If there is severe pain, the doctor will perforate the nail to release blood and decrease pressure. This instantly relieves the pain and avoids the risk of nail detachment. Illnesses that lead to nail discolouration are treated.

Pain

If home remedies for ingrown toenails are not effective, the doctor may perform minor surgery to partially or completely remove the nail.

Onychophagia (nail-biting)

If you have made a concerted effort but have been unable to stop, psychotherapy may be recommended.

Nasal Congestion

Nasal congestion is caused by local inflammation or irritation that narrows the nasal passages. It may occur with colds, sinusitis (inflammation of the sinus cavities of the face which serve a humidifying function), allergic rhinitis or a mechanical obstruction of the nasal passages.

The above conditions cause the following symptoms.

Cold: Primary symptoms
- Runny nose due to over-secretion of mucus in the upper airways.
- Sore throat and light cough.

Sinusitis: primary symptoms
- In many cases, fever and a bad cough.
- Children may not develop fever.
- Sensitivity to pressure on the cheeks and forehead.
- Yellow or greenish secretions from the nose or back of the throat.
- Headaches, toothaches, or earaches after the infection has settled in.
- Post-nasal drip in cases of chronic sinusitis.
- Nosebleeds near the end of the sinusitis attack.

Allergic rhinitis: primary symptoms
- Itchy nose and frequent sneezing caused by inflammation of the mucous membranes in the nasal cavity.
- Runny nose.
- Itchy, red eyes.
- Itchy throat caused by post-nasal drip.
- Possible nosebleeds.

Mechanical nasal obstruction: primary symptoms
- Semi-permanent nasal obstruction not caused by a cold or allergy.
- Disturbance of sleep, regular activities, or sports for as long as a few months.
- Possible snoring and throat irritation.

► In children, tendency to breathe through the mouth during sleep; possible nosebleeds.

WHAT ARE THE CAUSES?

Cold
► *Viral infection* (usually rhinovirus) in the nose and throat.

Sinusitis
► *Secondary bacterial infection* (sinusitis complicated by a bacterial infection).
► *Viral infection* due to complications of a cold or flu.
► *Cystic fibrosis.* This hereditary disease causes an over-secretion of mucous resulting in chronic digestive and respiratory problems.
► *Sensitivity to medication* such as aspirin. This is rare.

Allergic rhinitis
► *Allergy* to pollen, animals or dust.
► *Hay fever.* Chronic seasonal rhinitis due to pollen allergies.

Mechanical obstruction
► *Structural problem in the nose,* such as a deviated septum.
► *Adenoid vegetations in the nose* is one of the most frequent causes of nasal obstruction in children.
► *Polyps* (fleshy growths) inside the nose.

PRACTICAL ADVICE

Use a nasal decongestant. Available over-the-counter in drugstores, these medications can temporarily ease moderate congestion by shrinking the nasal mucous membranes, freeing air passage. Be careful: overuse can produce the opposite effect. If used for more than five consecutive days, you may become dependent on the medication and require its decongestive effects continually.

Try traditional home remedies. Breathing in the steam from a hot shower is highly recommended as a way to liquefy and expel mucous. Inhaling the vapors from a raw onion or rubbing the nose with menthol will also temporarily unplug the nasal passages. Certain spicy foods are also recommended, as they trigger a reflex that makes the nose run: mexican food with hot peppers or Tabasco sauce, for example, or spicy Indian dishes with curry, cumin, coriander and ginger. Adding a few cloves of garlic to your salad is also recommended, as well as drinking chicken broth, which may reinforce the body's immune system and dilute mucous in the nose with its hot vapours.

Be sure to get enough sleep. An air humidifier in your bedroom will make it easier to breathe at night. To avoid dispersing mould and bacteria throughout the air, use distilled water and clean the machine once a week. If you do not have access to a humidifier, place a large dish of water on top of a heater. Be sure to change the water frequently. Raise the head of the bed at night to ease nasal pressure and drain mucous.

Allergies and nursing

Nearly six million Canadians suffer from hereditary or environmental allergies. Allergies occur when the immune system mistakenly stimulates the body's defences against harmless substances such as pollen, cat hair, or dust. The substances provoking the reactions are known as allergens.

Family members are likely to suffer from the same allergies. If one parent is allergic to a specific substance, a child has a 30% to 40% chance of developing the same allergy. If both parents suffer from the same allergy, there is a 60% to 70% chance of it being carried on to the child. Cigarette smoke in a baby's environment increases the risk of allergy development. Breastfeeding a baby can delay the development of the allergy or reduce the intensity of reactions. It may even eliminate the risk of developing an allergy altogether.

Take zinc. Zinc is known to be beneficial for nasal function. It was used to treat the loss of smell and is now believed to provide effective protection against sinus congestion. Take 50 mg a day.

Nosebleeds

Allergies, colds, pollution, or exposure to strong chemicals can occasionally provoke light nosebleeds as well as nasal congestion. Nosebleeds may also occur due to fragile blood vessels in the nose. In this case, they are heavier and more frequent.

Preventing nosebleeds
Dry air, frequently caused by continuous heating systems, make nasal mucous membranes more susceptible to bleeding. Use a humidifier, especially during the winter months. If you are particularly prone to nosebleeds, take iron supplements to help compensate for lost blood. Vitamin C and B complex are also recommended, as they are necessary for the creation of collagen, which reinforces nasal mucous membranes. Secaris, a non-prescription ointment available in drugstores, prevents the nasal membranes from drying out and forming scabs, which eventually leads to nosebleeds. Salinex, a saline nasal humidifier can also help control the problem.

Stopping nosebleeds
If you have a nosebleed, sit up straight in a chair. Do not lie down, as this will cause the blood to run down the throat. Blow your nose once to get rid of any blood clots, then pinch the soft part of the nose immediately below the bone (not the tip) for three to five minutes. Breathe through the mouth.

If the cause of the nosebleed is located in the nose itself, a doctor can cauterize (seal by burning) the small surface vessels of the nasal mucous membranes.

Decrease your risk of exposure to allergens at home. There are a number of simple methods to protect yourself from allergens at home. Cover your mattresses with anti-allergenic slipcovers, replace feather pillows with synthetic foam ones, and revert to wood floors if you have carpeting. Dust regularly. Electronic filters on a central heating system help eliminate pollen, dust and animal hair. Ask for information at your doctor's office or medical clinic.

Get rid of dust mites. Parasites living in household dust are responsible for a number of allergies. Use an aerosol acaricide such as Acardust, available in mattress stores and most pharmacies. Spray the product on your mattresses, rugs, and cloth-covered armchairs and sofas to kill the mites. Air out the room for several hours before you allow a child to spend any time in it. Repeat this treatment every three months. Remember that dust mites can also live in stuffed animals and blankets. Put these articles in the freezer for 72 hours every three months to kill the mites as well as their larva and eggs.

Nasal congestion in infants

A newborn with a blocked nose will refuse to eat or sleep, causing many parents to run to the doctor. The baby's reaction is normal, however, because a blocked nose will prevent it from breathing while feeding. Parents can help relieve the congestion by drawing out mucous with a syringe or nasal aspirator. Afterwards, hold the baby in your arms with its head a little lower than its body and carefully administer a drop of saline solution in each nostril with a dropper. Lift the baby to an upright position.

Be careful:
For slightly older children with chronic nasal congestion, consult a doctor if the child is able to breathe only through the mouth. Leaving the mouth open all the time can cause problems in facial development and may result in language development problems in young children.

Improve air quality in the workplace. An air purifier at work may help, especially if your colleagues smoke. If the windows do not open, be sure to go outside and take a few breaths of fresh air during breaks. Find out what the humidity levels are in your building and whether the air conditioner filter is frequently changed.

Watch what you drink. Fermented alcoholic beverages such as beer and wine, among others, contain substances that dilate the blood vessels and cause mild congestion.

WHEN TO CONSULT?

► Your nose is very congested. Your eyes and forehead feel tender. You have a fever and are coughing.
► Yellow or greenish secretions are expelled when you spit or blow your nose.
► Your nose has been blocked for several months.
► Your eyes are itchy, you sneeze repeatedly, your throat is scratchy, and you feel tired.
► You experience heavy nosebleeds that last more than ten minutes, several times a day.
► Your child's nose is consistently blocked.

WHAT HAPPENS DURING THE EXAM?.

A simple medical examination involving a nasal cavity assessment with a rhinoscope is the only requirement for disorders affecting the nose. Rhinoscopes are similar to the instruments used for ear examinations.

If the doctor suspects an allergy, he or she may order skin tests (even for very young children). The doctor will place drops of different allergens on the forearm, scratching or pricking the skin lightly. If swelling occurs, this indicates an allergy. The doctor will determine the seriousness of the allergy by the degree of swelling.

WHAT IS THE TREATMENT?

Cold

In most cases, the only option is to wait until the cold has run its course and the body has successfully fought off the virus. Antibiotics are not effective against the common cold.

Sinusitis

If the condition lasts for a week or more, antibiotics are usually prescribed. If the sinuses are very congested, the doctor may also prescribe a topical corticosteroid nasal spray, which reduces inflammation in the nasal mucous membranes. The effects of this medication are progressive. In the meantime, decongestants can ease your discomfort.

In the rare severe cases where the sinuses become permanently blocked (often due to repeated infections), surgery is required to clean and widen the openings of the cavities. It is performed under general anesthesia.

Allergic rhinitis

The doctor will prescribe antihistamines to counter the effects of the histamine causing the sneezing and runny nose, as well as a corticosteroid nasal spray to treat the allergy itself and reduce inflammation of the mucous membranes. A nasal or oral decongestant can be temporarily added to provide more rapid relief. Investigation also includes skin tests performed by an allergist to determine the offending allergen.

Mechanical block

If the block is due to malformation of the nose itself, surgery is required (for example, in the case of a severely deviated septum). In cases of adenoid vegetations (most common in children), surgery is indicated to remove the fleshy growths blocking air passage. This simple procedure is performed in less than half an hour under general anesthesia.

Nausea

When people say they feel nauseated, queasy or sick to their stomach, they are describing that very unpleasant sensation indicating the urge to vomit. This urge results from a stimulation of the vomiting centre in the medulla oblongata (also known as the after brain or spinal bulb).

Nausea may be accompanied by the following symptoms:
- Increase in saliva.
- Vomiting.
- Headache.
- Abdominal pain.
- Fever.
- Stiffness in the back of the neck.

WHAT ARE THE CAUSES?

- *Digestive problems,* caused by gastro-duodenal ulcer, bile duct (liver) or pancreas problems, gallstones, appendicitis, food poisoning, poorly-managed diabetes, stomach surgery, alcohol abuse or overeating, intestinal obstruction (tumour, abscess, etc.), or irritable bowel syndrome.
- *Neurological phenomena or problems* such as migraines, unpleasant odours, inner ear disorders (for example, labyrinthitis), motion sickness, meningitis, Ménière's disease, or tumours.
- *Medication or chemical agents* such as chemotherapy, morphine, codeine, and drugs for Parkinson's disease.
- *Digitalis poisoning.* Digitalis is a heart tonic.
- *Psychological factors* such as fear, stress, anorexia, or bulimia.
- *Intense pain.*
- *Pregnancy.*

PRACTICAL ADVICE

Wait for it to pass. If your nausea is mild, simply slow down until you feel better. In many cases, nausea disappears once the sufferer vomits.

Do not force yourself to eat. Although eating a little can help ease mild nausea, never force yourself to do so if you do not feel able. You should, however, keep drinking liquids to avoid dehydration.

Relax. If you become nauseated when you feel stressed, try to relax.

Watch what you eat and drink. Whether or not you are vomiting, avoid the following items which are very difficult to digest: milk and dairy products, excessively sweet juice and drinks, red meat, sweets, fried food, and fresh vegetables.

If you are not vomiting, nibble and drink small amounts to steady your stomach (dry biscuits, unbuttered bread, fruit, tea, water, or un-sweetened fruit juice, for example).

If you are vomiting, avoid eating for 12 to 24 hours, but continue taking in fluids, consuming 1.5 litres of lightly salted drinks, such as soup stock or tomato juice. Begin with small amounts and gradually increase every 20 minutes. Avoid sweet drinks, as this will make your nausea worse.

After you stop vomiting, eat food your system can digest easily, such as light soups, bread and peanut butter, pasta, rice, potatoes, and fish. Have several smaller meals a day to avoid overworking the digestive system. Reintroduce your usual diet gradually.

Take medications. Anti-nausea medications such as dimenhydrinate (marketed under the name of Gravol, among other brands) can help ease nausea. Please note that this drug can cause drowsiness and should not be taken if you have to drive a vehicle.

WHEN TO CONSULT?

► Your nausea persists or increases.
► You are unable to stop vomiting.
► You have a stiff neck, abdominal pain, fever, or a headache.
► Your general condition is worsening.

WHAT HAPPENS DURING THE EXAM?

The doctor will take a history and perform a complete physical examination to determine the origin of the problem. He or she will take the patient's blood pressure and perform an abdominal and basic neurological exam. He or she may order blood tests, X-rays or ultrasounds.

WHAT IS THE TREATMENT?

If nausea is caused by an underlying disease, the appropriate treatment will be undertaken.

In some cases, nausea and acute vomiting require hospitalization so the patient can be intravenously rehydrated.

Several medications can be used to treat persistent nausea, including cisapride (Prepulsid) and metoclopramide (Maxeran), which contract the stomach and prevent its contents from coming up. Note that the latter drug is not recommended for elderly people since it may cause confusion. Prochlorperazine (Stemetil) is also an effective anti-nausea drug.

Nausea and Vomiting of Pregnancy

The nausea and vomiting of pregnancy (often called morning sickness) is characterized by loss of appetite and a distaste for food. It typically appears in the fourth week of gestation and gradually diminishes towards the end of the first trimester. This phenomenon affects at least 50% of pregnant women, with approximately 20% experiencing the symptoms beyond the first trimester.

Morning sickness is a very real phenomenon and all mothers-to-be should discuss it with their physician. Studies have revealed that in 83% of cases, the effects are bothersome enough to disturb daily activities, with one third of symptomatic women being compelled to rest.

These symptoms are in no way harmful to the fetus and generally indicate nothing but a normal pregnancy.

In 1% of cases, the vomiting is so unrelenting that it leads to weight loss, dehydration, and electrolyte imbalance. This is known as hyperemesis gravidarum.

The nausea and vomiting of pregnancy can occur at any time (not just in the morning) and may last throughout the day.

WHAT ARE THE CAUSES?

► *A variety of factors.* Although exact causes are not yet known, hormonal changes brought about by the fetus and placenta, digestive problems, and psychological factors (stress and fatigue) may be responsible.

► *Prenatal vitamins* contain high concentrations of iron that may irritate the stomach. They are therefore usually prescribed only after the first trimester.

PRACTICAL ADVICE

Eat small amounts frequently. Forget the rule about three meals a day and eat whenever you feel hungry. Because the production of

gastric juices increases during pregnancy, snack frequently throughout the day to neutralize the acid.

Eat what you want. Do not force yourself to eat something if it makes
you feel sick. The most important thing is to have something in your
stomach, so eat food you enjoy. Once the stomach is partially full, the
queasiness should abate, enabling you to eat some healthier food.

Try "anti-nausea" foods. Certain food items do not produce nausea
in pregnant women (*see list below*). You are sure to find at least a few
that you enjoy. Keep them handy.

- chips
- pickles
- brown rice
- celery sticks
- bread
- cakes
- juice
- crackers
- raw almonds (salted or unsalted)
- pretzels
- lemonade
- mushroom soup
- apples
- pasta
- sweetened cereals
- popsicles
- mashed potatoes

Avoid fatty, fried, or excessively rich food. For example, fried food,
butter, and mayonnaise are difficult to digest. They spend more time
in the stomach and frequently cause nausea.

Do not drink too much with your meals. Mixing liquids and solids stimulates the stomach and amplifies the sensation of being over-full, which
can lead to nausea and vomiting. Limit yourself to one or two glasses of
liquid per meal, but drink as much as you like between meals.

Try liquid nutritional supplements. If solid food nauseates you,
purchase some liquid supplements at the pharmacy.

Drink plenty of liquids. This is particularly important if you are
unable to keep solid food down. Drink water, soup stock, fruit or
vegetable juice, or sports drinks.

Get some rest. Fatigue worsens nausea and vomiting, so be sure to take a break from your activities and rest. You may need to take it easy for a couple of days.

Take vitamin B (pyridoxine) supplements. Taking 25 mg every eight hours may aid digestion. Exceeding the recommended dosage can increase nausea and give you a headache. Supplements are available over the counter at pharmacies. Speak to your doctor if you have any questions.

Take ginger supplements. Powdered ginger root can be found at health food stores and most pharmacies. Take 250 mg, four times a day, to calm the nausea and vomiting. Note that ginger soft drinks and ginger used for cooking do not have the same properties. Be careful: high doses of powdered ginger root can cause neurological damage to the fetus.

Wear an acupressure bracelet. These items stimulate the Neiguan pressure point, also known as the Pericardium-6 (P6), and can be bought without prescription at pharmacies and health food stores. Although their effectiveness has not been scientifically proven, they may help eliminate nausea and pose no danger to the mother or the fetus.

Drink herbal tea. Raspberry leaf, camomile or lemon balm (*Melissa officinalis*) tea can be soothing. These natural products are harmless, although their effectiveness has not been scientifically recognized.

Avoid poorly-ventilated environments. Pregnant women are sensitive to odour. Avoid places inundated with smells from cooking, cigarettes or perfume.

WHEN TO CONSULT?

► The advice listed above is not helpful.
► You are beginning to show signs of dehydration (dry mouth, lips and tongue, infrequent urination).

► You vomit four to six times a day and are losing weight.
► You are vomiting blood or experiencing abdominal pain.

WHAT HAPPENS DURING THE EXAM?

The doctor takes a history and performs a complete physical exam, including a blood analysis, if necessary.

WHAT IS THE TREATMENT?

If the vomiting persists, the doctor will prescribe Diclectin (doxylamine/vitamin B succinate), which several studies have shown to provide effective relief from the nausea and vomiting of pregnancy. This medication poses no risk to the mother or fetus, but should not be taken if the woman has to drive, as it can cause drowsiness. Diclectin is currently the only anti-nausea drug for pregnant women that is approved by Health Canada.

If the woman is suffering from gastroesophageal reflux (heartburn), the doctor may prescribe an antacid adapted for pregnant women.

If prenatal vitamins are responsible, the doctor may change the type of vitamins or halt treatment altogether.

Hospitalization may be required in severe cases. Treatment involves the administration of a rehydrating solution, medications to relieve the nausea, and the gradual re-introduction of solid food. In very rare cases, the woman is fed through a tube inserted directly into her stomach.

Night Sweats
and Cold Sweats

Excessive sweating, in the form of night sweats or cold sweats, is a sign of bodily distress that may indicate an underlying illness, emotional stress, or ill effects from certain lifestyle habits.

People suffering night sweats typically wake up in the middle of the night drenched in sweat from head to toe with their clothes, sheets and even covers saturated. Cold sweats can also occur at night and are accompanied by shivering and clammy cold skin.

WHAT ARE THE CAUSES?

Night Sweats

► *Room temperature too high, nightmares, sleepwalking or sleep apnea.*
► *Cold or fever.* Recurrent night sweats may be a sign that the body is fighting a viral infection, such as a cold, flu or mononucleosis, perhaps accompanied by a fever.

Cold Sweats

► *Estrogen deficiency.* Menopausal women sometimes experience cold sweats as well as hot flashes, especially at night.
► *Fear, anxiety or stress.* The release of adrenaline triggered by a strong emotion or pain can open the sweat glands and cause the blood vessels to contract, giving rise to sweats and a sensation of cold.
► *Hypoglycemia* (drop in blood glucose levels) can bring about cold sweats. This occurs in diabetics, persons who have undergone a gastrectomy (removal of all or part of the stomach), or those prone to hypoglycaemia.
► *Migraine headaches.* Cold sweats sometimes occur with the pain and other symptoms of migraine headaches.
► *Serious illnesses,* such as tuberculosis, AIDS, hepatitis, malaria, hyperthyroidism, leukemia and some lymphomas (e.g., Hodgkin's disease), are often accompanied by recurrent bouts of major sweating.

► *Myocardial infarction.* Cold sweats may be the first sign of a heart attack, although chest pain usually precedes them.

► *Internal bleeding* causes a drop in blood pressure, in turn causing other symptoms, including cold sweats.

► *Heat exhaustion* causes cold sweats and may bring about an increase in body temperature (hyperthermia).

PRACTICAL ADVICE

All types of sweating

Avoid alcoholic beverages, coffee and smoking before bedtime. They accelerate the heart rate and raise blood pressure and body temperature.

Avoid exercising before bedtime. Exercise and taking a sauna or whirlpool before bedtime raises the body temperature.

Avoid eating before bedtime. Take special care to avoid spicy foods and hot drinks.

Drink a lot of water. If you sweat profusely, replenish lost liquid by drinking 12 glasses of water a day—4 glasses more than the recommended average. Drink a glass of water just before bedtime.

Lower the thermostat. A room temperature of between 15 and 18 °C is ideal for sleeping. If necessary, use a fan or air conditioner and sleep with lightweight covers.

Apply powder occasionally before retiring to absorb moisture.

Shower before retiring at night. Take a lukewarm shower or spray yourself with cool rather than cold water. A comfortable temperature is more refreshing.

Take aspirin or acetaminophen if you are flush and have a fever, or are experiencing migraine pain. Take one or two tablets of acetaminophen (325 mg to 500 mg) four times a day, never exceeding 4 grams

440 ◁ **NIGHT SWEATS AND COLD SWEATS**

daily. For aspirin, follow the manufacturer's recommended dosage. Anti-inflammatories such as ibuprofen are not advised, as the problem is not caused by inflammation.

Rest. If you have mononucleosis, the flu or a cold, you need to rest, drink plenty of water, and eat properly.

Keep a journal. Record daytime and night time activities for a period of roughly two weeks to determine whether there is a relationship between specific events and your sweating episodes. This may help your doctor reach a diagnosis.

WHEN TO CONSULT?

► You have cold sweats and feel a general malaise after intense physical activity in warm and humid weather. Seek immediate medical attention.
► You have cold sweats accompanied by chest pain or a drop in blood pressure.
► Excessive sweating persists and your condition deteriorates.
► You suffer anxiety or have an illness that affects your immune system, such as AIDS or a lymphoma.

WHAT HAPPENS DURING THE EXAM?

The doctor will take a thorough history to determine the cause of the profuse sweating. He or she will perform a complete physical examination and order a blood work-up. If an underlying disease such as hyperthyroidism, tuberculosis, heart disease or AIDS is suspected, other laboratory tests will be required.

WHAT IS THE TREATMENT?

For menopausal women, the doctor may recommend hormone replacement therapy to alleviate the symptoms. The effectiveness of this treatment will be re-assessed after four or five years. Other treatments are determined by the cause: antibiotics are prescribed for bacterial infections, tranquilizers or psychotherapy for anxiety, and anti-migraine drugs for migraine-related sweats.

Numbness, Paralysis, and Cerebrovascular Accidents (CVA)

We are all familiar with that unpleasant sensation of numbness or "pins and needles" in a limb. Anything disrupting the transmission of information from the skin to the brain (or vice versa) can lead to numbness or paralysis. Although the phenomenon is usually temporary and has no serious consequences, it should be remembered that numbness can also indicate a serious disease, paralysis, or a cerebrovascular accident (CVA).

WHAT ARE THE CAUSES?

Benign numbness (examples)

- *A blow to the elbow or "funny bone"* can cause the elbow, lower arm, and in some cases, the last two fingers to go numb for a few minutes.
- *Temporary pinching of nerve or artery.* Sitting or lying in the same position or keeping your arms raised for an extended period of time can cause numbness in a limb (giving the impression it has "fallen asleep", or the sensation of "pins and needles").
- *Hyperventilation (rapid breathing).* Intense physical exercise or a panic attack can cause a general sensation of tingling around the lips and in the extremities. Hyperventilation is not dangerous and even those who suffer repeated episodes should not be concerned.

Numbness indicating a serious problem

- *Driving habits.* Resting the elbow on the ledge of the car door with two fingers on the steering wheel can cause persistent numbness of two fingers and eventually paralysis of the hand.
- *Carpal tunnel syndrome.* Repetitive movements of the wrist can pinch and irritate the nerve running through the carpal tunnel, a narrow conduit in the wrist. The hand becomes numb and weak, with the numbness frequently waking the sufferer during the night. People who play musical instruments, do repetitive

manual work, or spend long hours at a computer keyboard often develop this condition. Obesity is also a risk factor.

► *Herniated disc.* The rupture of an intervertebral disc and the resulting compression of nerve roots or the spinal cord causes pain and possibly numbness in the legs or arms, depending on the level at which the spine is affected.

► *Rheumatoid arthritis.* This inflammatory disease attacks the joints, causing deformities.

► *Osteoarthritis of the spine.* The erosion of the vertebrae affects the spinal cord or nerve roots.

► *Brain tumour.* A brain tumour can strike at any age. It may lead to numbness or paralysis in the opposite side of the body, accompanied by language and vision problems.

► *Spinal cord tumour.* This causes numbness or paralysis in the part of the body below the tumour.

► *Trauma.* Brain or spinal cord injuries due to an accident can lead to numbness or paralysis in one or more limbs.

► *Polyneuritis* describes a condition where the nerve endings of the feet or hands suffer toxic damage due to alcoholism or diabetes. It causes pain and numbness that slowly progresses up the limb over a period of months or years.

► *Multiple sclerosis* is the neurological disease most commonly responsible for paralysis in adults under the age of 50. The cause of the disease remains unknown. Occurring primarily in industrialized countries, it affects one person out of 500, mostly young women. Numbing or paralysis may occur in any part of the body, but in most cases the symptoms begin in the feet and spread up towards the abdomen over the space of a few days. The disease is episodic, characterized by periods of attack and remission.

► *Guillain-Barré disease* is characterized by numbness and paralysis that moves up the legs over a period of a few days. This rare disease can develop after an infection.

PRACTICAL ADVICE

Ease the discomfort of "pins and needles". The discomfort usually disappears quickly. Rub the area, and if necessary, take acetaminophen or ibuprofen. Prevent numbness by:

- ► Maintaining good posture.
- ► Taking care of your back and joints.
- ► Never carrying objects that compress the sciatic nerve (such as a wallet in your back pocket).
- ► Taking a break every 30 to 60 minutes if your work requires repetitive wrist movements.

Cerebrovascular accident (CVA)

Cerebrovascular accident (CVA), commonly known as a stroke, is the third cause of death after heart attack and cancer. It strikes quickly, manifesting in the numbing or paralysis of a limb, one side of the body, or the face. It may be accompanied by language or vision problems. The symptoms appear on the side of the body opposite to the brain hemisphere in which the CVA occurred.

CVAs have two causes:

Ischemia: If the blood clot forms in and obstructs an artery in the brain, it is known as a cerebral thrombosis. If the clot forms in another part of the body (usually the heart) and is carried to the brain, it is called a cerebral embolism.

Hemorrhage: This can occur if an artery in the brain bursts and blood leaks into the surrounding area.

In both cases, part of the brain tissue is damaged or destroyed. Prognoses vary, depending on the severity of the CVA: the symptoms may partially or totally disappear, the lesions on the brain may be permanent, or the patient might die. Quick consultation is crucial: new techniques can reverse a stroke with medication that dissolves the blood clot. Recurrent strokes are prevented with surgery, platelet aggregation inhibiting drugs (to thin the blood), or anti-coagulants (to prevent the formation of another clot).

► Eat well and do regular exercise to protect the heart and brain.
► Be on the lookout for high blood pressure, diabetes or high cholesterol. If you have any of these conditions, follow treatment.

Stay slim and don't smoke. Excess cholesterol caused by obesity and the high levels of nicotine caused by smoking shrink the arteries, creating the risk of numbness.

WHEN TO CONSULT?

► Half your body feels numb.
► Numbness in a part of your body lasts 5 to 20 minutes and is not due to bad posture.
► One side of your face or one arm is numb.
► You feel numbness in the feet that is slowly spreading to the abdomen.
► You experience a sudden loss of peripheral vision or vision in one eye and may also be having speech problems.

WHAT HAPPENS DURING THE EXAM?

The doctor performs a physical examination and interviews the patient to determine the causes. Family history and risk factors are particularly important, as is information regarding the length, frequency and circumstances of the symptoms. The doctor tries to determine whether the problem originates in a nerve, the spinal cord, or the brain.

Two tests are used to detect nerve problems:
► An electromyogram, involving small electric shocks to the fingers or toes to assess the patient's reaction.
► In ambiguous cases, the "somesthesic evoked potentials" test is used to measure the duration of nerve impulse transmissions from the extremities to the brain.

Two tests are used to identify problems in the spinal cord or the brain:
► Computerized axial tomodensitometry scan (CAT scan).

► Magnetic resonance imaging (MRI), for an even more thorough examination.

WHAT IS THE TREATMENT?

Carpal tunnel syndrome

The doctor may recommend wearing a splint overnight to keep the hand and wrist aligned. As a last resort, wrist surgery to cut the fibrous mass surrounding the median nerve can relieve pressure on the nerve and blood vessels.

Herniated disc

Treatment begins with rest and physiotherapy. If there is no improvement, surgery may be required.

Rheumatoid arthritis and osteoarthritis of the spine

Pain is treated with anti-inflammatories and locally-administrated cortisone injections. Controlling the inflammation helps avoid deformities.

Spinal cord tumour

If surgery is required, it must be undertaken as soon as possible.

Brain tumour

In 20% of cases, surgery is required, either to perform a biopsy or remove part of the tumour (if this does not present a high risk for the patient). Treatment is completed with radiation therapy and sometimes chemotherapy.

Trauma

If an operation is possible, it should be performed within eight hours of the accident to ensure the highest chance of re-establishing the transmission of nerve impulses and reversing the paralysis.

Polyneuritis

The underlying cause (diabetes or alcoholism) must be treated and controlled.

Multiple sclerosis

There is no specific treatment, although there are new drugs to help control the symptoms and progression of the disease.

Guillain-Barré disease

Patients are hospitalized. The patient may undergo plasmapheresis (filtering the blood to extract the antibodies causing the disease) or receive intravenous immunoglobuline injections.

Oily Skin

There are three types of skin: dry, normal (or combination), and oily. Oily skin is due to the overproduction of sebum by the sebaceous glands.

Oily skin has its advantages: it is less sensitive to irritation and skin diseases such as eczema. Moreover, although the claim has not been proven scientifically, it is generally believed that people with oily skin age better and develop fewer wrinkles than those with other types of skin.

While oily skin is considered to be a risk factor for acne, it is not always associated with the problem.

Oily skin presents the following characteristics:

► Blackheads down the middle of the face (forehead, nose, and chin).
► Thick texture.
► Dilated pores.
► Shiny skin.
► May be accompanied by red pimples (acne).

WHAT ARE THE CAUSES?

► *Heredity.*
► *Hormonal changes.* In adolescence, hormone level variations stimulate the production of sebum. Newborns often have oily skin for the first few months due to the effects of maternal hormones.
► *Rosacea* frequently triggers an overproduction of sebum, particularly on the nose.
► *Endocrine disorders.* A surplus of male hormones can cause oily skin, along with hairiness, a deep voice, and a tendency towards obesity. This can occur in both men and women.
► *Environment.* Hot and humid environments encourage the production of sebum.
► *Neurological disorders.* For unknown reasons, certain neurological disorders such as epilepsy and Parkinson's disease are frequently accompanied by oily skin.

PRACTICAL ADVICE

Clean your skin well. Very warm water effectively dissolves excess sebum. Begin with unscented soaps (such as Dove, Neutrogena or Aveeno) or cleansers that do not contain soap (Spectrojel, Keracnyl, Effaclar, Cleanance, or Cetaphil, for example) to dissolve and remove sebum without irritating the skin. If your skin remains too greasy, try products containing keratolytics like Effaclar K, Cleanance K or Reversa or Neostrata cleansing gel, which will dry the skin a little more. And remember that while soap can remove sebum, it cannot control its production.

Remove blackheads. Keep your skin clean by pinching the area very gently around the blackhead to remove it. Be sure to protect your skin from injury by covering your fingernails with tissue paper. Estheticians also provide this service. Keralytic and sebo-regulators (mentioned above) can also be effective blackhead treatments. Again, however, it is important to note that removing blackheads does not affect the rate of sebum production.

Choose your makeup carefully. Avoid oil-based products, using only water-based and non-comedogenic foundations and blush. Keep your makeup light and wear it as infrequently as possible. Remove your makeup with soap (Dove, Neutrogena, Aveeno), a cleanser (like Spectrojel) or, if your skin is very oily, cleansers containing salicylic acid or benzoyl peroxide.

Use masks. Mud or clay masks dry the skin and remove layers of dead epidermis. This is only a surface cleansing, however, and is not a long-term treatment for the overproduction of sebum or acne.

What about diet? Contrary to popular belief, no scientific studies have established a link between poor dietary habits and oily skin. Soft drinks, fast food, and chips play no role in the type of skin you have. Over-indulgence is never recommended, however.

WHEN TO CONSULT?

► You are self-conscious about your oily skin.
► You are developing acne.

WHAT HAPPENS DURING THE EXAM?

The doctor takes a history and performs a complete examination.

WHAT IS THE TREATMENT?

In cases of very oily skin, tretinoin or adapalene creams reduce the risk of acne and produce results in two to three months. If this treatment is not successful, the doctor may prescribe Accutane.

If the patient has acne, the treatment depends on the number of lesions present. If the lesions are infected, antibiotics (either topical or oral, depending on the severity) and the above-mentioned keratolytics may be prescribed. In very serious cases (where the lesions leave scars), the doctor may prescribe Accutane. This medication has certain side effects and can cause serious fetal deformities if taken by pregnant women.

Painful Legs

Pain in the legs can be nervous, muscular or circulatory in origin and develop suddenly upon exertion (acute pain), or more gradually (chronic pain).

WHAT ARE THE CAUSES?

Acute pain

▶ *Muscle tear or pull.* These types of injuries often occur upon exertion or after a movement that causes bleeding into the muscle tissue. The pain is usually severe at the outset and diminishes over time, although even minor efforts can cause the pain to recur.

▶ *Deep or superficial thrombophlebitis* occurs when a blood clot blocks circulation in the veins. Superficial thrombosis develops most commonly in varicose veins near the skin surface and is generally not dangerous. Deep vein thrombosis, on the other hand, involves a much larger blood clot that can dislodge and make its way to the heart and lungs. A blood clot in the lungs (pulmonary embolism) is often fatal. In these cases, the pain is diffuse and accompanied by a sense of heaviness, swelling and redness in the legs.

▶ *Acute arterial obstruction* occurs when a blood clot usually originating in the heart (due to atrial fibrillation, the most common type of arrhythmia) detaches and is carried through the arteries to the leg, causing pain, decreased sensitivity and mobility, and a sensation of cold.

▶ *Nocturnal leg cramps.* The cause of this painful but otherwise minor problem is unknown.

Chronic pain

▶ *Diabetes or alcoholism.* Both of these disorders can lead to the degeneration of nerves in the legs, resulting in pain or decreased sensitivity.

▶ *Atherosclerosis.* This gradual blockage of the arteries leads to decreased blood flow to the legs, especially during exercise. Pain after walking a certain distance most often appears in the calves, sometimes causing limping (intermittent claudication). Rest will relieve the discomfort.

▶ *Pinched nerve in the lower back.* The pain from a pinched lower back nerve originates in the spinal column and radiates all along the nerve down to one or both legs. Sciatica (pinching of the sciatic nerve) is the most common.

PRACTICAL ADVICE

Do not massage the leg. If the pain is caused by a deep thrombophlebitis, massage can dislodge the blood clot from the vein, possibly leading to pulmonary embolism.

Walk regularly. Regular exercise ensures good blood flow to the legs, thereby decreasing the risk of thrombophlebitis and atherosclerosis. One of the functions of the muscles is to help pump blood to the heart.

Strengthen your abdominal muscles. This protects your lower back and decreases the risk of a pinched nerve.

Use an orthopedic chair. This is another way to protect your back and avoid a pinched nerve.

Lose weight. Excess weight causes joint wear-and-tear, a greater susceptibility to stress fractures and unhealthy blood vessels.

Elevate the legs. People at risk of thrombophlebitis should raise their legs a few centimetres at night to increase blood flow to the heart.

Move around during long trips. When travelling in an airplane, bus, or train, move your legs frequently and walk around as much as possible to stimulate blood circulation. Although there is more room for your legs in a car, it is still important to stop every once in a while to stretch your legs. If your legs feel numb, stop every hour or two. Never sit with your legs crossed for long periods.

Wear support stockings. These help improve poor circulation and decrease the leg pain that goes with it. They do not, however, prevent recurrences of phlebitis.

Drink plenty of liquids. If you exercise on a regular basis, it is important to drink liquids (but not excessive amounts). Sports drinks contain potassium, electrolytes and glucose (sugar) to replace what the body consumes during prolonged exertion.

RICE for muscle pain. This acronym stands for Rest, Ice (no longer than 20 minutes at a time), Compression (compression bandage) and Elevation of the affected limb. This is a common-sense approach to muscle pain. Repeat this treatment three to four times a day.

Take quinine at bedtime for nocturnal leg cramps. Quinine is an anti-arrhythmic agent available by prescription that stimulates vein dilation, allowing blood to circulate more freely. In certain cases, quinine and vitamin E can reduce the frequency of nocturnal leg cramps. Consult your doctor to rule out possible contraindications.

Stretch the leg to relax nocturnal cramps. Stretch the leg muscle by flexing your feet. Contract and relax the calf muscle repeatedly. Perform this exercise three times a day to decrease the occurrence of nocturnal cramps.

Do not smoke. Smoking causes arterial spasms and thickens the blood, causing circulatory problems.

Avoid oral contraceptives. Birth control pills can increase blood coagulation. Women at high risk for thrombophlebitis or who have previously suffered from this disease should be particularly careful. Ask your doctor to recommend another contraceptive method.

Do not wear tight pants. A comfortable fit at the waist will decrease the risk of nerve compression in the lower back.

Avoid salt supplements if you are sweating. An overdose of salt dehydrates the muscles and provokes muscle pain.

WHEN TO CONSULT?

► You experience pain, heaviness and swelling in a leg for the first time. This is an emergency.

► You experience pain in superficial varicose veins.

► You suffer from chronic diabetes mellitus and have experienced recent muscle pains, accompanied by redness or sores.

► You have acute pain.

WHAT HAPPENS DURING THE EXAM

The doctor first rules out venous or arterial obstruction, which would require emergency medical treatment. He or she then compares the colour, temperature and size of the legs, looking for any swelling (edema) and a pulse.

The doctor will take a history of when and how the pain occurred. A Doppler ultrasound providing an image of the circulation in the leg may be used to confirm the diagnosis.

The physician will also take the opportunity to evaluate the overall health of your veins and arteries, identifying your risk factors and advising you on methods of prevention that will help avert future complications.

WHAT IS THE TREATMENT?

Acute pain

Muscular pulls and tears will heal with time. RICE will encourage speedy repair. The patient should resume exercise gradually.

Superficial thrombophlebitis is most often treated with warm compresses, leg elevation and anti-inflammatories.

Deep thrombophlebitis requires emergency anticoagulant treatment. This may be administered intravenously or through abdominal injections (Lovenox or Fragmin) for the first few days, followed by oral anticoagulants taken over a number of weeks to prevent blood clotting. In some cases, this treatment does not require the patient to be confined to a bed and can be administered at home.

Acute arterial obstruction requires rapid intervention. Antithrombin medication may be administered to dissolve the clot. In cases where the lack of circulation risks damage to the muscle, the doctor recommends surgery to remove the clot.

Chronic pain

The neurological pain related to diabetes is relieved with analgesics.

Atherosclerosis may require the dilatation of an obstructed lesion or its surgical bypass.

Sciatic pain may be treated with rest, muscle relaxants and physiotherapy.

Painful Sexual Intercourse (Women)

There are two types of pain women can experience during vaginal intercourse: pain upon penetration, and deep pelvic pain caused by the thrusting of the penis. In the latter case, the woman's discomfort can be so intense that she is forced to interrupt sexual intercourse, with the pain sometimes lasting into the next day. Painful intercourse may be accompanied by a burning sensation, irritation, strong odour, blood loss, abnormal vaginal secretions, or involuntary vaginal contractions at the moment of penetration (vaginismus). Whatever the cause, the pain can lead to a decrease in sexual desire if left untreated.

WHAT ARE THE CAUSES?

Pain upon penetration

► *Insufficient vaginal lubrication.*

► *Vaginal infection,* such as vaginitis caused by yeast or bacterial vaginosis. These are not sexually transmitted infections and are not contagious.

► *Fissure at the vaginal opening.* Although the cause is unknown, one theory suggests that a previous injury in this area may cause the skin to lose elasticity and tear more easily.

► *Irritation* caused by soap or vaginal douches.

► *Chronic skin conditions* affecting the genital area (eczema, lichen sclerosus, lichen planus, lichen simplex, etc.).

► *Vaginal atrophy* (in menopausal women). During their fertile years, women's ovaries secrete estrogen, a hormone that ensures lubrication, swelling, and elasticity of the vaginal tissues. With menopause, estrogen is no longer secreted, causing the vaginal mucous membranes to thin and become drier. The opening of the vagina also becomes smaller, which can contribute to pain with penetration.

► *Vulvodynia* is an irritation of the vulva characterized by a burning sensation, rough skin, and sometimes pain with urination. Although the cause is unknown, researchers believe it may result from a damaged nerve. Sexual intercourse is often unbearably painful for women with this condition.

► *Vulvar vestibulitis.* This inflammation of the vestibule (entrance) of the vulva is a complex condition that may be caused by an excessive amount of oxalic acid in vaginal secretions. It causes a burning sensation when the vaginal opening is stimulated.

Deep pelvic pain

► *Salpingitis.* This infection of one or both fallopian tubes is the primary cause of female infertility. It is often accompanied by abnormal menstrual bleeding and more intense cramps both during and between menstrual periods.

► *Endometriosis.* This condition involves the abnormal growth of the endometrium (tissue normally lining the uterus) outside the uterus, in the abdomen or, in some cases, the bladder. Although the exact cause is unknown, it is clear that the hormonal cycle affects the growth of this tissue. When a woman is menstruating, therefore, bleeding also occurs in the abdomen or bladder. Pain is also experienced according to the phases of the menstrual cycle. After salpingitis, endometriosis is the second highest risk factor for infertility due to fallopian tube problems.

Treatment of vaginitis

Some women feel guilty about refusing sexual intercourse because they feel pain with penetration. This can create feelings of apprehension about sex, sometimes evolving into anxiety, depression, and a loss of sexual desire that encourages the development of vaginitis. This condition is not a mental disorder and causes real pain that can be treated medically. If various treatments fail to alleviate the pain, however, desensitization therapy with a sex therapist or physiotherapist can be an effective complement to medical or surgical treatment (removal of the aggravating lesion). The latter does not cause any loss of sensation.

PRACTICAL ADVICE

Use a lubricant. If the pain is caused by insufficient vaginal lubrication, liquid lubricants will facilitate penetration. Traditional gel lubricants (such as K-Y Jelly) are not recommended as they only offer temporary relief and ultimately dry out the vaginal walls, making prolonged sexual intercourse difficult. Instead, use lubricants such as Astroglide or K-Y Liquid, available in pharmacies or specialty boutiques. Vaginal moisturizers that last for about three days (such as Replens or long-acting K-Y) are also available in biodegradable applicators. A longer period of foreplay before penetration also helps increase vaginal lubrication.

Find other ways to make love. Taking the focus off penetration helps give the woman peace of mind; kissing, caressing, and massage can be equally satisfying for both partners. Vaginal penetration may be possible again in the future.

Eliminate irritating soaps and vaginal douches. These products dry out the genital organs and disrupt the natural bacterial balance of the vaginal flora, possibly leading to infection. Even so-called "mild" soaps are irritating. You can use gentle, unscented cleansers like Cetaphil or SpectroJel, but water alone is usually sufficient.

Get a clear medical diagnosis. Pain during intercourse can be caused by any number of physical problems, some of which are serious. A doctor can treat the physical disorder and determine whether the woman has suffered any psychological or sexual repercussions from the pain. It is important to consult as soon as possible to avoid losing your sexual desire altogether or developing vaginitis. Do not let anyone tell you that the problem is "all in your head".

WHEN TO CONSULT?

► You feel pain every time you have sexual intercourse and derive no pleasure from lovemaking.

► Anticipation of pain during intercourse has led to a loss of sexual desire, decreased lubrication, or involuntary contraction of the vaginal muscles (spasms).

► You feel deep pelvic pain during intercourse and have to interrupt lovemaking. The pain persists afterwards.

► The pain is accompanied by vaginal itching, discharge, odour, or dryness.

► You experience pain with urination after sexual intercourse.

WHAT HAPPENS DURING THE EXAM?

The woman should consult within 24 hours of her last sexual contact, if possible. The doctor will interview the patient about the nature and location of the pain, as well as the woman's sex life in general. A clinical and gynecological exam will follow. Further tests, such as vaginal and uterine cultures or a uterine cytology (Pap) test may also be required.

In cases of deep pelvic pain, it is often difficult to arrive at a specific diagnosis. The doctor may order an ultrasound test (external examination of the organs); if this proves inconclusive, the next likely step is a laparoscopy (the insertion of fibre optic tubes through the abdominal wall to internally examine the abdominal cavity).

WHAT IS THE TREATMENT?

Pain upon penetration
Vaginal infections

Vaginal infections are not considered to be sexually transmitted (even though a woman may develop one when she changes partners). Doctors do not therefore treat the woman's partner unless symptoms have appeared on his genital organs.

Treatment of vaginitis caused by yeast infection consists of antifungal medication administered in the form of a vaginal applicator, suppository, or pill. If the condition is recurrent, the doctor may recommend cyclical (for example, once a week) oral suppressive treatments.

Bacterial vaginosis is treated with antibiotics. The patient may choose oral, gel, or cream form, according to her preference.

If vaginal infections recur frequently, cyclical or pain-suppressant treatment may be prescribed.

Fissure at the vaginal opening

Initial treatment by a sex therapist or physiotherapist will involve techniques to desensitize or protect the area. For some women, female condoms (available in pharmacies and specialty boutiques) can eliminate pain during sex. These small plastic pouches are inserted into the vagina with the edges protruding to completely cover the vulva. If the fissure does not heal, some doctors will recommend a surgical procedure known as vestibuloplasty (to repair the vestibule).

Chronic skin diseases

The doctor prescribes oral antihistamines for itchiness and local applications of cortisone to heal lesions.

Vaginal atrophy (in menopausal women)

Estrogen supplements are available in the form of pills, gel, skin patches, or vaginal rings (known as Estring), which release hormones directly into the vaginal wall and require replacement after three months. If women experience breast pain with high doses, estrogen is prescribed in cream form or administered with a vaginal ring.

Vulvodynia

A cold (not frozen) compress applied to the vulva can help ease the pain. The doctor may prescribe an antidepressant for its analgesic properties. Physiotherapy, acupuncture or other chronic pain treatments may also prove beneficial.

Vestibulitis

Every aspect of this complex condition must be treated. The doctor will begin by prescribing calcium citrate supplements (up to six tablets a day) and a diet low in oxalate (avoiding the following food items: rhubarb, prunes, peaches, spinach, cacao, peanuts, peppers, beans, beets, celery, parsley, zucchini, grapes and tea). Sex therapy completes the program. If no progress has been made after six months, vestibuloplasty may be suggested.

Deep pelvic pain
Salpingitis
A combination of antibiotics is used to treat this infection. Laser treatment can eliminate scarring in the pelvic cavity outside the uterus.

Endometriosis
Ovary function is interrupted to stop the abnormal growth of tissue outside the uterus. Several types of medication are available, including oral contraceptives, hormones that decrease ovarian stimulation, and Danazol (Cyclomen). As a last resort, the doctor may choose laser treatment to destroy the uterine lining and induce artificial menopause.

Pain in the arm can originate in the limb itself or in the spinal column. In the latter case, it may become more intense at night because of the bent position of the neck, which shortens the spaces between the vertebrae, possibly pinching a nerve.

Heart trouble can also cause pain to radiate into the arm. In such cases, the pain is diffuse, shooting, constant, and sometimes accompanied by tingling, numbness and weakness in the arm.

WHAT ARE THE CAUSES?

Problems in the arm

- *Musculotendinous fatigue* results from sedentary habits, the lack of a warm-up before physical activity, or overexertion.
- *Repeated movements.* Certain professions require repetitive movements of the arms or back over long periods of time (machine operators and people who work for hours at a computer terminal are particularly at risk). A number of leisure activities also present a risk (playing the violin or sports like tennis, for example). Repetitive movement of the joints, tendons (which attach the muscle to the bone), or muscles of the arm causes lesions and pain that can interfere with daily activities.
- *Trauma,* such as a broken bone.
- *Benign or malignant bone tumours* cause shooting pain that becomes more intense at night.
- *Arthritis or osteoarthritis of the shoulder, elbow or wrist.* Arthritis is an inflammatory disease, while osteoarthritis is degenerative. They can affect one or many joints, and the pain is frequently accompanied by swelling and redness. Episodes are intermittent, last a few days, and resolve on their own.
- *Shingles* is not a contagious disease. Caused by the virus responsible for chickenpox (herpes zoster), shingles can affect any nerve in the body, including those in the arm. The reactivation of the virus causes pain (often described as burning) and, 48 to 72 hours later, the development of small clear blisters along the path of the nerve.

Other causes

► *Insufficient oxygen supply to the heart.* In some cases, pain in the left arm is the only sign of an angina attack or myocardial infarction (heart attack). It may be accompanied by breathlessness, a feeling of tightness or heaviness in the chest, back and jaw pain, nausea, sweating, and general malaise. If caused by angina pectoris, these symptoms are less pronounced and the pain lasts only a few minutes, usually appearing during physical exertion and disappearing when effort ceases.

► *Herniated disc* (flattening and extrusion of a disc between two vertebrae) irritates the root of a nerve where it branches off from the spinal cord.

► *Spinal cord tumour* can compromise a nerve root.

► *Osteoarthritis of the spine* can cause inflammation in the root of a nerve extending down the arm.

PRACTICAL ADVICE

Do not "double up" on hot or cold treatments. Applying a heat-producing ointment and a heating pad at the same time, for example, can burn the skin.

Do not wear a sling on your arm for too long. This will impede circulation and lead to ankylosis.

Practice prevention. Warm-up exercises and stretching of the back, neck and arms before and after intense physical effort can help avoid injuries and musculotendinous pain. If your work requires prolonged effort using the back or arms, take frequent breaks.

Soothe the pain

► Put ice in a wet towel (or use a bag of frozen vegetables) and apply for 10 to 15 minutes at a time. Or, rub the ice compress/frozen vegetables on the sore area for a maximum of four minutes until the skin becomes numb to the touch (but not blue or white, which can indicate frostbite).

► If the pain in the arm radiates from a cervical spine lesion, apply heat (hot water bottle or heating pad) to the base of the neck for 15 to 20 minutes at a time.

► Supporting your arm with cushions, raise your arm to chest level, or wear a sling when moving around.

► Take a painkiller. Anti-inflammatories such as ibuprofen should be taken with meals to avoid stomach problems, following the manufacturer's recommendations. Never take anti-inflammatories if you are allergic to aspirin, since the two medications are molecularly similar. Acetaminophen can also help ease the pain. Take one or two tablets (325 mg to 500 mg) four times a day, never exceeding 4 grams daily. If the pain is difficult to control, take both medications together.

WHEN TO CONSULT?

► Pain in your arm suddenly appears during physical exertion and disappears when you are at rest. Go to the emergency room. If this is accompanied by breathlessness, pain in the chest, nausea, sweating, and general malaise, call an ambulance.

► You feel an unusual pain in your arm.

► Your arm has been hurting for two days and the pain has stopped you from performing your daily activities.

► Your arm or hand is numb.

► You have fallen or suffered a trauma and your arm is deformed or swollen. You can neither move it nor hold it straight. You likely have a fracture.

WHAT HAPPENS DURING THE EXAM?

If the doctor suspects the problem originates in the arm, electromyography (small electrical shocks to test sensitivity levels) and X-rays will be ordered, as well as more complex tests such as radioscopic and tomographic scans. A joint tap may be required for diagnosis if arthritis is suspected.

If the doctor believes the pain is due to a problem in the cervical spine, he or she will order radioscopic, tomographic, and magnetic resonance imaging (MRI) scans to obtain the most complete information possible. A myelogram (a process to detect abnormalities by injecting contrasting liquid) is used to scan for compressions or spinal cord tumours.

WHAT IS THE TREATMENT?

Trauma
The doctor will refer the patient to a physiotherapist, osteopath or acupuncturist, depending on the nature of the injury. In cases of fracture, a cast is usually required and, if the bone is displaced, surgery may be necessary.

Tumours
The patient receives the care and treatment appropriate to the stage of the cancer.

Arthritis and osteoarthritis
Treatment for arthritic conditions must be supervised by a doctor, as it includes the use of cortisone, local infiltrations of painkillers, or anti-inflammatories. If several joints are affected, cortisone may be taken orally, which causes side-effects that must be closely observed.

Shingles
Taking antiviral drugs within 72 hours after the development of the first blisters can reduce the severity of the condition. The doctor may also prescribe an ointment to ease any pain that persists after treatment. It should be noted, however, that even though the symptoms will disappear, the virus itself cannot be eliminated.

Herniated disc
Surgery may be required in severe cases. Most of the time, traditional treatment (physiotherapy, anti-inflammatories, cervical collar, exercises, etc.) is preferred.

Pallor

"Pallor" describes lightness of the skin in comparison to its usual colour. A healthy glow to the complexion is caused by blood flow just beneath the skin; when blood flow decreases, the face becomes paler. There are, of course, natural variations in skin colour: blondes, red-heads, and the elderly usually have pale complexions, for example. The individual's general health is also a factor.

WHAT ARE THE CAUSES?

- *Emotional or physical stress.* The body responds to stress by contracting the blood vessels just under the surface of the skin, diverting circulation to the vital organs (heart, liver, kidneys, and brain) and causing pallor.
- *Lack of physical activity.*
- *Iron-deficiency (anemia).* A lack of iron causes the blood to become less concentrated, resulting in pallor. It is usually accompanied by fatigue and shortness of breath. This type of anemia is often caused by an iron-poor diet that is most common to vegetarians, alcoholics, and elderly people with poor eating habits. It is also observed in pregnant or nursing women, as well as growing children, all of whom require high levels of iron. Blood loss resulting from heavy menstrual flow, bleeding hemorrhoids, fibroma of the uterus, or digestive problems (caused by overuse of aspirin or anti-inflammatories) may also lead to anemia and therefore pallor.
- *Heat exhaustion.* When exposed to heat, the body protects the vital organs by reducing blood flow under the skin surface. Inadequately hydrated marathon runners or elderly people, for example, become extremely pale, sweat profusely and feel faint after lengthy exposure to hot temperatures.
- *Myocardial infarction (heart attack)* is characterized by sudden pallor accompanied by palpitations, shortness of breath and chest pain.
- *Cerebrovascular accident (stroke).* Paleness is generally accompanied by speech problems or paralysis.

PRACTICAL ADVICE

Increase the amount of iron in your diet. Iron-rich foods like green vegetables are particularly important if your body requires higher levels of iron (you are pregnant, nursing, or going through a growth spurt, for example). Take iron supplements as needed. Multivitamins are generally not necessary, although they can be good for elderly people with unbalanced diets.

Abstain from alcohol. Do not take a shot of alcohol to pick you up after an emotional shock or suffering heat exhaustion. This can lower your blood pressure and increase paleness.

Do not take aspirin. If you are suffering from anemia due to blood loss, aspirin and other blood-thinning medications will increase the rate of bleeding and may cause a stomach ulcer.

Move around. If you are chronically pale, improve your blood circulation by exercising at least twice a week for 15 to 20 minutes each time. Simple activities like walking are perfectly acceptable ways to stay active.

If you are suffering from heat exhaustion, lie on your back and lift your legs. This is the safest way to direct blood flow back to the brain, but you can also put your head between your knees while standing or sitting. Drink cold liquids, take off any excess clothing, and rest in the shade. Your discomfort, dizziness and pallor should quickly disappear.

Be a well-informed vegetarian. If you decide to eliminate meat from your diet, do some research on what types of food will help maintain iron levels in your new regime. Take iron supplements if necessary.

WHEN TO CONSULT?

▶ You suddenly become pale, have palpitations, sweat profusely, feel short of breath, and experience chest pain or indigestion. Go to the emergency room immediately. This may be an attack of angina pectoris or a myocardial infarction (heart attack).

► You are pale, feel tired, and become short of breath quickly.
► Your friends and family have noticed that you are pale.
► You suffer significant blood loss.
► You believe that a child or an elderly person has heat exhaustion.

WHAT HAPPENS DURING THE EXAM?

The doctor will take a history and perform a physical examination, possibly checking the patient's medications. Blood tests, other laboratory tests, or an electrocardiogram may be required.

WHAT IS THE TREATMENT?

The disorder will determine the treatment. If the underlying problem is anemia, the doctor will increase the patient's iron intake through diet or supplements. Oral contraceptives may reduce menstrual flow and make a woman's periods more regular. If the pallor is caused by anemia resulting from blood loss due to a uterine fibroma or benign/malignant intestinal tumour, surgery may be necessary. Treatment for heat exhaustion includes rehydration. If the patient is suffering from a myocardial infarction, there are a number of medications to ease the pain and stop its progression.

Men frequently find it embarrassing to consult a doctor about problems affecting their genital organs. Certain conditions, however, are quite bothersome and can be easily treated by a medical professional.

Skin of the penis, groin area, and scrotum
- Itching.
- Redness.
- Secretions.
- Discomfort during erections.
- Warts or pimples.

Testicles and scrotal lumps
- Soft or moderately hard lumps.
- Pain.
- Fever.
- Increase in size of testicles, difficulty urinating.
- Large pimples.

WHAT ARE THE CAUSES?
Skin of the penis, groin area, and scrotum
- *Irritation of the scrotum* (sac containing the testicles). Hot weather, obesity or athletic activity may cause excessive perspiration that leads to redness and itching. Scented products, soaps and fabric softeners are also irritants.
- *Pubic lice.* Commonly known as "crabs", this parasite is transmitted through sexual contact (intercourse is not necessary) and lodges in the pubic hair, causing intense itching. Visible to the naked eye, they are easily detectable and generally appear 10 to 14 days after sexual contact.
- *Mycosis* (Tinea cruris). Yeast proliferates in humid environments, making the groin and the area under the foreskin of uncircumcised men vulnerable to infection. Diabetics are particularly at risk.

The infections cause redness, itching, secretion and, in rare cases, strong odour.

▶ *Condyloma.* Also known as genital warts, the incubation period of this sexually transmitted infection can last several months. The condition is sometimes difficult to identify because the lesions can be microscopic in size or look like pimples. They may also cluster to form a cauliflower shape. Genital warts have been linked to cervical cancer in women.

▶ *Sebaceous cysts* on the scrotum are whitish or yellowish in colour and of moderately hard consistency. They occur because of blocked sebaceous glands and may be accompanied by a yellowish discharge. They present primarily an aesthetic problem.

▶ *Shrinking of the foreskin* (phimosis). The skin of the foreskin can lose its elasticity, causing discomfort or pain during erection. There are a number of possible reasons.

▶ *Herpes.* This sexually transmitted viral infection causes the appearance of bullae (blister-like sores) that rupture and dry, leaving redness and scabs.

▶ *Cancer of the penis.* Fortunately, this disease is very rare. It first appears as a red sore on the penis. Any sore that does not heal should be checked by a doctor.

Testicles and scrotal lumps

▶ *Spermatic cysts* (spermatocele) occur when sperm leaks out of the vas deferens and accumulates to form a cyst. These relatively soft masses (occasionally reaching the size of a golf ball) are usually located above the testicles. While painful in some cases, they are not cancerous and present no cause for alarm. Consult a doctor if you are unsure.

▶ *Epididymitis.* The epididymis is a coiled tube located to the side of the testicles. In men under 35, the inflammation of this organ is usually caused by gonorrhea or chlamydia infection. In older men, it is generally the result of a urinary infection and is accompanied by difficulty urinating. The condition causes the scrotum to enlarge significantly (sometimes to the size of an orange), as well as pain, fever and redness.

▶ *Abscess.* An accumulation of pus resembling a large pimple can appear inside or on the surface of the scrotum (the sac containing the testicles). It is most common in men who have developed an infection after surgery in this area (such as a vasectomy). In some cases, it is accompanied by a fever.

▶ *Abdominal muscle tension.* Strain on the abdominal muscles (linked to the testicles) due to obesity or exertion can produce pain in the groin area.

▶ *Post-vasectomy granuloma.* Even several years after the cutting of the vas deferens in a vasectomy operation, there may be small sperm leaks. The auto-immune system perceives it as a foreign body, causing intermittent and intense pain in the scrotum.

▶ *Hernia.* A portion of the abdominal wall can collapse into the scrotum and increase its size.

▶ *Varicose veins in the scrotum* (varicocele). The dilation of the veins of the scrotum appears as a poorly-defined and relatively soft lump, usually located above the left testicle. It may cause a feeling of heaviness in the testicles and is sometimes linked to infertility.

PRACTICAL ADVICE

Take painkillers. To ease the pain, take one or two acetaminophen tablets (325 mg to 500 mg), four times a day, not exceeding 4 grams

Self-examination of testicles

Testicular cancer is most common in men between 20 and 35 years of age, affecting 4 men in 100,000. Performed once a month, self-examination of the testicles in theory allows young men to screen for the disease.

Palpate the testicle between the thumb (placed on the upper side) and the index and middle finger (placed under the testicle).

While a hard lump is not necessarily cancerous, it is nevertheless wise to consult a doctor. Testicular cancer is easily treated if detected early.

daily. Anti-inflammatories are also helpful. Follow the manufacturer's recommended dosage and take both medications at once, if the pain is difficult to manage.

Don't touch the warts or lumps. This may cause infection and pain.

Reduce irritation. After any activity that causes excessive sweating, take a shower as soon as possible. Use unscented soaps and dry yourself thoroughly. Sprinkle your underwear with baby-powder or apply Zincofax to the irritated area.

Make laundry and garment choices carefully. If you have sensitive skin, avoid using liquid or sheet fabric softeners and rinse your clothes twice. Do not wear tight underwear and never wear them to bed. Wash your sports clothes after every activity, especially if you play regularly.

Treat pubic lice. Once you have confirmed their presence, use special shampoos or soap sold over-the-counter in drugstores. Wash all your underwear in hot water.

For yeast infections, let the skin breathe. Because yeast cannot survive in the open air, the best treatment is to let the skin breathe for a few hours every day (this will also prevent recurrences). Antifungal creams can also be used to accelerate healing.

Be sure that they really are genital warts. Soak a facecloth in vinegar and apply it to the affected area for at least two minutes. If the lesions are warts, the vinegar will turn them white. If this is the case, see your doctor. Have safe sex: tell your partner about your infection and always wear condoms.

Stay in shape. Weight loss will stop your thighs from rubbing together, reduce the amount of yeast in the groin area, and help avoid pain in the groin. For pain in the scrotum, wear a jock strap (special underwear that supports the testicles, available in pharmacies).

Regular underwear made from strong, supportive material can also help.

Clean a baby's penis with care. Ideally, a baby boy's penis should be delicately retracted during washing to ensure proper hygiene. In some boys, however, the foreskin has significantly less elasticity, and using force to pull it back can tear the skin. If it cannot be retracted gently, then do not retract it at all, as it will not seriously affect hygiene. If you choose to have your son circumcised, it should be done before puberty or the beginning of sexual activity.

WHEN TO CONSULT?

► Itchiness persists despite your attempts to rectify it.
► You have recurrent yeast infections.
► You have condyloma (genital warts).
► You notice one or more lumps inside the scrotum.
► Your testicles have increased in size.
► You feel intense pain and have a fever.

WHAT HAPPENS DURING THE EXAM?

The doctor will perform a complete examination. If necessary, he or she will order specialized tests, such as a urine analysis or testicle ultrasound.

WHAT IS THE TREATMENT?

Mycosis

If the yeast infection reappears despite several treatments with anti-fungal creams, the doctor will perform tests to determine whether diabetes is responsible. Circumcision may be necessary.

Condyloma

Several treatments are available, including podophyllin, a liquid used to burn the warts. If ineffective, the doctor may apply liquid nitrogen or trichloroacetic acid with a cotton swab, a treatment requiring several sessions. A more radical procedure using an electrical current or laser to burn off the warts may be performed in the doctor's office. Due to the relatively long incubation period of condyloma, the use of a condom for at least six months after the disappearance of the warts is recommended in all cases.

Sebaceous cysts
These cysts pose no danger to a man's health, but may be surgically removed for aesthetic reasons.

Shrinking of the foreskin (phimosis)
In most cases, circumcision is the only treatment. The foreskin is removed under local or general anesthesia, freeing the glans.

Herpes
Anti-viral creams may be prescribed. This recurrent disease is sometimes difficult to manage and the virus cannot be eradicated from the body.

Cancer of the penis
Treatment involves surgery to remove the lesion and, in some cases, radiation therapy. In extremely rare cases, the penis is amputated.

Spermatic cysts
These cysts are surgically removed only if they are extremely painful.

Epididymitis
This inflammation is treated with antibiotics. If caused by a sexually transmitted infection, the man's partner must also be treated.

Abscess
Abscesses are surgically drained.

Pain in the groin
There is no specific treatment, other than losing weight to avoid putting strain on the muscles and exercising regularly to strengthen them.

Post-vasectomy granuloma
These generally disappear within a few days without complications.

Hernia
Minor surgery is required.

Varicose veins in the scrotum (varicocele)
When varicocele becomes a source of severe discomfort and disrupt the patient's daily activities, ligation surgery is performed. Ligation may also correct the problem in many cases of infertility (after one year and three sperm analyses showing sluggish sperm).

Problems Caused by Contact Lenses

Contact lenses are foreign objects to the eyes, no matter how comfortably they fit. Not only must they be perfectly adjusted to the wearer's vision, they must also be cleaned and manipulated with care. Most problems arise because of improper adjustment, contamination from touching, or damaged lenses.

Common problems include:

► Conjunctivitis (pink eye)
► Inflammation of the transparent membrane (conjunctiva) coating the area surrounding the cornea (transparent curved membrane covering the iris, the coloured circle of the eye) and the inside of the eyelids.
► Manifests as redness, irritation, burning sensation, and increased secretions.
► May be chemical, irritative, or allergic (giant papillary conjunctivitis).

Keratitis

► Inflammation of the cornea.
► May cause pain or sensitivity to light.

Corneal ulcer

► Acute bacterial infection of the cornea causing pain and, possibly, diminished visual acuity and permanent scarring of the cornea.

WHAT ARE THE CAUSES?

Conjunctivitis

► **Errors or accidents** while using cleaning solutions, disinfectants, or moisturizers can cause chemical conjunctivitis. Confusing the wrong product for eye drops is a common mistake made by shortsighted people. Leaving the products open or lending them to someone else can lead to contamination.
► **Broken lenses** cause irritative conjunctivitis.

▶ *Deposits* Allergic reactions (allergic conjunctivitis) can be triggered by deposits of denatured proteins (lumps) in old cleaning solutions, impurities, or lipids from handling lenses with dirty hands. The inflammation increases the amount of secretions, worsening the problem.

Keratitis

▶ *Infected cleaning solutions* disinfectants, or moisturizers can cause chemical keratitis.

▶ *Broken lenses* cause irritative keratitis.

▶ *Prolonged wear* unsterilized or extended-wear lenses, or a bad fit can cause hypoxia (lack of oxygen), leading to keratitis. It is most common in extended-wear lens users, who wake up with swollen eyes in the morning and develop red blood vessels around the cornea.

▶ *Oral herpes* (herpetic keratitis). Touching your eyes after touching a cold sore can cause herpetic keratitis, a very painful condition. The herpes virus can affect all three layers of the cornea and cause permanent damage. Consult immediately.

Corneal ulcer

▶ *Bacterial infection of the cornea.* Bacteria can enter the cornea through a cut or scratch in the epithelium (protective outer layer of the cornea) caused by irritation or hypoxia.

PRACTICAL ADVICE

Remove your lenses if you feel any discomfort. If the pain disappears, your lenses are most likely the problem and must be replaced with new ones or glasses. If the pain persists for more than a few hours, see a doctor.

If you are concerned, consult immediately. If you wait, it may get worse. Your doctor will refer you to an ophthalmologist, if necessary.

Never use cortisone eye drops to ease the pain. If you have herpetic keratitis without knowing it, these eye drops (sold over-the-counter in pharmacies) will actually encourage the proliferation of the herpes virus. See a doctor first.

Remove your lenses before going to bed. Even extended-wear lenses should be taken out.

Replace your contact lenses regularly. Cracks may develop after a year or two and, while invisible to the naked eye, can lead to irritation. Gas permeable contact lenses only have to be replaced every five years or so. Wear disposable lenses to ensure cleanliness.

Maintain proper hygiene. Wash your hands with soap and water before rubbing the lenses with cleaning solution and clean your carrying case frequently. Once a week, use the protein-dissolving tablets recommended by your eye specialist.

Develop a routine. Always store your lenses, cleaning products and case in the same place; when you clean your lenses, always perform the steps in the same sequence.

Do not go swimming with your lenses. Remove your lenses before swimming in lakes or rivers to avoid contamination and wear tight-fitting goggles in the pool or ocean.

Use the recommended solution. Never moisturize or clean your lenses with saliva, as it contains bacteria that may lead to infection. Tap water is equally risky, particularly if you are travelling.

Be sure you are using the right solution. Some solutions are more irritating than others and you may be using one that is incompatible with your lenses. Ask an eye specialist for advice.

Do not play lab chemist. Never mix solutions, or try to concoct a home recipe with salt and water. This can cause infection.

Rinse burning eyes. If you have forgotten to neutralize the peroxide cleaning solution, your eyes will burn when you insert your lenses. Remove them and rinse your eyes well with saline solution or water.

Stay well-hydrated and be aware of your environment. If your lenses feel worse indoors than out, your environment may be the problem. Rugs, fluorescent lights, cigarette smoke and air conditioning can dry out the eyes and make your lenses uncomfortable. Drink plenty of liquids and use a humidifier to avoid dehydration.

Blink frequently. Staring at a computer screen for hours can dry out the eyes. Blink regularly to keep them moist.

Hair and makeup tips. Avoid getting your lenses dirty. Apply hairspray before inserting your lenses, and eye makeup after the lenses are in.

Wear glasses during housework. It will prevent cleaning products from coming into contact with your lenses.

Keep your glasses and lens case handy. You never know when you will need to remove your lenses.

Never lend your cleaning solution or contact lenses. It will reduce the risk of contamination.

WHEN TO CONSULT?

► You follow all the advice listed above, but your contact lenses have been bothering you for more than a day.
► You feel pain in your eyes.
► You suspect you may have herpetic keratitis.

WHAT HAPPENS DURING THE EXAM?

The physician asks a number of questions about the type of lenses the patient wears, how long he or she has been wearing them, the type of solution used, as well as the cleaning procedure. The lenses are checked for scratches, cracks, and deposits, and the eye is examined with a slit lamp and microscope to rule out conjunctivitis and ulcers.

WHAT IS THE TREATMENT?

Conjunctivitis (pink eye)

► Chemical conjuncivitis: change the cleaning solution.

► Irritative conjunctivitis: replace the lenses.

► Allergic conjunctivitis: deep-clean the lenses, wear them less frequently, and use disposable lenses for everyday wear. The doctor may prescribe non-steroidal anti-inflammatory eye drops.

Keratitis

► Chemical keratitis: change the cleaning solution.

► Irritative keratitis: replace the lenses.

► Hypoxic keratitis: replace with gas permeable lenses and wear them less frequently. Always remove extended-wear lenses at night.

► Oral herpes (herpetic keratitis): take antiviral medication to control herpes. If the virus has affected all three corneal layers, scars may form and cause vision problems. In serious cases, cornea transplants are necessary.

Corneal ulcer

This is treated with strong doses of antibiotics. In serious cases, the patient may require a corneal transplant.

Laser treatment

If the patient cannot tolerate wearing lenses, the doctor may perform laser surgery to repair vision.

The prostate gland is approximately the size of a walnut. It is located beneath the bladder and crossed by the urethra, a canal through which urine passes from the bladder to the end of the penis and out of the body. The prostate also marks the point where the spermatic canals join the urethra.

Although it is not involved in the mechanisms of erection or ejaculation, the prostate plays an essential role in male fertility by secreting the liquid necessary for sperm mobility and nutrition.

The symptoms of prostate infection include fever, shivering, difficulty urinating, and a sensation of burning with urination. Other prostate problems are grouped under the general term, "prostatism". They are listed below:

► Difficulty instigating urination.
► Weak urinary flow.
► Inability to empty the bladder completely.
► Constant need to urinate.
► Urinary incontinence.
► More frequent urination.
► Stomach pain when urinating, in some cases.

WHAT ARE THE CAUSES?

► *Benign prostate hypertrophy (prostate adenoma).* After the age of 30, the prostate begins to enlarge. This is a normal phenomenon, although not yet well understood. It is known that testosterone (male sex hormone) plays a role in the hypertrophy. As it enlarges, the prostate may compress the urinary canal, causing prostatism. Between 25% and 30% of men will suffer from this condition at some point in their lives, but only 10% will need medical treatment.

► *Prostate cancer.* It is estimated that 9% of men over the age of 50 are at risk of developing this type of cancer, with 3% of them losing their lives to it. For reasons unknown, black men and men with a family history of prostate cancer are at a higher risk. The signs include prostatism and, in some cases, blood in the urine.

► **Prostatitis** is an inflammation of the prostate, usually due to a urinary tract sexually transmitted infection. The following symptoms will appear: high fever (39 °C - 40 °C), shivering, lower abdominal and lower back pain, frequent need to urinate, difficulty urinating, a sensation of burning with urination and ejaculation. In some cases, there will be blood in the sperm.

PRACTICAL ADVICE

Avoid drinking after dinner. One of the most unpleasant aspects of prostatism is the need to visit the bathroom several times during the night. Reducing your liquid intake after dinner can help prevent this annoyance.

Don't worry. As we age, our kidneys gradually increase the production of urine at night. Everyone over the age of 50—both men and women—frequently need to get up in the middle of the night, whatever their previous habits.

Avoid certain foods. Food that irritates the bladder (such as coffee, tea, cola, chocolate, or spicy items) can aggravate the symptoms of prostatism.

Practice safe sex. The best way to avoid getting a sexually transmitted infection is to be safe. Wear a condom.

Prevention is better than cure. Starting at age 50, men should visit their doctors for a yearly prostate cancer screening. This involves a digital rectal examination and, in some cases, a blood test to assess the levels of prostate specific antigen (PSA). Men in the highest risk group (family history or black) should talk to their doctor about the advantages and disadvantages of beginning testing at the age of 40.

WHEN TO CONSULT?

► You have symptoms of prostatism.
► There is blood in your urine.
► You have the symptoms of an infection.

WHAT HAPPENS DURING THE EXAM?

The doctor will take a history and perform a physical examination (including a digital rectal examination). Blood and urine tests, a measurement of urinary output, or an abdominal ultrasound may also be necessary. In some cases, the doctor will order an ultrasound guided biopsy.

A prostate ultrasound (through the rectum) and a specific prostatic antigen (SPA) test may be required to assess cell proliferation in the prostate.

WHAT IS THE TREATMENT?

Hypertrophy of the prostate (prostate adenoma)

The treatment depends on the severity of the symptoms. If mild, the doctor may simply recommend regular medical supervision. If they are quite bothersome, a number of medications, including alpha-blockers, 5-alpha reductase inhibitors, or finasteride inhibitors, can effectively reduce symptoms with very few undesirable side effects.

If the problems are persistent, surgery to remove the hypertrophied area of the prostate may be necessary. This operation has no effect on virility and sexual intercourse is still possible. It may, however, affect ejaculation by causing some or all of the semen to flow into the bladder. This is a harmless phenomenon and does not necessarily prevent conception.

Certain hospitals offer a new laser vaporization technique, whereby the cells in the hypertrophied section of the prostate are heated to a high temperature, causing them to vaporize. This treatment allows a fast return to regular activities.

Prostate cancer

Many treatments are possible, depending on the size of the tumour, as well as the patient's age, general physical condition, and preferences.

Complete prostatectomy involves removing the entire prostate gland. This treatment can cause sexual dysfunction (erectile dysfunction, inability to ejaculate) and urinary incontinence.

External radiation therapy leaves the prostate in place and destroys the malignancy by exposing the affected area to radiation. This may cause rectal irritation and diarrhea, which will disappear when the treatment is discontinued.

Prostate cancer requires testosterone to develop. To deprive the cancer of its fuel, the production of this hormone by the testicles can be blocked with drugs. This treatment can prolong life, but is reserved only for very advanced cases, as it does not rid the body of the disease.

In some advanced cases, the testicles must be removed. Once testosterone can no longer be produced, the cancer is unable to grow. In many cases, the tumour will actually shrink and remain stable for several years.

Prostatitis

Intravenous antibiotic and anti-inflammatory treatment will clear up the infection. A prescription for oral antibiotics will follow, to be taken for a longer period of time.

Swelling or puffiness of the upper and lower eyelids is very rarely serious. Sufferers complain of the following symptoms:

► Puffiness of the eyes, particularly in the morning.
► Sometimes accompanied by redness and itching.

WHAT ARE THE CAUSES?

► *Lifestyle,* such as alcohol abuse, eating salty food before going to bed, or lack of sleep.
► *Allergies* to feather pillows, sheet fabric, or face cream, for example.
► *Certain diseases,* such as blepharitis (inflammation of the eyelid), orbital cellulitis (infection of the orbital tissues), kidney infections, thyroid problems, or chalazions (small, benign tumours on the eyelids).
► *Aging and hormonal changes.* Aging causes the skin to irreversibly lose elasticity and accumulate around the eyes. Hormonal changes just before and during menstruation sometimes cause water retention, which can lead to puffy eyes.

PRACTICAL ADVICE

Use compresses. Apply lukewarm compresses to the eyes four times a day, or wash your face with cold water. This will stimulate blood circulation and reduce swelling.

Never pinch your eyelids. This will aggravate the edema.

Massage lightly. Gentle pressure with your fingertips around the eyes can stimulate circulation.

Use a mask. Masks filled with cold water or soothing gel are available in drugstores and should be worn for a few minutes first thing in the morning. Chilled teaspoons also work.

Soothe your eyes with teabags. Place damp, chilled teabags on your eyelids for 15 minutes to reduce puffiness. The tannic acid in the tea constricts the blood vessels, reducing inflammation.

Take diuretics. Non-prescription diuretics can be very helpful if you frequently experience bloating a few days before your period. Note, however, that diuretics can lower blood pressure, so make sure to get yours checked before taking this medication.

Wear makeup. Upper eyelid puffiness can be disguised by applying a darker cover-up than your skin tone under regular makeup. The same technique can be used to hide bags under the eyes.

Prevent puffiness. If your eyes are often puffy first thing in the morning, there are a few things you can do:
- Raise the head of your bed to stimulate blood circulation.
- Avoid drinking before going to bed, as this will worsen any existing swelling.
- Avoid salty food before going to bed.
- Use water-based foundation makeup instead of oil-based (the latter can irritate the delicate skin around the eye).
- Use pillows made from synthetic fibres if you are allergic to feathers or down.
- Use hypoallergenic creams if you are allergic to face creams.

WHEN TO CONSULT?
- Your eyes have been puffy, red, and irritated for over a week.

WHAT HAPPENS DURING THE EXAM?
The doctor can generally reach diagnosis and recommend treatment after a complete eye examination.

WHAT IS THE TREATMENT?
Antihistamines are prescribed to treat allergies.
Blepharitis is treated with antibiotic ointment on the eyelids.
Orbital cellulitis is treated with oral antibiotics.

If the problem is caused by a chalazion, minor surgery may be performed if medication proves ineffective. The procedure involves the drainage of the swollen sebaceous gland. It is performed under the eyelid and leaves no scar.

If the problem is primarily aesthetic (such as premature aging), blepharoplasty may be recommended. This is a minor procedure that removes excess eyelid tissue.

Pupil Dilation

The pupil (the small black spot at the centre of the eye) is the orifice through which light enters the eye. It is controlled by two muscles: the dilator and the contractor (sphincter). Abnormal dilation of the pupil (mydriasis) can occur in one or both eyes. When only one is dilated, there is cause for concern.

Symptoms associated with abnormal dilation of the pupil include:
► Blurred vision at close range.
► slightly or not at all.
► Diplopia (double vision) accompanied by pain and, sometimes, drooping eyelids. The last two symptoms may indicate serious neurological problems.

WHAT ARE THE CAUSES?
Dilation of both pupils
► *Certain medications,* such as eye drops to eliminate redness, various pill-form atropine or belladonna based medications, ophthalmic preparations to treat various eye diseases, or patches to combat motion sickness and nausea.
► *Contact with certain toxic plants.*
► *Certains drugs*, such as marijuana and cocaine.

Dilation of one pupil
► *Genetic origin.* In about 10% of the population, the pupils are different sizes at birth. Known as "anisocoria", this phenomenon is not associated with any other symptoms and presents no cause for concern.
► *Certain medication,* such as eye drops to eliminate redness or those with an atropine or belladonna base. Touching the eyes after handling any substance containing atropine or belladonna will also have this effect.
► *Migraine* due to ocular pain.
► *Glaucoma.* Pupil dilation is accompanied by pain, eye redness, blurred vision, nausea, and vomiting.

► *Adie's Syndrome.* This condition is often a symptom of a larger neurological syndrome or associated with a viral infection. One of the pupils is abnormally dilated and contracts more slowly in the light than the other, causing blurred vision at close range and dizziness in the light.

► *Neurological conditions.* A cranial nerve disorder, vascular deformity (aneurysm), or tumour are all possible causes, however rare.

PRACTICAL ADVICE

Go to the emergency room. If one of your pupils is more dilated than the other and you present other symptoms like eye redness or an unusual headache, consult a doctor right away. You may have glaucoma or an aneurysm in a brain artery. Quick medical intervention can save your eye, or even your life.

Do not ignore the problem. It is especially important to see a doctor if one or both eyes are painful and red and your vision is blurred.

Never use drugs with a base of pilocarpine (or any of its substitutes) without a doctor's advice. These drugs, frequently used to treat glaucoma, cause the pupil to contract. They present a certain risk, however, since they can also mask the presence of another even more serious condition. Never use them without prescription or before consulting an ophthalmologist.

Bring photos to the doctor's office. A few close-up shots of yourself taken over the last ten years will help the doctor verify whether the dilation of one or both of the pupils is a recent development.

Have your medications checked. If both your pupils have been dilated for more than one day, your doctor will help you identify which medication is causing the problem. Tell him or her about any prescription medications you are taking, as well as any over-the-counter preparations, such as drops to eliminate redness.

WHEN TO CONSULT?

► You are experiencing eye pain.
► One of your eyelids is drooping.
► One or both of your eyes is red.
► You have used eye drops or taken some medication and both your pupils are dilated. The dilation may be a normal reaction and resolve within a few days. Wait one week before consulting, unless you also have one of the four symptoms listed above.

WHAT HAPPENS DURING THE EXAM?

The physician uses different types of light to check for redness and test the reflexes of the pupil and eye movement. He or she will also verify whether the patient has been in contact with any toxic plants. The patient's vision will be assessed through reading exercises, and if necessary, the doctor will order X-rays.

WHAT IS THE TREATMENT?
Medications

The patient must eventually stop taking the medication that is causing the condition. The physician will suggest alternatives.

Contact with toxic plants

Pupil dilation caused by contact with toxic plants is not serious and will disappear with time.

Migraine

Treatment includes lifestyle changes as well as painkillers or triptan medications. The pupil will return to normal after the migraine attack.

Glaucoma attack

Laser treatment and ophthalmic drops are the only options. If left untreated, the attack may lead to an irreversible loss of vision in the affected eye.

Adie's syndrome
There is no specific treatment. The symptoms will fade with time.

Neurological disorder
Surgery is required to correct the vascular abnormality or remove the tumour.

Rapid Pulse

A normal heartbeat at rest measures between 60 and 80 beats per minute. Any pulse exceeding 100 beats per minute is known as "tachy-cardia", which can be a harmless normal phenomenon, depending on the cause. Tachycardia can either go unnoticed, or manifest in a pounding heart (palpitations).

Note that a rapid pulse does not automatically indicate high blood pressure. In cases of anemia or heart attack, for example, the heart beats more quickly to compensate for low blood pressure.

WHAT ARE THE CAUSES?

- *Physical exercise* causes the pulse to accelerate in proportion to the intensity of the activity. This is completely normal. The heart rate slows down again once the individual stops exercising.
- *Sedentary lifestyle.* People who lead sedentary and inactive lives will experience an increase in heart rate upon the slightest physical exertion. This is due to the unusual increase in oxygen consumption, which leads to shortness of breath.
- *Tea, coffee, cola, and chocolate* all contain caffeine, which increases the heart rate.
- *Stress,* either physiological (serious disease, injury, surgery) or psychological (family or financial problems, change of jobs, nervousness).
- *Cigarettes and other tobacco products* have a double effect. On the one hand, they induce the heart to beat more quickly and use more oxygen. On the other, they decrease the amount of oxygen carried to the heart.
- *Certain medications,* including decongestants and bronchodilators such as salbutamol (Ventolin) or theophylline, used to treat asthma and other bronchial ailments.
- *Drugs and alcohol,* as well as stimulants and amphetamine derivatives that excite the central nervous system.
- *Wolff-Parkinson-White syndrome* is a congenital abnormality of the cardiac electrical conduction system (causing a "faulty

connection"). Uncommon and generally harmless, the condition is usually discovered in adolescents and young adults who complain of sudden weakness, fainting during intense physical exertion, and episodes of tachycardia.

► *Paroxysmal tachycardia* may be atrial or ventricular, depending on which chambers of the heart are beating more rapidly. If the tachychardia is atrial, the upper chambers of the heart beat at 95 to 150 beats per minute; if ventricular, the heart rate can go as high as 160 to 190 beats per minute. This abnormality in the cardiac electrical conduction system is most common in young people and characterized by episodes of regular, rapid (160 to 190 beats per minute) heartbeat, lasting anywhere from a few minutes to a few hours. The increased heart rate occurs suddenly and unexpectedly (with no apparent trigger factors) and returns to normal just as abruptly. Paroxysmal tachycardia may be triggered by mild physical effort (bending over to tie your shoes, for example), or an emotional shock. In some cases, there is no discernable cause.

► *Atrial fibrillation.* This condition affects heart rhythm and often causes an irregular, usually rapid heartbeat because of the erratic contractions of the atria. It may lead to brain or pulmonary embolism (sudden obstruction of a vessel by a blood clot). Atrial fibrillation is usually brought on by heart trouble, although it is sometimes caused by thyroid dysfunction, lung disease, or alcohol abuse. It is most common in elderly people.

► *Ventricular tachycardia.* This type of tachycardia (140 to 220 beats per minute) is very serious and caused by a short-circuiting in the ventricle (lower heart chamber) that commonly occurs during a myocardial infarction (heart attack). Various types of heart disease and heart failure may also be responsible.

► *Anemia.* A significant decrease in the number of red blood cells that transport oxygen can lead to a rapid pulse.

► *Respiratory disease* such as asthma, pneumonia, bronchitis, and chronic emphysema (dilation of the pulmonary alveoli) disrupt oxygen exchange in the alveoli, causing the heart to beat more rapidly to compensate for the lack of oxygen.

▶ *Overactive thyroid gland (hyperthyroidism)* or, in rare cases, endocrine problems. Excess thyroid hormones speed up the metabolism in the same way a thermostat set to a high temperature consumes more energy. This can cause different forms of tachycardia.

PRACTICAL ADVICE

Just say no. Reduce your consumption of products containing caffeine (coffee, tea, cola, chocolate) as well as drugs and alcohol. Better yet, eliminate them altogether.

Quit smoking. In just a few days after quitting, you will notice your heart rate has slowed down. With time, you will experience less shortness of breath and have better stamina for physical exertion. Scientific studies have also shown that quitting smoking is one of the most effective ways to reduce the risk of cardiovascular disease.

Maintain a healthy weight. In most overweight people, the slightest physical effort results in tachycardia as the heart is forced to pump blood more rapidly to ensure proper oxygenation to the entire body. A healthy weight is important for a healthy heart, but be careful, as excessively strict diets can have serious side effects as well, including tachycardia. Have a doctor supervise your weight-loss program.

Improve your stamina. The only way to improve your cardiovascular health and energy levels is to regularly take part in activities that require endurance. Go walking, work in the garden, work out at the gym, or play sports several times a week.

Control your stress level. Stress is a necessary part of everyday life, keeping us active and dynamic. Too much stress, however, is bad for your health. Keep stress at a reasonable level by using relaxation techniques, taking time off, exercising regularly, and being organized at work.

See a doctor. A number of prescription medications are available to treat persistent tachycardia (beta-blockers, some calcium channel inhibitors, and anti-arrhythmic drugs).Your doctor will evaluate your condition and determine whether one of these medications is appropriate.

Try the vagal maneuver. If you are experiencing an uncomfortable episode of paroxysmal tachycardia (a sudden increase in heart rate), stimulating the vagal nerve (which runs along the thorax and is responsible for calming the cardiac system) can help. The vagal maneuver sends false messages to lower heart rate. Cough repeatedly, attempt to breathe out through the nose while blocking it, or bear down as though trying to have a bowel movement.You can also try massaging the carotid arteries (in the neck) one at a time, until you feel better. Placing firm pressure on your eyes with your hands can also ease the symptoms. To avoid falling, any of these maneuvers should be performed sitting down. Do one of these exercises for ten seconds and repeat two or three times.

WHEN TO CONSULT?

► Your pulse exceeds 100 beats per minute or you can feel your heart pounding rapidly when you are relaxed and at rest.
► Your pulse does not return to a normal, stable rate after you stop exercising.

WHAT HAPPENS DURING THE EXAM?

The doctor will interview the patient to uncover the reasons for the increased heart rate (a medication, for example), as well as perform a physical examination to check the state of the heart. He or she may order blood tests and an electrocardiogram (recording heart activity) while the patient is at rest and during exercise (walking on a treadmill).

The doctor may also ask the patient to use a Holter monitor, a small, portable device that records heart activity over a 24-hour period (the apparatus is about the size of a walkman).The patient presses a button, the machine displays the symptoms, and the patient takes note of the information for the doctor. The patient's heart activity and blood pressure may also be tested in various inclined positions on an adjustable examination table. Cardiac activity can also be directly monitored by inserting a catheter into the arm or femoral artery (in the thigh) under local anaesthesia. This examination is called electrophysiological endocavity exploration.

Paroxysmal tachycarida is more difficult to identify and may require the introduction of a heart catheter (through a vein) to measure electrical activity and discover the trigger mechanism.

WHAT IS THE TREATMENT?

Sedentary lifestyle, stimulants, psychological stress, cigarettes and other tobacco products, alcohol and illicit drugs

Changing lifestyle habits will improve the situation.

Medications

The doctor may change the prescription.

Wolff-Parkinson-White syndrome (congenital abnormality of the cardiac electrical conduction system)

The doctor will observe the patient to ensure the condition is being well controlled. A number of treatments are possible, including anti-arrhythmic drugs (to control irregular heartbeat), the implantation of a pacemaker, or surgical removal of the area causing the "short-circuit" (see chapter on Slow Pulse).

Paroxysmal (atrial or ventricular) tachycardia

Because this condition is most common in younger individuals with otherwise healthy hearts, there is usually no cause for concern. Generally, the most serious effects are nothing more than the unpleasant sensations experienced during an episode. Anti-arrhythmic drugs may be prescribed to prevent or interrupt the palpitations. Newer fulguration techniques such as radiofrequency ablation (using energy of a specific frequency) or cryotherapy (using electrode catheters inserted into the heart cavities) can provide permanent relief by destroying the tissue responsible for the tachycardia inside the heart chambers. In most cases, only one treatment is necessary.

Atrial fibrillation

The doctor will prescribe medication such as anti-arrhythmic drugs to control heart rate. Anticoagulants may also be prescribed to prevent embolisms.

Ventricular tachycardia

The doctor will apply standard treatment for myocardial infarction (*see chapter on Slow Pulse*), or treat the ventricular tachycardia specifically with anti-arrhythmic drugs, the implantation of an internal defribillator (which delivers electric shocks to interrupt the abnormal heartbeat), fulguration techniques, or heart surgery.

Anemia

The underlying ailment is treated. The most common causes of anemia include malnutrition, chronic kidney failure, and gastrointestinal bleeding.

Respiratory disease

Treatment of a reversible respiratory problem will restore heart rate to normal. If the disease is chronic, however, the patient must modify his or her lifestyle and, above all, quit smoking.

Hyperthyroidism

Beta-blockers are prescribed to prevent heart symptoms caused by excess thyroid hormones, and radioactive iodine is used to destroy the overactive portion of the thyroid gland.

Rash

"Rash" is a general term to describe a recent eruption of lesions on the skin.

There are three main types of rash: inflammatory, infectious, and that caused by skin disease.

Sufferers may develop one or more of the following symptoms:

- Erythema (redness)
- Itching (pruritis).
- Burning sensation.
- Scaly skin.
- Fissures (possibly weeping).
- Scabs.
- Erosion or ulceration (small cavity or hole in the skin).
- Macula (small, flat spots on the skin, less than 1 cm in diameter).
- Papule (small raised bumps, less than 1 cm above skin surface).
- Red patches (raised bumps, more than 1 cm above skin surface).
- Vesicles (small blisters, less than 1 cm in diameter, filled with clear liquid).
- Bulla (larger blister, more than 1 cm in diameter, filled with clear liquid).
- Pustules (pus-containing blisters).

WHAT ARE THE CAUSES?

Inflammatory rashes (allergies or irritation)

- **Contact dermatitis** describes an allergic reaction of the skin after contact with substances such as poison ivy or irritants such as soap. Symptoms of contact dermatitis usually include vesicles, redness and itching. Scaly skin, weeping fissures and scabs sometimes develop.
- **Diaper rash** is an irritation caused by urine and stool. It occurs most often in babies with diarrhea or poor hygiene (infrequent diaper changing). The baby's buttocks become red, raw, and painful, sometimes developing skin erosions.

► *Intertrigo* is generally brought on by a combination of obesity and humidity and describes irritation in the folds of skin under the chin, on the neck, in the armpits, the groin and under the breasts. Sufferers of this type of dermatitis develop weeping red patches, scaly skin, erosion and a burning sensation. It is sometimes complicated by a yeast infection (candida albicans), leading to the appearance of small white pustules around the perimeter of the other lesions.

► *Drug reactions.* Allergic or toxic reactions in the form of skin lesions and itching can develop a few hours or days after ingesting medication. In mild cases, there is itching although the mucous membranes (of the eyes, mouth and genital organs) are spared, and there is no fever. In very serious cases, the mucous membranes are affected and the sufferer develops bullae and a fever. This requires emergency treatment.

► *Urticaria (hives)* can be caused by biochemical or allergic reactions. There are a number of possible triggers, the most common being medication, insect bites, or certain foods (eggs, nuts, fruit or seafood, for example). Hives can also be triggered by exercise and emotional stress, or may appear secondary to infections like hepatitis, mononucleosis, or rubella (German measles). In some cases,

Cellulitis: A Medical Emergency

"Cellulitis" is not the same as "cellulite", the unaesthetic orange-peel effect in certain areas of the body (a totally benign condition). Rather, cellulitis is an infection of sub-dermal tissue, usually due to the entrance of bacteria through an abrasion (rubbing or scratch) on the skin.

The rash takes the form of a hot, swollen, and tender red patch of skin, possibly accompanied by fever and chills. Consult a doctor immediately: if left untreated, cellulitis may lead to septicemia (blood poisoning).

Oral, intravenous or intramuscular antibiotics will control the infection and avoid the development of septicemia.

the cause is unknown. They appear in the form of itchy papules and patches resembling insect bites (white centre surrounded by red). They vary in size, the larger ones often joining to form irregular raised patches, and may move around the body from hour to hour. They are sometimes accompanied by swollen mucous membranes (lips, tongue, eyelids, genital organs), and in rare cases, life-threatening edemas on the larynx. In cases caused by allergies, the sufferer may also develop rhinitis or asthma. Although hives may become chronic or recurrent, the problem usually only lasts a few hours.

Infectious hives (virus, bacteria, fungus, or parasites)

▶ *Oral herpes (cold sores) and genital herpes.* Caused by the herpes simplex virus, this contagious and chronic infection can affect any area on the skin, although eruptions most commonly occur on the lips, face, or genital organs. After the first attack, the virus remains in the nerves of the affected area, causing periodic recurrences. The first eruption of genital herpes generally appears three to ten days (sometimes as long as 21 days) after sexual contact with an infected person. Lesions are accompanied by intense itching or burning and disappear within five to fifteen days. Recurrences are preceded by a short period of uncomfortable tingling. For the first few days, the lesions are red and painful with vesicles on the surface that eventually dry into a thin, dark scab. In both types of herpes, the first eruption can be very severe and last up to two weeks, although recurrences are mild because the body gradually develops antibodies. The virus can be transmitted even when the lesions are not present.

▶ *Erythema infectiosum* (also known as "fifth disease"). A mildly contagious virus that causes bright redness in the cheeks of otherwise healthy children and lasts anywhere from a few days to four weeks. There are generally no other symptoms, although in some cases, it may be associated with a rash on the arms and legs (pale pink maculae forming swirling patterns).

▶ *Chickenpox, rubella, roseola, and measles.* These contagious viral illnesses, generally affecting children, are usually transmitted through saliva droplets or mucous from the nose or throat of an infected person. They are most contagious during the incubation period (5 to 21 days) and first few days after the skin lesions appear.

▷ Chickenpox manifests as salmon pink maculae that turn into vesicles resembling water droplets. The maculae first appear on the torso and spread to the rest of the body. As the infection progresses, the lesions become papules and pustules that eventually form scabs. Itching, headache, fever, and nausea may precede or accompany the rash.

▷ Rubella (or German measles) manifests in reddish papules that first appear on the face and neck, subsequently spreading to the torso. The eruption lasts for six or seven days and is usually accompanied by a moderate fever, headache, sore throat and swollen glands behind the ears and in the neck.

▷ Roseola causes a sudden high fever lasting three to four days until pink maculae appear, particularly on the neck and torso. The rash disappears within two to three days.

▷ The measles manifests as bright red papules on the face and neck that spread down through the rest of the body over three days. The rash lasts 10 to 14 days and is accompanied by a high fever, runny nose, dry cough, sensitivity to light, watery eyes, and in some cases, nausea and vomiting.

► **Warts** are contagious and caused by different forms of the papilloma virus. They most often occur as well-defined, rough growths on the hands, feet, genital organs and face.

► **Shingles (herpes zoster)** is caused by the chickenpox virus. Once a person has had this childhood disease, the virus remains in the nerve cells and sometimes reactivates when the immune system is weak. Shingles manifests in one to three days of intense pain, followed by the appearance of vesicles or bullae on a red base that trace the path of a nerve down one side of the body. The lesions then form scabs and sometimes leave scars. If the nerve is severely damaged, the pain may persist and become chronic, particularly in the elderly.

► **Impetigo.** This contagious bacterial skin condition appears in bullous or nonbullous form. Bullous impetigo is the least common and manifests in vesicles or bullae that break easily. Both forms of impetigo manifest as scabby, honey-yellow lesions most common-ly affecting the face (around the mouth and nose) and skin folds. It may be a symptom of another skin disease such as scabies or pediculosis.

► **Scarlet fever.** In most cases, this contagious group A streptococcus bacterial infection initially manifests in a fever, sore throat, redness of the mucous membranes inside the mouth, and swollen throat glands, followed by a deep red erythema and eventual flaking of the skin on the entire body or only the arms and legs.

► **Tinea** (ringworm, jock itch or athlete's foot) is a fungal infection that can affect the scalp, beard, body (particularly the groin), feet or nails. It may cause hair loss (on the head or face), pustules, or round, crusty, reddish/pinkish patches. A tinea infection in the groin area (jock itch) affects the inner thighs, but not the genitals. Foot tinea (athlete's foot) is the most common form. Propagating in humid environments, it causes the skin between the toes to whiten and crack. If left untreated, the infection can spread to the heel and side of the foot, causing redness. It may also spread to the sole of the foot and cause redness and flaking.

► **Scabies** is an infectious skin condition caused by a mite called the Sarcoptes scabiei, transmitted by close physical or sexual contact between humans, or less frequently, through contact with animals. The period between contact and the appearance of symptoms is two to four weeks. The female mite enters the body by making an incision in the skin and moves around to lay its eggs. In some cases, symptoms include papules or vesicles in the armpits and on the wrists, nipples, buttocks, and genitals. Scabies causes very uncomfortable and intense itching all over the body (excluding the head), particularly at night.

► **Pubic lice** (commonly known as crabs). This parasitic infection is transmitted sexually, or sometimes through contact with infected bedding, towels or clothes. Pubic lice have six legs and are the size of the head of a pin. Developing within two to three weeks, they burrow into the hair of the pubic area, anus, armpits and eyebrows and feed off the host's blood, causing itching in the infected areas.

Rashes caused by skin disease

► *Atopic dermatitis (atopic eczema).* This chronic hereditary skin disease usually begins in childhood. It causes dry skin, intense itching, red patches, flaking, weeping vesicles, and scabs on the eyelids, ears, neck, elbows and knees. Sufferers may also have asthma and hay fever. Irritants such as cleaning products, certain types of cloth or dye, and cosmetics, or low humidity levels are often aggravating factors.

► *Lichen planus* is a skin disease of unknown origin. Its characteristic deep red papules—sometimes grouped together in large patches on the wrists, ankles, and the mucous membranes of the mouth and genital organs—cause itching and may leave brown spots on the skin after healing.

► *Miliaria rubra (prickly heat).* This benign condition occurs when sweat ducts become blocked due to heat and humidity. The characteristic vesicles, surrounded by a reddish areola, are usually concentrated on the torso.

► *Psoriasis.* This chronic hereditary skin disease can appear at any age. Eruptions may be triggered by a streptococcus throat infection or certain medications (lithium or cortisone, for example), but in most cases, have no apparent cause. Sufferers develop red, flaky patches on the knees, elbows, face, scalp, and genitals. Itching manifests in one third of all cases.

PRACTICAL ADVICE

Be cautious with contagious diseases. The infected person should be isolated for a few days while he or she rests and receives proper nutrition and liquids. Sufferers should take recommended doses of acetaminophen. Caution: never give aspirin to children (even baby aspirin), as it can cause Reye's syndrome, a fatal liver disease. Wash your hands carefully, wear gloves to be sure not to touch the sufferer's skin, and never drink from the same glass as an infected person. Pregnant women must be especially careful and may want to avoid contact altogether.

Ease the pain, inflammation, and itching. Take one or two acetaminophen tablets (325 mg to 500 mg) four times a day, never exceeding four grams daily. Apply wet compresses or take lukewarm baths (with baking soda, if you wish). Take non-prescription antihistamines such as Benadryl and use gentle, unscented soaps. Wear loose clothing made of cotton or other natural fibres. Avoid caffeine, spicy foods and alcohol, which increase the itching. Refrain from scratching, as this can spread the rash and make the symptoms worse. Calamine lotion soothes the itching caused by chickenpox, but is ineffective for other conditions. Be careful: never use calamine lotion containing an antihistamine (such as Caladryl). There is a risk of contact dermatitis, as it is very difficult to control the amount of antihistamine absorbed by the skin.

Apply moisturizer. If the lesions are dry, apply an unscented moisturizer. In some cases (atopic dermatitis, prickly heat, and diaper rash), non-prescription 0.5% hydrocortisone cream is recommended to ease the symptoms and moisturize the skin.

Treat infectious bacterial diseases (such as impetigo or shingles). Use over-the-counter antibiotic creams such as Baciguent.

Choose your soap carefully. Unscented soaps such as Dove, Neutrogena, or Ivory are recommended. In cases of bacterial infection, use antiseptic soaps like Hibidil or Phisoderm.

Have your child vaccinated. Vaccines against measles, rubella and chickenpox (a recent development) are effective. There are no vaccines for roseola or scarlet fever.

WHEN TO CONSULT?

► Consult immediately if you develop a rash accompanied by fever, nausea, vomiting, or difficulty breathing.
► The symptoms are persistent and very uncomfortable.
► You are worried.

WHAT HAPPENS DURING THE EXAM?

The doctor takes a history and performs a general examination. Skin samples (scrapings, biopsy, etc.) and blood tests are sometimes required.

WHAT IS THE TREATMENT?

Inflammatory rashes (allergies or irritation)

Contact Dermatitis

Avoid the substance provoking the rash. Corticosteroid creams may be prescribed to control the allergic reaction or irritation.

Diaper rash

In severe or persistent cases, the doctor may prescribe mild corticosteroids, moisturizers or protective creams.

Intertrigo

Mild creams containing mild dermocorticoids, possibly combined with antifungals are effective, although the inflammation may recur. If appropriate, the patient's obesity should be treated to prevent recurrences.

Drug reaction

The symptoms should disappear with a change of prescription.

Hives

Eliminating the cause is the best treatment. If the trigger cannot be identified (allergy tests are often ineffective in non-acute cases), the doctor will prescribe short, medium, or long-term antihistamine treatment to control the symptoms. Oral or, in severe cases, intravenous corticosteroids may also be recommended.

Infectious hives (virus, bacteria, fungus, or parasites)

Oral herpes (cold sores) or genital herpes

Although the virus remains in the body and causes recurrences, cold sores do not require treatment as the lesions resolve on their own. However, anti-viral ointments or petroleum jelly may ease the symptoms. In some cases, oral anti-viral medications are prescribed. Genital herpes is treated with oral (or occasionally cream) anti-virals (acyclovir, phamcyclovir or valacyclovir), while cream and oral analgesics are prescribed to ease the pain. In very severe cases of genital herpes, the anti-viral may be administered intravenously.

Erythema infectiosum (fifth disease)
No treatment is necessary; the rash will disappear on its own.

Chickenpox, rubella, roseola and measles
In most cases, no treatment is necessary. However, in cases of adolescent or adult chickenpox, the doctor may prescribe an oral anti-viral medication, since the symptoms are much more severe than in childhood. The medication must be administered within 24 to 48 hours after the rash appears.

Warts
In two-thirds of cases, the warts disappear in one or two years without treatment; although they can be eliminated with a non-prescription salicylic acid preparation (several treatments may be required). The doctor may also remove the wart with liquid nitrogen, electrodessication surgery (burning), curettage (scraping), or laser (CO_2). Ano-genital warts (condyloma acuminatum) are treated with trichloroacetic acid, podophyllin or Aldara.

Shingles
Anti-virals can diminish the rash and acute or chronic pain only if taken less than 72 hours after the first lesions appear (the medication is no longer effective after four days). This treatment is particularly indicated for patients over the age of 50, since they run a much higher risk of chronic pain.

Impetigo
Impetigo is treated with antiseptics and/or antibiotics (in oral or topical form). The dosage is determined by the number of lesions.

Scarlet fever
Oral antibiotics are prescribed.

Tinea
The doctor will prescribe antifungal cream or pills, depending on the extent and location of the infection.

Scabies
Topical treatments such as lindane and permethrine are prescribed. Pregnant women and young children will be given a sulfur-based preparation.

Pubic lice (crabs)
Over-the-counter antiparasitic creams or shampoos (containing lindane or permethrine) are effective.

Rashes caused by skin diseases
Atopic dermatitis (atopic eczema)
Corticosteroids, immunosuppressants, sometimes antibiotics (to prevent bacterial infection of the lesions) and antihistamines can help ease the eruptions. Dry skin must be moisturized in short, lukewarm baths and with moisturizing creams.

Lichen planus
Treatment varies according to the severity of the rash. Dermocorticoid creams in combination with oral corticosteroids or light therapy (ultra-violet irradiation of the affected area) may be prescribed.

Miliaria rubia (prickly heat)
No medical treatment is required. If the patient avoids the heat, the rash will disappear in a few hours or days.

Psoriasis

Psoriasis is treated with creams and ointments (containing tar, corti-costeroids, or anthralin, for example) or with oral or injectable med-ications (such as methotrexate, etretinate, or cyclosporine). Light therapy and photochemotherapy may also be beneficial for serious cases. Photochemotherapy involves treating lesions with molecules activated by laser light.

Recurrent Problems Affecting the Mouth

The mouth can be the site of various types of recurring problems and disorders. Dryness (sometimes associated with a sore throat) and bad breath are only two of the most frequent complaints. Another common annoyance is recurring aphtha (canker sores), which can appear in large numbers simultaneously on the gums, tongue or inside of the cheeks. Although generally benign, canker sores can be quite painful and may be contagious if viral in origin. Candida albicans, also known as thrush, causes blotches in the mouth, throat, and even on the bronchial tubes. Uncommon in most healthy people, this yeast infection generally occurs in newborns, the elderly, and people undergoing chemotherapy or radiation therapy. Another example is leukoplakia, a pre-cancerous condition causing the whitening of areas in the oral mucous membrane of long-term smokers.

WHAT ARE THE CAUSES?

Dryness of the mouth
- ► *Stress* can impede the production of saliva.
- ► *Dehydration.*
- ► *Aging,* which causes a decrease in saliva production.
- ► *Medications,* such as antidepressants and antihistamines.
- ► *Sjögren's syndrome.* This disease destroys the salivary glands, making it impossible for the body to produce saliva.

Bad Breath
- ► *Stress* changes the composition of saliva.
- ► *Smoking* leaves an unmistakable odour on the breath.
- ► *Poor oral hygiene,* cavities and gingivitis (inflammation of the gums).
- ► *Fasting* causes the breath to take on the odour of acetone.
- ► *Cryptic tonsils.* In some people, the cavities on the surface of the tonsils are larger than average and accumulate deposits of food and saliva that cause white blotches to form on the tonsils.

▶ *Your imagination!* Many people think they have bad breath, but actually do not.

Aphtha (canker sores)

▶ *Unknown causes,* in 80% of cases. Canker sores may be viral or bacterial in origin. The patient may have a genetic predisposition. Fatigue and stress are possible triggers, as well as iron, folic acid, vitamin B_{12} and zinc deficiencies. They may also develop from oral trauma (after a dental procedure, for example), inflammatory

The normal mouth and benign anomalies

Many people get worried when they examine the inside of their mouths because they don't quite know what they should see. Normal colouring for the inside of the mouth varies from shades of pink to red. The raised bumps at the base of the tongue are taste buds. The red spots scattered over the surface of the tongue are benign dilations of small veins.

"Geographic tongue" is a completely harmless anomaly of unknown origin. In such cases, the taste buds disappear on certain parts of the tongue, creating smooth patches surrounded by white lines. The tongue may be more sensitive in the smooth areas, but mild analgesics can be taken to relieve the pain.

"Hairy tongue" is a condition that develops when the taste buds become more prominent than usual. This prompts the bacteria normally present in the mouth to create a pigment that turns the tongue a shade of brown. This is also a benign condition and normal colour can be temporarily restored by brushing the tongue.

People who respond to stress by tensing their jaws and grinding their teeth (frequently during sleep) are often afflicted with lesions on the inside of their cheeks. This phenomenon is known as bruxism and can be relieved with relaxation techniques. If pain occurs, a removable dental prosthesis can be worn at night to stop the upper and lower teeth from grinding. Ask your dentist.

digestive tract diseases (such as Crohn's disease), the use of certain drugs (barbiturates and anti-epileptics), or the fluctuations of the menstrual cycle.

PRACTICAL ADVICE

Dryness of the mouth and bad breath

Drink liquids. Drinking large amounts of water and fruit juice is highly recommended, especially if you are taking antidepressants or antihistamines.

Eat well. Choose a variety of food, with large helpings of fruit and vegetables.

Drink tea and coffee in moderation. These beverages cause dehydration, just like alcohol.

Use mouthwash sparingly. The alcohol and flavours contained in mouthwash may irritate the oral mucous membranes. Use it only as often as you brush your teeth, after meals and before going to bed.

Be physically active and do relaxation exercises. Both can minimize the effects of stress.

Use artificial saliva. This medication is available over-the-counter in spray form and is especially indispensable for people suffering from Sjögren's syndrome or receiving radiation therapy.

Canker sores

Take painkillers. Taken before meals, analgesics can relieve the pain and make eating easier. Take one or two acetaminophen tablets (325 mg to 500 mg), up to four grams a day. Anti-inflammatories are also helpful. Follow the dosage recommended by the manufacturer. If the pain is difficult to control, take both types of medication.

Avoid food that is too hot, spicy or salty. These types of food can exacerbate the pain.

Avoid treatments that claim to accelerate healing. It has never been proven that milk of magnesia, chamomile, vitamin C, vitamin E, yogurt, lemon, or mouthwash containing diluted hydrogen peroxide have any healing properties. Similarly, the direct application of tea bags or ice cubes to the ulcer is not known to be effective.

Never apply salt directly to an ulcer. This will increase the burning sensation and may aggravate the problem. Rinsing your mouth with salt water, however, may provide some relief.

Do not burn the ulcer. Do not apply aspirin or silver nitrate to the canker sore as it causes pain and does nothing to speed up the healing process.

Use over-the-counter products. Orabase, a gelatin applied on the canker sore to protect it from air and food particles, will ease the pain. Amosan, a mouthwash, is also effective. Avoid viscous xylocaine (for example, Oragel). This is a topical analgesic that numbs the reflexes and may cause choking when you eat.

Be careful not to spread the virus. Your canker sore may be contagious so don't take any chances while you have one: avoid sharing your glass, cup, eating utensils, toothbrush, and refrain from kissing anyone.

Be patient. Canker sores heal by themselves in seven to ten days.

WHEN TO CONSULT?
- You are generally run-down. You feel feverish and tired. You are losing weight and have difficulty eating.
- Bumps or swelling on your neck are apparent to the touch.
- You feel like there is a foreign object in your throat.
- Your mouth or throat is covered with white spots or a whitish membrane.
- You have had a mouth ulcer for more than ten days.

WHAT HAPPENS DURING THE EXAM?

Most problems can be identified through manual palpation of the head and neck and a visual examination. If a throat examination is required, it will be performed by endoscopy, which involves the insertion of a soft or rigid tube containing a fiber-optic beam. If necessary, the doctor orders a blood analysis, laboratory tests or X-rays. Biopsies are ordered if there are lesions (such as leukoplakia or a tumour).

WHAT IS THE TREATMENT?

Bad breath, dryness of the mouth and recurring sore throats can be successfully treated by keeping the body hydrated, maintaining a healthy diet, getting proper rest, regular physical exercise, learning how to relax, and quitting smoking. If cryptic tonsils cause chronic sore throats as well as bad breath, they may be surgically removed. Candida albicans is eliminated with a prescription antifungal medication. For persistent canker sores, the cause determines the treatment. In addition, cortisone-based medication (such as Kenalog Orabase) may be prescribed to relieve inflammation. The doctor may also ask the pharmacist to prepare a medicated mouthwash (containing antihistamines, antifungals, cortisone and antibiotics).

Restless Legs Syndrome

Restless legs syndrome (RLS) describes a discomfort of the muscles in the lower limbs that creates an irresistible urge to move the legs. This is a common condition also known as Ekbom syndrome or akathisia.

This phenomenon occurs primarily when the legs are at rest (lying in bed or sitting in a movie theatre, for example). It is most common in people over 30 and the rate of occurrence increases with age. For unknown reasons, women are slightly more at risk than men. The condition causes intermittent and benign reflex movements of the legs and in most cases, is not associated with any particular illness.

Restless legs syndrome usually presents in the following manner:
- Discomfort or tingling, twitching sensations under the skin of the thighs and calves.
- An irresistible compulsion to move the legs.
- In rare cases, pain.

WHAT ARE THE CAUSES?

- *Organic disorders.* While commonly believed to be a vascular disturbance, recent studies show that RLS is instead caused by fibre irritability in the nervous system. There is often a family history of the disorder.
- *Risk factors.* The syndrome may arise at any time, although certain factors have been associated with its appearance, including fatigue, stress, certain medications (particularly neuroleptics used to treat depression), tobacco (according to certain studies) and stimulants (coffee, tea, chocolate, alcohol).

PRACTICAL ADVICE

Do not worry. Restless legs syndrome is a benign condition with no adverse health consequences. It is similar to a twitching eyelid or blushing.

Stand up and walk around for a few minutes. This is the best way to relieve the discomfort.

Take a hot bath to relax your muscles. Particularly if you are stressed or exhausted.

Massage. Massaging the legs (with or without massage oil) effectively decreases muscle tension.

Modify your lifestyle. If you suffer from RLS, decreasing your consumption of stimulants (tea, coffee, chocolate and alcohol), quitting smoking and learning relaxation techniques to manage stress should improve your condition.

In serious cases, take painkillers. If the problem regularly affects sleep for you or your partner, acetaminophen or anti-inflammatories before bed may relieve the symptoms. Take two acetaminophen tablets (325 mg to 500 mg), or follow the manufacturer's recommendation for anti-inflammatories. This may help decrease the frequency of leg movements during the night.

WHEN TO CONSULT?
► The practical advice outlined in this chapter does not help and RLS is seriously compromising the quality of sleep for you or your partner.

WHAT HAPPENS DURING THE EXAM?
The doctor takes a history and performs a physical exam. Diagnosis is usually easy to establish and additional tests are rarely required.

WHAT IS THE TREATMENT?
Three classes of medication can be used to treat restless legs syndrome.

Benzodiazepines and propoxyphene
Your physician may prescribe a benzodiazepine (to relax the muscles). Analgesics such as propoxyphene have also been successfully used to relieve the aches and discomfort of restless legs syndrome. Warning: do not take a larger dose or take it for longer than

prescribed by your doctor and be sure not to take propoxyphene in combination with other medications that cause drowsiness.

Antiparkinsonian drugs
Even though restless legs syndrome is in no way related to Parkinson's disease, antiparkinsonian drugs may soothe the discomfort if the above medications offer no relief.

Sciatic Pain

The sciatic nerve is the largest in the human body and has a number of roots. Beginning in the upper buttocks, the nerve runs down the thigh to the knee, where it splits into two. One branch (the external popliteal sciatic nerve) innervates the muscles of the shin, while the other (the internal popliteal sciatic nerve) controls the calf muscles. The sciatic nerve is responsible for motor skills and sensitivity in the lower legs.

In most cases, sciatic pain, or sciatica, is caused by compression, irritation or damage to one (or in rare cases, two or more) of the sciatic nerve roots.

The pain manifests in one of the following ways:

- ► Usually, the pain shoots from the hip or buttocks down to the area just below the knee.
- ► The pain may radiate down to the foot.
- ► The pain may start in the lower leg, moving down to the foot.
- ► The pain may be felt in one or both legs.
- ► There may be numbness or tingling in the painful area.
- ► There may be loss of sensation in the leg (muscle weakness).
- ► The sufferer may have difficulty moving the foot and toes.
- ► In rare cases, the sufferer has difficulty raising the foot to walk.
- ► The sufferer may experience urinary or anal incontinence, in extremely rare cases.
- ► Erectile dysfunction (or impotence), in extremely rare cases.

WHAT ARE THE CAUSES?

- ► *Herniated disc.* This is the primary cause of sciatica. A herniated disc occurs when part of the lumbar disc (the cushion between two vertebrae) protrudes from its natural cavity, compromising one or more sciatic nerve roots. Excessive physical effort (such as lifting a heavy object), certain contact sports (hockey or football, for example), or even regular movements can displace the disc. Pregnant women are also at risk, because of the excess weight they are carrying. As well as affecting the sciatic nerve, herniated discs also cause back pain. In very rare cases, the disc can affect the roots of nerves controlling the genital organs and sphincter muscles, causing urinary or anal incontinence and even erectile dysfunction.

- **Central spinal stenosis.** Degenerating spinal support structures can cause the inside of the spinal column to shrink, compressing and irritating the roots of the sciatic nerve and impeding the blood circulation that normally provides nourishment to these roots. This condition usually causes pain in both legs, whether the sufferer is walking or standing still.
- **Lateral spinal stenosis.** In this condition, degenerating spinal support structures cause the shrinking of the orifices through which the sciatic nerve roots branch out. Compression and irritation of the nerve root cause pain, usually in one leg, that manifests either while walking or at rest.
- **Trauma.** For example, a car accident causing a pelvic fracture can injure the sciatic nerve.
- **Cancer.** A tumour in the spinal column or pelvis, or a cancer in metastasis (spreading throughout the body) can compress one or many roots of the sciatic nerve.

PRACTICAL ADVICE

Take a painkiller. To ease the pain, take two tablets of acetaminophen (325 mg to 500 mg) every four hours, never exceeding 4 grams daily. Anti-inflammatories are also helpful; follow the manufacturer's dosage recommendations. Take both medications if the pain is difficult to control. Be careful: some medication is contra-indicated for pregnant women, particularly during the first trimester. Speak to your doctor.

Lie on your back. Lie on your back and bring your knees to your chest, so that the entire surface of your back touches the floor. Keep your back as straight as possible. Use a pillow under your head, if it helps. Stay in this position for a few minutes until the pain subsides.

Lie in a foetal position. Lie on your side with your head and knees curled into your chest. Or lie on your back with your hips and knees bent at a 90-degree angle, your feet resting on a chair. Stay in this position until you feel better.

Apply heat to the painful area. Warm up the area by covering it with an electric blanket, hot compress, or by taking a hot bath. Keep the area warm for 20 to 30 minutes. Repeat several times a day, as needed.

Get a massage. Massage releases natural analgesics called endorphins, which makes it an effective way to ease the pain. Have someone gently massage the painful area (the lower back and buttocks), but be sure he or she does not apply too much pressure, as this can cause pain.

Move around. Staying in bed for several days will do nothing to help the pain. Moving around can help recovery, so continue doing at least some of your daily activities.

Slowly resume physical activity. Once the sciatic pain has subsided, resume as much regular physical exercise (walking, for example) as you can tolerate. Regular exercise helps prevent attacks and eases the pain more quickly. Ask your doctor to suggest a regime for you.

Avoid intense physical effort. Taking part in intense physical activity you are not trained for can lead to a herniated disc.

WHEN TO CONSULT?

► You feel intense pain.
► The pain lasts for more than three weeks.
► Your leg feels weak.
► You are suffering from urinary or anal incontinence or erectile dysfunction.

WHAT HAPPENS DURING THE EXAM?

The doctor interviews the patient and performs a physical examination. He or she may also order spinal X-rays, axial tomodensitometry

(CT scan), or magnetic resonance imaging to identify the cause of the sciatica. Electromyography (E.M.G.) tests are sometimes ordered to assess the damage to the sciatic nerve roots. Blood tests may also be required.

WHAT IS THE TREATMENT?

Herniated disc

If a lumbar disc protrudes from its cavity, it generally moves back into position by itself. Nevertheless, a herniated disc requires the moderation of physical activity for a few weeks, or in rare cases, a few months. Analgesics, anti-inflammatories or cortisone injections can be prescribed to ease the pain. If the sciatica has not cleared up after four to six weeks, the doctor may recommend physiotherapy (ultrasounds, weak electrical currents, massage, etc.) to help ease the pain and speed recovery (specific exercise regime). In less than 5% of cases, surgery is required to remove a lumbar disc.

Pregnant women with herniated discs are usually referred to a physiotherapist for pain relief. The problem usually corrects itself after childbirth.

Central and lateral spinal stenosis

Analgesics or cortisone injections are prescribed. In some cases, surgery is needed to reduce the degree of stenosis.

Trauma

Surgery may be required to stabilize a fracture. If not, painkillers or physiotherapy (or a combination of the two) is prescribed. The more severe the trauma, the higher the risk of chronic sciatic pain.

Cancer

The appropriate treatment is immediately undertaken.

Sensitivity to Light (Photosensitivity)

Everyone, to some degree, experiences sensitivity to light (for example, when leaving a darkened cinema). The eye must adapt to the change in brightness, resulting in discomfort at times. This discomfort is natural. Fair-skinned, blue-eyed individuals are particularly sensitive to light.

One particular phenomenon known as photophobia requires medical attention. Photophobia is defined as an intolerance of light severe enough to induce pain.

Other accompanying symptoms include headaches, dizzy spells and eye irritation.

WHAT ARE THE CAUSES?

- ► *Eye disorders,* such as conjunctivitis, blepharitis (inflammation of the eyelids), uveitis (inflammation of the inner layer of the eye), or glaucoma. A foreign object in the eye or an abrasion (scratched eye surface) can also trigger photosensitivity. In fact, any eye problem can cause some degree of photosensitivity.
- ► *Systemic illnesses.* Measles can give rise to minor keratitis (inflammation of the cornea). Uveitis and, consequently, photophobia, may accompany arthritis and other inflammatory diseases.
- ► *Certain drugs.* Most eye drops cause some degree of photophobia. Moreover, some individuals who take beta-blockers to manage high blood pressure may experience photophobia.
- ► *Contact lenses* can cause microscopic lesions to the eye that, in the long term, expose it to the risk of photophobia.
- ► *External factors.* A particularly warm, dry wind, exposure to certain gases such as tear gas) and cayenne pepper can trigger photophobia. Not to mention smog. When the air is warm and dry, the sun's rays are directed downwards in a straight line and are immediately absorbed by the earth. On particularly humid days, however, when there is dust in the atmosphere, the rays strike these particles and are

refracted directly into the eyes. Hence the tendency for them to sting somewhat even on a hazy day when the sun's rays seem filtered.

▶ *Cataracts* do not necessarily cause photophobia (as there is no pain), although certain types result in significantly heightened sensitivity.

PRACTICAL ADVICE

Avoid rubbing your eyes. Rubbing your eyes only aggravates the situation.

Identify the cause and take remedial action. For example, remove the foreign body or take out contact lenses if they are the culprit.

Apply cold compresses to relieve the pain. Analgesics may also offer pain relief. Do not, however, take drugs without knowing their specific indications or side effects. Always seek the opinion of an expert.

Wear sunglasses. There are excellent anti-UV lenses available. Choose a frame that also protects your eyes from the sides of the face. The colour of the lens is not particularly important, although orange lenses are recommended for winter sports, as they give a clearer image of the terrain, accentuating the contours in the snow. Polarized lenses cut the glare of the sun and are especially practical for water sports, skiing and other winter sports.

WHEN TO CONSULT?

▶ Symptoms occur suddenly.
▶ The onset of symptoms is moderate, but is ongoing for two to three days.
▶ You are undergoing treatment for an ocular condition and are experiencing pain.
▶ You wear contact lenses and experience photophobia.
▶ You are prone to glaucoma and experience eye pain and diminished vision.
▶ You suffer from arthritis or an inflammatory disease and have recently developed an eye disorder.

► You are diabetic and have noticed a change in your vision or eye discomfort. Diabetics should have ophthalmological exams annually.

WHAT HAPPENS DURING THE EXAM?

The doctor will perform a thorough eye exam. In most cases, he or she will be able to identify the cause and recommend the appropriate treatment.

WHAT IS THE TREATMENT?

Eye disorders

Antibiotics will be necessary if there is an infection. Anti-inflammatories can be used to treat inflammation. Glaucoma is treated with medications that reduce pressure inside the eye.

Systemic diseases

The doctor will treat the underlying disease causing keratits, uveitis, or photophobia. In some cases, eye damage is irreversible and smoked lenses should be worn to protect the eyes.

Medications

If the patient's medication is causing pronounced photophobia, the doctor may modify the prescription.

Contact lenses

If contact lenses are the culprit, they cannot be worn for as long as the problem persists. In most instances, there is no recurrence.

Cataracts

Surgery is required to replace the crystalline lens with an artificial one.

Shivering

Shivering is defined as general, irregular, and transient trembling caused by a sensation of cold. In most cases, especially when briefly endured, it merely indicates that the body is cooling down. If other symptoms (fever, headache, muscle pain) are also present, however, an infection or underlying disease may be indicated.

WHAT ARE THE CAUSES?

- *Cold.* This is the main cause. When the body becomes cold, all the muscles contract to warm it up. The contraction of the muscles under the surface of the skin causes goosebumps and shivering, which, if uncontrollable, may indicate the early stages of hypothermia.
- *Infectious diseases,* such as the flu, gynecological or urinary infections, pneumonia, bronchitis, or sinusitis. In most cases, a fever appears approximately fifteen minutes after the shivering begins. An attack by a virus or bacteria not only raises the body temperature but also causes the blood vessels to contract, giving the sufferer the impression of cold, clammy skin. Headaches and muscle pain may also appear in cases of viral infection. In the elderly, shivering and confusion may be a sign of infection, even in the absence of fever.
- *Malaria or typhoid fever,* usually contracted in foreign countries, cause fever and shivering.
- *Diabetes.* Diabetics are particularly subject to infection and may experience shivering when a sore fails to heal.
- *Drug intoxication.* Heroin, cocaine, ecstasy, PCP (Phencyclidine hydrochloride), or any other illicit drug can cause shivering, fever, an altered state of consciousness, agitation, and convulsions.
- *Drug allergies.* Shivering is often accompanied by rashes, fever, and in some cases, edema.
- *Underlying diseases,* such as cancer.
- *Sudden stress,* or a "close shave", such as almost being hit by a car.

PRACTICAL ADVICE

Control the symptoms. Take one or two acetaminophen tablets (325 mg to 500 mg, four times a day, never exceeding 4 grams daily) to control shivering, lower body temperature and soothe sore muscles and headaches. Anti-inflammatories can also help; follow the manufacturer's recommended dosage (if prescribed doses are not followed, the symptoms may return). If this does not significantly reduce your temperature, the infection may be serious and require medical attention.

Give children acetaminophen. Ibuprofen is an anti-inflammatory that even adults should take with caution. Children's fevers should be treated with acetaminophen. Calculate the doses at 15 mg for every kilogram of body weight and administer them every four hours, never exceeding five doses a day. If ineffective, use ibuprofen (30 mg per kilogram of body weight per day, spread over three or four doses every six to eight hours). Never give ibuprofen to a dehydrated child, as this can cause liver damage.

Never give aspirin to a child. Even baby aspirin should be avoided. In the presence of a viral infection (particularly, but not exclusively, chickenpox), aspirin can cause Reye's syndrome (a serious neurological, kidney and liver disease primarily affecting children). As fever is a common symptom of infection, aspirin should be avoided in all cases. Acetaminophen is the recommended medication. After the age of 14 the child can be given aspirin if he or she has had the chickenpox or been vaccinated.

Do not use rubbing alcohol. A rubdown with this product can cause the skin to absorb the alcohol, possibly leading to poisoning. It also does very little to relieve shivering.

Drink plenty of liquids. If the fever or hypothermia is accompanied by shivering, it is very important to remain properly hydrated.

Avoid alcohol. Alcohol affects mental capacity, can cause loss of consciousness or falling, and masks other potentially dangerous symptoms. In cold weather, for example, people who have drunk alcohol feel warm even though their bodies are actually losing heat rapidly.

Never take medications that were not prescribed for you. Even if you suffer from the same disease, do not take antibiotics or any other medication prescribed for another person without a doctor's advice.

Relax. Try to relax if you are feeling especially stressed. Provide comfort and a sympathetic ear to anyone who has recently suffered an emotional shock.

Take a bath. Room temperature baths can help get rid of the shivers.

Get some rest. Your immune system becomes more and more vulnerable to the flu virus as fatigue accumulates.

WHEN TO CONSULT?

► Your child is shivering, running a fever, irritable and lethargic. He or she does not respond to the proper doses of acetaminophen or ibuprofen. Consult immediately—your child may have meningitis or encephalitis. A body temperature of over 40°C can provoke convulsions in a child.
► You shiver constantly.
► Shivering and fever persist for more than an hour after treatment.
► Your temperature has remained above 39°C for more than 48 hours, despite medication.
► Shivering is accompanied by respiratory problems, coughing and pain.
► You shiver so intensely that your teeth chatter.
► You are shivering and suffer from a disorder that affects the immune system, such as diabetes, cancer, lymphoma or leukemia.
► You are shivering and have had a hip or cardiac valve replacement (shivering may be a sign of infection).
► You are shivering and taking oral corticosteroids (cortisone weakens the immune system).

➤ You begin to shiver after being bitten by a dog or cat.
➤ You are shivering and have undergone treatment for cancer, or been in remission for less than five years.

WHAT HAPPENS DURING THE EXAM?

The doctor takes a history and performs a complete physical examination, looking for other symptoms such as pain, coughing, or fever. Blood tests may be ordered. In cases of drug intoxication, special tests assess the level of drugs in the patient's blood or urine.

WHAT IS THE TREATMENT?

Infectious diseases
The doctor may prescribe antibiotics.

Malaria or typhoid fever
These diseases are treated with the appropriate medication. To prevent them in the first place, take a prophylactic drug both before leaving and after coming back from a tropical country.

Drug intoxication
In cases of drug intoxication, the patient requires hospital supervision of kidney, liver and heart function until he or she regains consciousness.

Drug allergies
In the six hours after ingestion, the substances are removed from the body by stomach pump or (preferably) the administration of activated charcoal, which absorbs the contaminants and prevents them from spreading further through the system.

Underlying diseases
The disease will determine the treatment.

Shortness of Breath Due to Heart Disease

Dyspnea—shortness of breath—develops due to a number of conditions, including lung disease, anemia, anguish (emotional or mental distress), or poor physical condition. It is also a symptom of various forms of heart disease.

In these cases, dyspnea is usually not a chronic problem, but a new condition that has only developed over recent days, weeks or months. Sufferers who become short of breath with exertion usually breathe normally again when at rest. If shortness of breath develops in the absence of exertion (sometimes even waking the sufferer), an even more serious heart condition is indicated. Fatigue, chest pain, palpitations and fainting are other frequent symptoms of heart disease

WHAT ARE THE CAUSES?

► *Heart failure.* If not controlled, coronary artery disease, high blood pressure, or other heart conditions may evolve into heart failure. Heart contractions become weaker because the walls and muscles of the heart are too rigid and cannot relax. Unable to pump enough blood to the body, the weakened heart does not fully release its contraction, causing increased blood pressure in the lungs that in turn leads to dyspnea, the primary symptom of heart failure. Sufferers generally tend to use more pillows at night to ease breathing. They may also experience fatigue, expectorate blood, and develop edema in the legs and feet. If left untreated, the heart may suddenly give out, causing intense congestion known as acute pulmonary edema. The symptoms are extreme shortness of breath and a feeling of smothering. This requires immediate emergency consultation.

► *Angina pectoris* is one manifestation of coronary artery disease. It is caused by the obstruction of the coronary arteries, which results from a progressive cholesterol accumulation over a number of years. During an angina attack, the sufferer usually experiences dyspnea and intense chest pain (heaviness or pressure), often developing with exertion, but, in some cases, when the patient is at rest or sleeping. Diabetics suffering from angina do not experience chest pain, although they do become short of breath. In many cases, the symptoms of angina pectoris act as an early warning sign for heart attack and require immediate medical consultation. People with one or more of the risk factors for coronary artery disease (smoking, high cholesterol, high blood pressure, diabetes, obesity or sedentary lifestyles) must be particularly cautious. High-risk groups also include people with a family history of early coronary artery disease or previously diagnosed heart conditions.

► *Arrhythmia.* This general term refers to any abnormal heart rhythm caused by problems with the electrical signals inside the heart, from the most benign (caused by stress or certain medications) to the most severe. Tachycardia (accelerated heart rhythm) frequently leads to dyspnea, heart palpitations, dizziness and sometimes fainting. Bradycardia (slow heart rhythm) leads to weakness, dizziness, dyspnea and faintness. Arrythmia may accompany pre-existing heart conditions.

► *Valve disease.* Proper blood circulation is ensured by four valves inside the heart: the tricuspid, pulmonary, mitral and aortic valves. Patients with a heart murmur (sign of a defective valve, perceptible through a stethoscope) or those who suffered from rheumatic fever at a young age risk developing valvular stenosis (shrinking) or regurgitation (leaking) of one or more valves later on. In severe cases, dyspnea that initially only occurred with exertion begins to develop during rest or even sleep, as well. In some cases, patients also experience heart palpitations, faintness and chest pain.

PRACTICAL ADVICE

Be vigilant. It is normal to become short of breath after climbing a set of stairs quickly. However, if you become abnormally short of breath with exertion, while at rest or sleeping, consult a doctor immediately, or go to the emergency room if the condition is intense and persistent. Even in the absence of chest pain, dyspnea may be a sign of heart disease or an incipient heart attack.

Adopt a healthy lifestyle. Quit smoking: you will live longer and decrease your risk of coronary artery disease. Maintain a healthy weight by eating well (follow the Canada Food Guide) and exercising daily. Thirty to forty minutes of fast walking, at least three or four times a week, is a step in the right direction.

Get a checkup. After the age of 40, a complete medical checkup for men often includes tests for diabetes, high blood pressure, and cholesterol. Female hormones offer some protection to women from coronary artery disease prior to menopause.

WHEN TO CONSULT?

- ► You become abnormally short of breath with exertion, particularly if this is a new development.
- ► Shortness of breath develops when you are at rest, or wakes you up at night.
- ► You are diabetic and have recently become unusually short of breath.
- ► You have risk factors associated with coronary artery disease.
- ► You currently suffer from heart disease, or have suffered from heart disease in the past.

WHAT HAPPENS DURING THE EXAM?

The doctor takes a detailed history and performs a complete physical examination. He or she checks for lung disease, anemia, mental distress, and determines the patient's overall physical condition. Blood tests, electrocardiograms (recording the heart's electrical activity), heart and lung X-rays, and cardiac ultrasounds may be required. A treadmill test (perhaps involving nuclear medicine tests) may be ordered if coronary artery disease is suspected.

The doctor may also refer the patient to a cardiologist, who may order further in-depth testing (heart catheters or coronary angiography).

WHAT IS THE TREATMENT?

Heart disease cannot be cured. The aim of treatment, therefore, is to slow the progression of the disease, ease the symptoms, improve the patient's quality of life, and, if possible, allow him or her to live a long, productive and enjoyable life. Medications are usually prescribed for life.

Heart failure

This insidious disease requires the patient to carefully follow treatment. In most cases, the doctor prescribes combined medications (angiotensin converting enzyme inhibitors, certain types of diuretics, digoxin, beta-blockers, or calcium channel blockers). Sometimes, coronary artery dilation, coronary bypass or valve replacement surgery is required, depending on the origin of the heart failure. In very serious cases, heart transplant surgery is necessary. Some people are able to eliminate their symptoms by controlling their blood pressure.

Arrhythmia

The doctor may recommend implanting a pacemaker to correct symptomatic bradycardia. Tachycardia is treated with anti-arrhythmic drugs or, in serious cases, surgery to interrupt the arrhythmia or implant a defibrillator.

If heart medication has caused the arrhythmia, the prescription is modified.

Coronary artery disease

Nitroglycerine (in pill or spray form) provides rapid relief from shortness of breath and angina. The patient must visit the doctor again if his or her need for the medication is increasing. If the patient has taken three successive doses of nitroglycerine in five-minute intervals and the symptoms have not disappeared, he or she must go to the emergency room.

Angina attacks are prevented with medication (nitrates, beta-blockers, calcium channel blockers) and, in severe or difficult cases, coronary artery dilation or bypass surgery is required.

Aspirin is an essential treatment to reduce the risk of heart attack.

Valve disease

Surgery to replace or repair the defective valves may be required, as well as a life-long prescription for anticoagulant medication.

Shoulder Pain

The shoulder is one of the most complex joints in the human body, which also means it is one of the most fragile. Overuse or misuse of the joint easily leads to injury and, of course, pain.

Shoulder pain may:
► Occur when the arm is moved upward.
► Prevent movement or lock the shoulder.
► Radiate towards the neck or the fingers.
► Spread quickly if caused by inflammation, since all the structures of the joint then come into direct contact with one another.

WHAT ARE THE CAUSES?

► *Tendinitis and bursitis* (with or without calcium deposits) are the most common complaints of those who consult for shoulder pain. Tendinitis is an inflammation of the tendons attached to the joint, while bursitis affects the bursa protecting the tendons. The conditions are usually caused by repetitive movement (such as sawing wood, playing golf, pitching a baseball, or working with the arms elevated). In some cases, constant rubbing against the acromion, a shelf of bone in the shoulder-blade, leads to erosion of the tendons and rupture of the rotator cuff (covering the head of the humerus). This is known as "impingement syndrome". Tendinitis and bursitis are inflammatory conditions that cause increasing pain as the arm is raised or pulled back (for example, to put on a shirt); they may be accompanied by calcium deposits (a type of internal scarring).

► *Trauma.* Breaking a fall with the arm frequently leads to trauma of various kinds, from simple fractures, to partial dislocations of the shoulder (partial popping out of the joint, although still held by the tendons), to complete dislocations, and dislocations accompanied by a fracture or torn tendon.

► *Arthritis* is an inflammatory disease attacking and sometimes destroying one or several joints.

- *Osteoarthritis* is caused by the erosion of joints during the normal aging process.
- *Capsulitis* is caused by a shrinking of the capsule (membrane surrounding the shoulder) after inflammation, making it impossible to raise the arm. It frequently affects young women in their thirties (probably due to repetitive movement).
- *Bone or lung cancer.* In cases of lung cancer, pain can radiate to the shoulder.

PRACTICAL ADVICE

Avoid painful movements. Performing the motions you find painful may delay healing or aggravate your condition.

Rest the joint. Immobilize your shoulder in a sling, remembering, however, that you must not do so for more than one to two weeks. While using it, perform the following exercises as often as possible: with your arm free, fold your fingers into your hand, then straighten and spread them as far as possible. Straighten your arm, and let it hang down as you bend forward. Repeat 5 to 10 times. These exercises are also recommended for the days immediately following the accident to stimulate blood circulation and lower the risk of ankylosis ("frozen shoulder").

Apply ice first. Apply a bag of ice wrapped in a towel several times a day for three days in 20-minute intervals. This will reduce swelling and pain.

Then apply heat. Heat should only be applied when the acute stage has passed. A hot water bottle wrapped in a towel or a heating pad stimulates blood circulation and directs waste products away from the painful area.

Alternate heat and cold. After the first three days of cold treatment, give the circulation in the shoulder an extra boost by applying five minutes of heat followed by five minutes of cold. Repeat three times, three times a day.

Do not resume regular activities immediately. Once the problem has been treated, return to your regular routine slowly. Remember that your joint is still fragile and can be easily re-injured.

Never lift or carry weights at shoulder level, as this is very bad for your shoulder joint.

Alternate activities. If baseball makes your shoulder sore, try bicycling for a few days.

Take painkillers. To ease the pain, take one or two acetaminophen tablets (325 mg to 500 mg) four times a day, never exceeding 4 grams daily. Anti-inflammatories are also helpful; follow the manufacturer's dosage recommendations. Take both medications if the pain is difficult to manage.

Maintain your flexibility. After the acute stage has passed, do the following exercise: let your arm hang along the side of your body, then gently swing it back and forth, keeping the elbow straight.

Strengthening exercises. Once your shoulder has healed, do the following exercises after warming up and stretching.
► imagine you are drying your back with a towel, one hand holding the edge of the towel at shoulder-height, the other at hip-level. Make full, complete movements, alternating the position of the arms.
► keeping your bent elbows against the body, put an elastic band around your two wrists and pull them apart. Repeat 30 times, 3 times a day.

WHEN TO CONSULT?
► You have had an accident. Your shoulder is sore, does not move normally, or is obviously misshapen.
► The pain in your shoulder is not related to movement, but constant and an impediment to sleep.
► Pain in your shoulder becomes worse when you move your arm.

► You have followed our practical advice for three weeks and the pain persists.

WHAT HAPPENS DURING THE EXAM?

In the case of trauma, X-rays are used to eliminate causes such as arthritis, osteoarthritis, or cancer (bone or lung).

If initial treatment is not effective, the doctor may order more in-depth examinations using a diagnostic ultrasound, arthrography (X-rays with liquid contrast) or magnetic resonance imaging (MRI).

WHAT IS THE TREATMENT?

Tendinitis and bursitis

These conditions are treated with rest, anti-inflammatories, physiotherapy and steroid infiltrations. The inflammation generally disappears after three or four weeks. Recurrences are common and depend on the stage of bone erosion. Surgery may be necessary to stop the impingement of the rotator cuff and remove calcium deposits.

Arthritis

Arthritis is treated with anti-inflammatories and cortisone infiltrations (no more than two or three a year, as cortisone can destroy healthy joints).

Osteoarthritis

As long as the joint can still move, treatment generally focuses on pain management. Once the joint has completely worn out, it can be replaced with a prosthesis.

Capsulitis

This condition usually lasts 12 to 18 months and resolves on its own or with the help of physiotherapy. In some cases, cortisone infiltrations are administered.

Trauma

Some joint dislocations can be manually replaced; if not, surgery is required. Tendon or capsule tears must be repaired. The latter is a major procedure and contra-indicated for the elderly due to the low success rates in this age group. In the case of a fracture that only slightly displaces the bone, the patient wears a splint for two weeks. In very severe cases, the doctor inserts a screw, plate, or prosthesis, and the patient wears a sling or splint for a few weeks. In other instances, the patient wears a cast to hold the bone in place.

Skin Discoloration

Skin discoloration is caused by a pigmentation disorder. Hyperpigmentation is responsible for the development of dark or brown patches of skin, while hypopigmentation leads to the appearance of pale or white patches.

Hyperpigmentation is generally caused by chloasma (also known as melasma) or lentigo. Hypopigmentation is usually the result of one of three disorders: vitiligo, pityriasis versicolor or pityriasis alba. None of these conditions are contagious.

These diseases present in the following manner:

Chloasma (also known as melasma)
- Large brownish patches, appearing most frequently on the face (more rarely on the arms).
- Dark patches become more apparent during the summer due to sun exposure.
- Condition lasts a few months to several years.
- May spontaneously disappear.
- Especially common in women who are pregnant or undergoing hormone replacement therapy.

Lentigo
- Small beige or brown spots.
- Usually appear in areas most often exposed to the sun (face, shoulders, arms, back of the hands, legs).
- Do not spontaneously disappear.
- Tend to increase in number and size with time.
- Also known as "age spots".

Vitiligo
- White patches of varying sizes appear on the face, hands and in the genital area.

► In some cases, patches develop all over the body.
► Condition is usually permanent and may become more pronounced over time.
► In rare cases, patches may spontaneously disappear and recur.

Pityriasis versicolor

► Small blotches, usually pink and dry at first, accompanied by itchiness.
► After a few weeks, the blotches whiten and the itchiness resolves.
► Generally develop on the back, chest, arms and shoulders.
► May spontaneously disappear and recur.
► Usually occurs in the summer.

Pityriasis alba

► Small whitish and dry blotches.
► Generally disappear at puberty.
► Usually located on the upper body (face, arms and shoulders).
► In rare cases, is accompanied by itchiness.
► Tends to disappear and recur.
► Usually affects children between the ages of 6 and 12.

WHAT ARE THE CAUSES?

Chloasma (melasma)

► *Triggering factors.* While medical research has not yet discovered the origin of this skin disease, it has been able to identify certain trigger factors, such as hormone changes associated with pregnancy (chloasma is also known as the "mask of pregnancy"), the birth control pill and hormone replacement therapy for menopausal women. Exposure to the sun may also be a trigger, as it is known to stimulate pigment cells. Certain drugs (in particular, anti-epileptic medications) affect the chemical reaction of skin cells.

Lentigo

► *Repeated exposure to the sun.* Over-exposure to the sun for several years can alter the chemical composition of skin pigment and lead to the development of lentigo. Although the condition is most common in people over the age of fifty, people as young as thirty are also at risk. The earlier lentigo appears, the higher the risk of skin cancer.

Vitiligo

► *Heredity.* Vitiligo is a chronic auto-immune disease involving the self-destruction of the skin's pigment cells. General heredity (uncles, aunts, siblings, etc.) is responsible for 30% of cases.

► *Triggering factors.* In many cases, heredity does not play a role. For some, a white vitiligo patch will develop in the area of a minor skin trauma such as a cut, burn, or severe sunburn. Intense emotional trauma (profound grief, loss of a job, or divorce, for example) is another possible trigger. Vitiligo may also accompany other immune system diseases like diabetes (type 1), pernicious anemia, or Addison's disease.

Pityriasis versicolor

► *Pityrosporon orbiculare.* This yeast, normally present on the skin, is in the same family as the yeast responsible for dandruff. It multiplies more quickly in hot and humid environments, particularly in people between the ages of 20 and 45. The specific trigger factor is not yet known.

Beauty Marks and Tanning Salons: Words of Warning

If you notice that your moles or beauty marks have changed colour, texture, or size, see a doctor.

It is also important to consult if new moles appear, particularly if they are very dark or an irregular shape.

Skin self-examinations for early detection of new moles or irregularities are now recommended as an effective way to prevent skin cancer.

Tanning salons? Avoid them. UV rays are harmful, whether they come from a sun lamp in a salon or the sun itself.

Pityriasis alba

► **Eczema.** Medical experts generally believe that this condition is an uncommon form of eczema that temporarily disturbs the skin's pigmentation. Pityriasis alba is sometimes associated with other types of eczema.

PRACTICAL ADVICE

Don't worry. There is no cause for concern and the condition is not contagious, whether the blotches are dark or light. Both vitiligo and pityriasis versicolor are quite common, affecting approximately 2% of the population.

Relieve the itching. A simple moisturizing cream is usually enough to soothe the itch. Calamine lotion is contraindicated because it dries the skin.

Protect yourself from the sun. Darker or lighter patches of skin are more sensitive to the sun. Avoid excessive exposure, particularly between 10 a.m. and 3 p.m., when the sun's rays are at maximum intensity. Wear adequate clothing and a hat, use sunscreen, and stay in shaded areas as much as possible.

Use at least SPF 15 sunscreen. Purchase sunscreens containing parsol 1789, parsol MCX or mexoryl (they may be found in combination). These substances provide effective protection from ultraviolet (UV) rays linked to skin cancer. Sunscreen should be used even on cloudy days in spring, summer and fall, since both ultraviolet A (UVA) and ultraviolet B (UVB) rays penetrate cloud cover. In winter, wear sunscreen on milder days when more skin is exposed. Use specially made products for children.

Treat pityriasis versicolor. Products with a base of selenium sulfide or zinc pyrithione effectively clear away the blotches caused by this condition. These compounds are easily available in anti-dandruff shampoos such as Head and Shoulders, Selsun, or Nizoral. Apply the product on the entire upper body (from neck to waistline). Leave on for 15 to 20 minutes and rinse. Repeat once a day for a week. To avoid recurrences, apply preventive treatments once a month.

WHEN TO CONSULT?
► Dark or light patches or red blotches appear on your body.

WHAT HAPPENS DURING THE EXAM?
After taking note of the pertinent information, the doctor performs a clinical exam. This is usually sufficient for diagnosis.

WHAT IS THE TREATMENT?
Chloasma (melasma)
Treatment requires three elements: sunscreen, a whitening agent, and time.

Sunscreen will prevent the spread of the dark patches, while the whitening agent (a cream with a base of retinol, hydroquinone, or concentrated vitamin C) will bleach the skin.

If these treatments are ineffective, camouflaging creams may be used. Special clinics can teach the patient tricks to hide the patches.

In some cases, laser treatment may be advised. This may not be covered by government medical insurance.

Lentigo
There is no easy treatment to remove age spots, although products with a base of retinol, hydroquinone, or concentrated vitamin C will make them fade somewhat. They can be covered with makeup, and if they are extremely bothersome, the patient can opt for laser treatment, although the process is tedious and expensive. It is very important to avoid exposure to the sun and follow doctor's orders because this condition is often an early indicator of skin damage that is associated with skin cancer.

Vitiligo
Cortisone cream has been used effectively in a number of cases. PUVA phototherapy, a combination of UVA rays and medication (psoralen) is available in the dermatologist's office or in some

hospitals. This treatment may restore the pigment to normal or near-ly-normal levels, although the white patches may recur later on. The doctor may prescribe creams to temporarily colour the skin.

Pityriasis versicolor

For persistent problems, an antifungal cream or spray-on lotion will be prescribed. In severe cases, the doctor may resort to oral antifungal treatment.

Pityriasis alba

There is no specific treatment, since the blotches generally disappear on their own when the child reaches puberty. In the meantime, a mild cortisone cream will soothe the itchiness.

Skin Lesions

In most cases, skin pigmentation marks are harmless and not contagious. Certain lesions are potentially dangerous, however, particularly moles or beauty marks that have been transformed into malignant skin cancers by the destructive rays of the sun.

Skin lesions are grouped into three broad categories.

Moles or beauty marks
- Generally appear at puberty.
- Amount largely determined by heredity.
- Appear as flat or elevated lesions of varying size and colour.
- Are found anywhere on the body, though rarely on the genitals or soles of the feet.
- May have harmless protruding hair.
- May become darker, thicker, raised, and in some cases, unsightly with age.
- May persist for long periods (10 to 40 years), then spontaneously disappear or considerably shrink.
- Are generally benign, but may evolve into malignant cancer.

Brown spots
Senile lentigos
- Commonly known as "age spots".
- Appear between the ages of thirty and forty.
- Occur on the face, forearms, back of the hands, chest and shoulders.
- Are accompanied by wrinkles (skin is often thick or leathery).
- Are frequently grouped together where the skin is more fragile.
- Quantity, colour, size and location determined by extent of sun exposure.
- Are generally benign, but may evolve into malignant cancer.

Hyperpigmentation spots
- May appear during pregnancy (the so-called "mask of pregnancy")

or in women taking birth control pills. In these cases, the condition is temporary.
► More common in individuals with dark skin.
► In some cases, appear on scar tissue.
► Benign.

Seborrheic Keratosis
► Wart-like lesions (the size of the nail on your baby finger) with a dry and irregular surface.
► Initially beige in colour, they darken with sun exposure.
► May appear anywhere on the body.
► Benign.

Lesions secondary to yeast infections
► Pale, peeling lesions.
► May occur all over the body or in only one or two areas.
► Do not darken or tan
► Become red if irritated.
► Benign.

Angiomas or port-wine stain
There are four main types (as well as a number of other, more rare forms)

Common port-wine stain
► Flat lesions of varying sizes.
► Small lesions frequently appearing on the eyelids, neck or forehead.
► Large lesions frequently developing on the cheeks or (rarely) the thorax.
► Are present at birth or appear later in life.
► Red or purplish in colour, these spots are benign (the problem is primarily aesthetic).

Senile angiomas or cherry-red spots
► Quite common.

► Small red spots that may grow bigger.
► Usually start appearing around the age of thirty.
► May appear anywhere on the body (although generally not on the face).
► Benign.

Hemangiomas or strawberry naevus
► Present at birth; disappear around age four or five.
► Elevated.
► Reddish.
► Get bigger in the first month.
► May appear anywhere on the body.
► Benign.

Pyogenic granulomas
► Small tumours developing secondary to a small wound (such as a cut, mosquito bite, or vaccination causing itching and scratching).
► Elevated.
► Bleed readily and abundantly if accidentally caught on clothing.
► Red or purplish in colour.
► Benign.

WHAT ARE THE CAUSES?
Beauty marks
► *Heredity.*
► *The damaging rays of the sun.*

Brown spots
Senile lentigos (age spots)
► *The damaging rays of the sun.*

Hyperpigmentation spots
► *A combination of factors,* including the sun, birth control pills, pregnancy, dark skin and perfume.
► *Wound or scar* exposed to the sun.

Seborrheic keratoses
▶ **Heredity.**

Lesions secondary to yeast infections
▶ **Yeast infections.**

Port-wine stains
Common port wine stain
▶ **Congenital or hereditary.**
▶ **Abnormal accumulation of embryonic blood vessels.**

Cherry red spots
▶ **Hereditary.**

Strawberry naevus
▶ **Congenital.**
▶ **Very rare malformation of the blood vessels.**

Pyogenic granulomas
▶ **Abnormal healing or scarring of a wound.**
▶ **Subsequent abnormal blood vessel development.**

PRACTICAL ADVICE

Avoid tanning salons. These are even more dangerous than the sun's rays.

Protect lesions from the sun. During your treatment, protect the lesions from the sun; even three or four hours of sun exposure will damage the lesion and leave you right back where you started. Wait until you have finished treatment to go out in the sun.

Do not play with your moles. Constant or frequent irritation can cause a number of problems.

Protect yourself from the sun. Start young. If you have many moles or beauty marks, you carry a 15% higher than average risk of developing melanoma (the most virulent form of skin cancer). If it is impossible to completely avoid the sun, wear ample clothing to cover the body, a hat, sunglasses and strong sunscreens (at least SPF 30) on exposed parts of the body. Remember that no sunscreen provides 100% protection and that it should be applied at least 15 minutes before going outside to give the skin time to absorb the cream. If swimming, keep your T-shirt on until you enter the water.

Learn the ABCDE's of moles. Certain qualities or changes in the aspect of a mole are an early indication of trouble. Keep on the lookout for:

A asymmetry (not completely round);
B a border that is irregular or changing;
C colour change or blackness;
D diameters greater than 6 mm; and,
E rapid evolution (one to three months).

Perform a monthly self-examination. Use a mirror. Be particularly vigilant when examining your back, as this is the most difficult area to observe regularly. Remember that melanoma can develop from pre-existing moles or appear out of nowhere. Document any change with periodic photos or videos of your back and skin. Record the dates so you can compare.

Apply dandruff shampoo on secondary yeast infections. Selsun Blue, Head and Shoulders, and Nizoral are equally effective. Apply, wait 15 minutes and rinse, repeating daily for 15 days. The lesions should eventually disappear. If they do not, consult your doctor. Do not follow treatment during the summer (these lesions do not tan and will be more visible after you have absorbed some of the sun's rays).

Epilation of a hairy naevus. This procedure is completely safe. Electrolysis is also an option, although a little less effective.

WHEN TO CONSULT?

► A mole or age spot becomes asymmetrical and its borders fluctuate or become irregular. It becomes partially or completely black.

- The diameter of your mole has increased beyond 6 mm (the size of a pencil eraser) over a period of one to three months. The lesion bleeds easily, burns, itches, or transforms into a cyst or open wound. These are signs of melanoma, one of the most virulent forms of skin cancer. Consult a doctor immediately.
- Your mole is aesthetically or practically inconvenient (often cut or irritated by activities like shaving).
- Your child has a port-wine stain.
- You have pale, persistent skin lesions that do not darken in the sun.

WHAT HAPPENS DURING THE EXAM?

Suspicious moles or lesions are biopsied and sent for laboratory analysis to reach a precise diagnosis. Some lesions, however, only require a simple dermatologic examination. In rare cases of deep and complicated port-wine stains, CT scans, Doppler, or ultrasound can help determine whether there is any risk.

WHAT IS THE TREATMENT?
Beauty marks
Moles that are poorly located (constantly rubbing on clothing, for example) or simply unattractive can be easily removed under local anesthesia. They will then be analyzed, just to be safe. Some lesions can be cauterized or removed by elliptical incision (closing of the resulting wound with stitches). Melanoma is malignant and requires urgent surgery and the appropriate follow-up.

Brown spots
Some senile lentigos (age spots) are treated with liquid nitrogen. Laser treatment is also effective, although the cost is still prohibitive. In both cases, the treated lentigos heal in the form of a white plaque. Age spots may also be treated with tretinoin (vitamin A) gel and a de-pigmentation agent such as Ultraquin or Eldoquin (4%), although this requires patience since it takes from six months to two years to complete. Applying Neostrata HQ lotion may accelerate the process somewhat. Glycolic acid or other chemical peels are

possible alternatives. Limiting sun exposure after treatment is the best way to achieve long-term effects.

Lesions secondary to yeast infections respond well to Nizoral, Head & Shoulders and Selsun Blue. Nizoral tablets (Antifungal medication) are also an effective treatment. Sporanox is an oral treatment for yeast infections resistant to traditional approaches.

Port-wine stains

If port-wine stains do not resolve spontaneously, they should be treated as soon as possible, as they will grow with the child and become more complicated to treat with age. Most disappear completely with laser treatment. Cherry-red spots can also be treated by laser. Strawberry hemangiomas do not require treatment, as they disappear before the child reaches the age of four.

Pyogenic granulomas may resolve spontaneously. In most cases, however, they must be surgically removed, as they may cause unnecessary heavy bleeding. The procedure involves a simple excision under local anesthetic.

Slow Pulse

The pulse is evidence of the contractions of the heart muscle and can be measured by placing gentle pressure with the fingers on the artery of the inner wrist or the carotid artery in the neck. (If it is difficult to feel the pulse in these areas, it can be taken where the femoral artery passes through the groin area.) At rest, the pulse is generally 60 to 80 beats per minute. A heart rate slower than 60 beats per minute is known as "bradycardia", a form of arrhythmia that can be literally translated as "slow heart". While medical intervention may be necessary in some cases, a slow pulse may also be a perfectly normal phenomenon, in some cases even helping you live longer. A slow pulse does not necessarily indicate low blood pressure.

WHAT ARE THE CAUSES?

- *Serenity and relaxation.* A person who is absolutely calm, meditating, or sleeping will have a slower heart rhythm.
- *Very good physical condition*. People who do regular, rigorous physical activity such as cross-country skiing, running, or competitive bike racing may have a lower heart rate than average.
- *Autonomic nervous reaction.* Fear, pain, prolonged standing (particularly in hot and humid environments) may abnormally stimulate the autonomic nervous system, which is responsible for the unconscious regulation of the organs. A number of symptoms may develop, including sudden bradycardi, rapid drop in blood pressure, vision problems (like a black veil falling over the eyes), yawning, sweating, and, in many cases, brief loss of consciousness.
- *Medications* for coronary artery disease (angina pectoris, myocardial infarction) significantly slow down the heart rate. The following drugs have this effect: antihypertensives to lower blood pressure, certain anti-arrhythmic drugs to regulate heartbeat, and some cardiotonics (those derived from digitalis) to strengthen cardiac muscle tone. Other types of medication (for example, lithium salts for emotional disturbances) can slow the pulse as well, although this is not a desirable side effect in such cases.

► *Congenital abnormalities* of the heart conduction system, also known as atrioventricular blocks, may cause bradycardia. In most cases, there are no other consequences.

► *Coronary sinus problems.* The coronary sinus is located in the atrium (upper cavity of the heart) where it meets the ventricle. It sends out electrical signals that stimulate heart rhythm. Malfunction of the sinus may result in no heartbeat for a few seconds, followed by rapid and irregular beating, sometimes causing loss of consciousness when the sufferer sits or stands up (it may also occur after a person has been lying down for a few hours). Although coronary sinus disease is often caused by aging, it can also result from heart disease, long-term high blood pressure, or any disease affecting the muscles of the heart (cardiomyopathy).

► *Heart attack* (myocardial infarction). The coronary arteries form a network of vessels that nourish the heart muscle with blood. If they harden or contract due to cholesterol deposits (or other causes), the heart receives less blood, which may result in infarction. At first, the pulse will increase to compensate for heart failure. If the infarction is severe and there is a nearly complete lack of oxygen, the heart will have difficulty performing and begin to beat more slowly before stopping completely. In most cases, an infarction is accompanied by pain in the chest, left arm and throat, extreme pallor, heavy sweating, fear of imminent death, and sometimes nausea and vomiting.

The Pacemaker

This term most commonly refers to a miniature computer implanted under the skin and connected to the heart with electrodes. This device constantly analyzes electrical activity in the heart and provides stimulation to trigger contractions when necessary. It is usually employed in severe cases of bradycardia (such as those caused by coronary sinus disease).

► *Hypothyroidism* slows down the functions of the entire body.
► *Hypothermia and severe malnutrition (anorexia).* These conditions can affect the electrical impulses stimulating the heart and slow the heartbeat significantly.

PRACTICAL ADVICE

Take any sign of myocardial infarction seriously. If you have symptoms that resemble a heart attack, ask for help and call 911 immediately. Do not wait, as early treatment is crucial. Ambulance workers will provide care to protect your heart until you get to the hospital.

Watch out for drug interactions. Always be conscious of whether the drugs you are taking can cause bradycardia and the way your different medications interact. If you are beginning a new drug treatment (either prescription or over-the-counter), ask your doctor or pharmacist to tell you if the medication can cause bradycardia on its own or in combination with your other prescriptions.

Do not stop prescribed treatment without a doctor's advice. Consult your doctor before stopping the use of any drug that causes bradycardia, as he or she will be able to prescribe an alternative.

Do not take medication prescribed for another. Although your symptoms may be the same, it can be dangerous to take medication that has been prescribed for another person.

WHEN TO CONSULT?

► Your pulse is lower than 50 beats per minute and accompanied by dizziness and weakness, particularly when you stand up.
► You have lost consciousness or feel faint; you are very tired and may feel confused; you have been short of breath for some time.

WHAT HAPPENS DURING THE EXAM?

The doctor will take a history and perform a physical examination to check the heart. He or she may also order electrocardiogram (EKG) tests, to be administered both while at rest and during exertion (walking on a treadmill).

Other tests may be necessary. Holter monitoring involves continuous ambulatory monitoring of the patient's heart activity for a 24-hour period. The inclined-plane test checks for variations in the pulse rate as the patient takes different positions on an adjustable inclining table. The doctor may also administer a local anesthetic (into the arm or through the femoral vein in the thigh) to check heart activity. This technique is known as electrophysiological endo-cavity exploration.

WHAT IS THE TREATMENT?

Autonomic nervous reaction
If possible, the best treatment is to avoid unpleasant situations that bring on this reaction. Otherwise, a number of medications can stop the heart rate from slowing down too much, particularly if there is a risk of losing consciousness while driving, for example. However, results are still somewhat controversial and a great deal of research remains to be done. In some cases, a pacemaker is recommended.

Medication
The doctor will change the prescription if necessary.

Congenital abnormalities of the heart conduction system
In most cases, bradycardia has no medical consequences, does not affect the sufferer's normal activities, and requires no treatment.

Coronary sinus problems
People who have problems with their electrical conduction system require a pacemaker to avoid potentially dangerous bradycardia (loss of consciousness while driving, falling, etc.) along with a prescription for anti-arrhythmia drugs to treat rapid heartbeat.

Heart attack (myocardial infarction)
At the hospital, the patient receives oxygen, nitroglycerine (sublingual melting tablets, oral spray or intravenous), and aspirin

(an antiplatelet agent preventing blood clots). Other medications are also administered intravenously or orally. The type of surgery depends on the severity of the infarction. Coronary angioplasty, for example, involves dilating a blood vessel to its original size, whereas aorto-coronary bypass surgery revascularizes the heart muscle by rerouting the blood around the obstruction. The latter is accomplished by means of a grafted vein from the leg or an artery from the patient's chest.

Hypothyroidism
This condition is treated with medication (thyroid extracts).

Hypothermia, and severe malnutrition (anorexia)
In both cases, a slow pulse is merely a symptom of the overarching condition. The doctor will do his or her best to save the patient's life.

Snoring

Snoring is a respiratory noise that occurs during sleep and varies in volume and intensity from person to person, or even in the same individual, depending on the circumstances. Snoring is produced by the vibrations of the uvula and the soft palate as air passes by. The uvula, a small, pointed flap of muscle attached to the palate, can be seen at the back of the mouth.

When the air we inhale reaches the back of the throat, it goes through a narrow passage and speeds up as it moves toward the trachea and lungs. This acceleration creates a negative pressure, sucking the uvula and soft palate back. This rapid, back-and-forth movement is what causes snoring. It is a generally harmless phenomenon that does not bother the sleeper, although it can be a source of conjugal or social tension. For unknown reasons, men tend to snore more than women.

WHAT ARE THE CAUSES?

► *Excess body weight.* Accumulated fat reduces the already narrow passage for air in the back of the throat, increasing the likelihood of snoring.
► *Individual throat structure.* In some people, the space behind the uvula is smaller, the tongue larger, or the pharynx longer and perhaps narrower.
► *Menopause* is frequently accompanied by a loss of tone in the muscles and tissues, including the throat. This laxity increases the risk of vibration and, combined with the weight gain that often accompanies this period of life, may lead to snoring.
► *Nasal obstruction* can be caused by nasal congestion, a deviated septum, nasal polyps, or hypertrophy (enlargement) of the turbinate bones. The latter are the spongy bones inside the nasal cavity (also comprised of mucous membrane) that humidify and filter the air as it enters the nose. Any of these conditions can obstruct the passage of air and lead to snoring.

► *Adenoid vegetations.* Two- and three-year-old children who habitually breathe through the mouth may develop adenoid vegetations at the back of the palate, blocking the passage of air.

► *Smoking.* The mucous membranes of a smoker's nose and throat are swollen and irritated, which affects breathing.

► *Sleeping on the back* causes the tongue and other tissues to slide toward the back of the mouth and throat, obstructing the respiratory passage.

► *Tranquilizers, sleeping pills, and other drugs.* All medications that cause drowsiness and muscle relaxation increase the risk of vibration.

► *Large meals accompanied by alcohol* relax the muscles, increasing the likelihood of vibration.

► *Aging.* Tissues lose their tone with age.

► *Certain diseases,* such as hypothyroidism or strong respiratory allergies.

PRACTICAL ADVICE

Avoid consuming alcohol. Particularly at night before you go to bed.

Be cautious with medications that cause drowsiness. If you tend to snore, do not take sleeping pills or certain antihistamines, which cause the muscles to relax even more during sleep. If necessary, speak to your doctor.

Lose excess body weight. Although it can be difficult, losing weight can make your snoring problem disappear.

Sleep on your side. Put tennis balls right behind your back to force yourself to stay in this position (wear a sweater to protect your skin). Although effective, this technique will wake you up every time you try to turn onto your back.

Treat nasal congestion. Clear nasal passages and easier breathing lower the risk of snoring.

Stop smoking. Even if you are unable to quit completely, simply cutting down could help your problem.

Use "BreatheRight", a small piece of metal covered with an adhesive strip. Applied to the nose at bedtime, it pulls the nostrils back, opening the nasal cavities for better passage of air. They are sold over the counter in pharmacies.

WHEN TO CONSULT?

- ► You do not feel rested when you wake up in the morning. If you snore a lot, you are probably making continuous efforts to breathe during the night, which may disturb your sleep.
- ► You experience daytime drowsiness. This is a sign of sleep apnea, which is often difficult to distinguish from simple snoring.
- ► Your snoring is becoming intolerable for the people close to you.

WHAT HAPPENS DURING THE EXAM?

The doctor checks for nasal obstructions, examining the septum (the division separating the nose into two equal sections) to see if it is straight. He or she may also perform an endoscopic exam whereby a small, flexible tube equipped with fibre optics is inserted into the nose to view the pharynx, check for polyps and determine whether the turbinate bones are hypertrophied. If the snoring is caused by an underlying ailment (such as hypothyroidism or a severe allergy), the doctor refers the patient to the appropriate specialist.

WHAT IS THE TREATMENT?

A change of lifestyle (weight loss, quitting smoking, drinking less alcohol, sleeping on the side, etc.) may be enough to correct the problem. If the septum is deviated, it may be corrected. Adenoids may be removed surgically.

The Continuous Positive Airway Pressure (CPAP) device increases positive air pressure in the nasal passages, reducing snoring. It propels air through a mask that the patient wears while asleep and can be adjusted to fit the patient's needs.

A partial resection of the soft palate and uvula may also be performed through laser surgery. This is an out-patient treatment, lasts only 15 to 20 minutes and is done under local anesthesia by an Ear, Nose and Throat Specialist. According to the sleeping partners of those who have undergone such a procedure, there is a complete or nearly complete disappearance of snoring in 70% of cases; it remains a serious problem in only 5% of cases. The Canadian Society of Otolaryngology does not recommend laser surgery in cases of sleep apnea.

Sore throat

What is commonly called a sore throat can be more precisely defined as pain in the larynx (the organ between the vocal cords), pharynx (the back of the mouth), or the mouth cavity itself. It may be accompanied by fever, swollen lymph nodes, nasal congestion, difficulty swallowing, redness, and/or white spots on the tongue or throat. The pain varies in intensity. Because the possible types of sore throat are so numerous, only the most common are listed here.

Repeated irritation or trauma
► Latent, chronic or intermittent pain sometimes accompanied by inflammation and redness in the throat.

Infection
► Intense and gradually increasing pain accompanied by inflammation, redness, fever, and sometimes white spots on the tongue, throat, or inside of the cheeks.

Epiglottiditis
► Infection occurring primarily in children.
► Characterized by acute inflammation of the larynx, pharynx, and epiglottis (the part of the throat that closes the larynx upon swallowing). This inflammation blocks breathing, sometimes to the point of causing asphyxiation.

Cancer
► Latent pain at first, increasing over a period of days to become localized and persistent.
► Generally accompanied by pain in the ear, a change in the voice, difficulty swallowing, blood in the phlegm, a lump in the throat, and unexplained weight loss.
► Occurs primarily in smokers, almost exclusively after the age of forty. Marijuana (pot) smokers are even more susceptible to throat cancer, since the smoke they inhale is much hotter than cigarette

smoke and held in the mouth for longer. Moreover, marijuana is frequently contaminated with toxic substances.

WHAT ARE THE CAUSES?

Repeated irritation or trauma

- **Nervous habits** such as repeated clearing of the throat or spitting eventually irritate the mucous membranes of the throat.
- **Snoring** causes the soft palate to vibrate, leading to a throat inflammation that may cause pain during the day.
- **Cigarettes, alcohol, or gastroesophageal reflux.**
- **Allergies.**
- **Immune system disorders** occur when the immune system is unable to distinguish between the body's own cells and foreign cells. Scleroderma is a disease affecting the collagen fibres of the epidermis, leading to hard, inflexible skin, pain, and difficulty swallowing.

Infection

- **Viruses** cause the majority of infectious sore throats (for example, tonsillitis, mononucleosis).
- **Bacteria** (streptococcus) or fungus (Candida albicans causing pharyngitis or laryngitis). Thrush is a fungal infection particularly common in babies, resulting in white spots covering the tongue, pallet, and inside of the cheeks. Bacteria and fungi may also cause redness in the throat.
- **Abscess** caused by a poorly treated or untreated infection. An abscess in the throat or on the tonsils can cause pain and fever. In most cases, the abscess cannot be seen, although the inside of the throat and neck are red and swollen.

Epiglottiditis

- **Bacteria** (Haemophilius influenzae).

Cancer

- **Heredity.**
- **Genetic mutation.**
- **Cigarettes and alcohol.**

PRACTICAL ADVICE

Avoid screaming or otherwise straining your voice. This can irritate the throat or cause you to lose your voice.

Avoid clearing your throat or spitting constantly. This can aggravate an irritation by contracting the throat and letting in too much air, leading to dryness.

Avoid spicy food and cinnamon or mint chewing gum. They can also further irritate your throat.

Avoid brushing your tongue or tonsils with a toothbrush. This can cause additional trauma.

Do not smoke, and avoid smoky environments. Cigarettes and second-hand smoke are irritants and will make your sore throat worse.

For children

Do a basic check-up. Take the child's temperature. Using a tongue depressor, press the child's tongue down gently and shine a flashlight down his or her throat to check for inflammation.

Is your child less energetic or active? Inactivity in a child is often a sign that he or she is becoming ill.

Be sure the child is well hydrated. Give your child plenty to drink.

Do not smoke in the child's environment. Second-hand smoke may be causing your child's sore throat.

Be sure your child washes his or her hands regularly. Keeping the hands clean is an effective way to protect against the spread of bacterial infections.

Be sure your child blows his or her nose regularly. Repeated sniffing and swallowing phlegm can irritate the throat.

Ease the pain. Give your child an appropriate dose of acetaminophen: 15 mg for every kilogram of body weight, every four to six hours, up to five doses a day. Do not give aspirin to children, as this can lead to Reye's syndrome, a serious neurological disease (viral in origin) that causes liver, kidney and brain damage.

Go back to the doctor if the child does not get better. If the child's condition becomes worse, he or she may be suffering from epiglottiditis.

For adults
Do a self-exam. Using a tongue depressor and a flashlight, check for inflammation or white spots in the throat.

Determine potential causes and eliminate them, if possible. For example, if gastroesophageal reflux is causing your sore throat, eliminate coffee, alcohol, spicy foods and other similar irritants from your diet.

Take painkillers, get some rest, and stay hydrated. Analgesics will soothe the pain, while rest and hydration will help you get better. It is particularly important to drink a lot of liquids.

Inhale steam and eucalyptus vapours. Eucalyptus is a natural lubricant that will help soothe the pain caused by irritation. Boil water with eucalyptus and breathe in the rising steam. Eucalyptus is available over-the-counter in pharmacies or natural food stores.

Inhale camphor vapours. This will help clear your nasal and respiratory passages, providing some relief.

Gargle with salt water to dislodge phlegm from inside the throat. Boil water, remove from the heat, then add enough salt to flavour the water. Let it cool to a lukewarm temperature and gargle. Never use mouthwash (it will increase the irritation) or rubbing alcohol (it is poisonous).

Eliminate possible allergens. Get rid of rugs, carpeting, dust, or anything else than may be causing your allergy.

WHEN TO CONSULT?
For children
► The baby has white spots on the tongue, inner cheeks, and/or in the throat.
► The pain lasts more than 48 hours, possibly becoming more intense.
► The younger the child, the earlier the consultation should be.

For adults
► The symptoms are associated with complications such as fever and difficulty swallowing or eating.
► The pain lasts more than four to eight weeks.
► The pain is chronic and latent, and you are a smoker.

WHAT HAPPENS DURING THE EXAM?
Children
The doctor will take the child's vital signs (temperature, pulse and respiratory rhythm). If epiglottiditis is suspected, he or she will order a throat X-ray.

Adults
The doctor will examine the ears and nose and verify the degree to which the nasal passages are congested, as well as the general state of the mouth cavity. The examination may also include checking the pharynx and palpating the neck to determine whether the lymph nodes are swollen. If a streptococcus infection is suspected, he or she will take a sample from the throat. If mononucleosis is a possible cause, blood tests will be ordered. The doctor may ask the patient to return in 24 to 48 hours to assess the progression of the disease.

WHAT IS THE TREATMENT?

Repeated irritation or trauma

Treatment aims to ease the pain. It may involve sucking on ice cubes or eating cold food, as well as prescribed painkillers. Anesthetics for the throat are prescribed, if appropriate. If gastroesophageal reflux is the cause, the doctor may prescribe medication to reduce, neutralize, or simply measure the levels of acid in the stomach. In cases of allergy, topical or oral steroids (cortisone), or antihistamines are prescribed. Treatment for immune system disorders targets the symptoms.

Infection

Oral antibiotics are prescribed for a period of three to ten days. Certain antibiotics must not be taken with dairy products as they prevent the body from absorbing the medication. It is very important to alert the doctor to penicillin allergies. Infectious mononucleosis requires rest, and, in certain cases, cortisone and antibiotics to bring down the swelling in the throat. Fungal infections are treated with Antifungal medication. Abscesses are treated with oral or intravenous antibiotics. In some cases, they are drained.

Epiglottiditis

If not treated quickly, epiglottiditis can be fatal. The number of deaths due to this infection has decreased, however, since the introduction of the Haemophilius influenzae vaccine. Once the infection has taken hold, the patient is treated with intravenous antibiotics for seven to ten days. Preventive intubation (inserting a tube in the trachea to facilitate breathing) for three to seven days may also be required.

Cancer

The treatment depends on the precise location of the cancer and the size of the tumour, as well as the age and general condition of the subject. In most cases, a combined treatment of chemotherapy and radiation therapy, or radiation therapy and surgery is undertaken.

Speech Disorders

Like other so-called higher functions (e.g., intelligence and memory), language (verbal comprehension and thought expression) is controlled by the brain and may be affected on the level of comprehension, expression, or both. Speech depends on a number of structures that facilitate pronunciation. Language problems or speech disorders are most often neurological in origin. If the onset is sudden, it is most often the result of a vascular disease. If it is a gradual process, a neurodegenerative disease is likely the cause.

WHAT ARE THE CAUSES?

► *Cerebrovascular accident (CVA).* A CVA (stroke) is usually caused by the blocking of an intracranial blood vessel or, more rarely, a hemorrhage (bleeding). Strokes can result in one or all of the following symptoms: speech impairment, paralysis, numbness on one side of the body, and sudden loss of vision.

► *Transient ischemic attack (TIA).* A TIA can result from an embolism caused by a clot fragment or decreased circulation in the carotid artery of the neck (which nourishes the brain). The symptoms resemble those of a stroke but are short-lived, generally lasting less than an hour and no more than a day. There are no after-effects.

► *Neurodegenerative diseases* such as Alzheimer's disease and other forms of dementia.

► *Cranial injury.*

► *Migraine headaches.* Some migraine sufferers may experience paralysis or language problems. While such symptoms are indeed alarming, they will disappear with the migraine.

► *Brain tumour.*

► *Inflammatory or infectious neurological diseases,* such as multiple sclerosis, encephalitis, or cerebral abscesses, can affect the areas responsible for language or speech.

► *Tumour of the tongue or throat.* In these cases, the impairment is mechanical in origin, not neurological.

PRACTICAL ADVICE

Be vigilant, but remain calm. Speech disorders do not always indicate a serious condition. Everyone at some time or other has trouble finding the right words and such occasional memory lapses do not necessarily reflect a neurological disorder. You should, however, take note if these small problems suddenly become more regular and extend beyond merely forgetting the details of an anecdote. If you find they are becoming more frequent and seriously impeding the expression of your thoughts, contact your doctor immediately.

Make sure any health problems are under control. Health problems such as hypertension, diabetes, smoking and hypercholesterolemia (high blood cholesterol levels) can increase the risk of stroke. See your doctor regularly, take medication as prescribed, and follow his or her lifestyle recommendations.

Call for emergency medical help right away. Most stroke or TIA victims arrive at the emergency room three hours after the episode. The sooner you receive medical attention, the greater the chances of avoiding any after-effects. Seek medical attention promptly even if the speech problem goes away on its own, as there is a risk that the next recurrence will have more serious consequences.

Take aspirin as a preventive measure. It has been scientifically proven that long-term use of aspirin reduces the incidence of recurrent vascular problems. Discuss the benefits of aspirin with your doctor and whether taking it is appropriate in your case.

WHEN TO CONSULT?

► You have a sudden episode of impaired speech, paralysis, numbness on one side of the body or loss of vision. Call for emergency medical help right away.
► Your speech is impaired after a head injury.
► You experience impaired speech for several minutes and it goes away on its own.
► Your speech or language problems are gradually worsening.

WHAT HAPPENS DURING THE EXAM?

The doctor will take a history and perform a physical examination, possibly recommending various tests such as a brain CAT (computed axial tomography) scan, Doppler ultrasound, electrocardiography, electroencephalography, MRI (magnetic resonance imaging) test, as well as laboratory tests (requiring blood samples).

WHAT IS THE TREATMENT?

CVA

When the patient gets to the emergency room, he or she will be given anti-platelet medication such as aspirin to prevent recurrences. If the sufferer arrives within three hours of the symptoms' appearance, thrombolytics (drugs that help dissolve the clot causing the blood vessel obstruction) may also be administered.

If the CVA affects speech or language, the patient will be referred to a speech-language pathologist. Speech/language pathology exercises have proven highly successful in helping stroke victims regain proper speech function.

TIA

Anti-platelet medication such as aspirin is the cornerstone of treatment, which focuses on preventing recurrences. Anticoagulants are also sometimes used. Surgery may be necessary for patients whose carotid artery is almost completely obstructed (more than 70%).

Neurodegenerative diseases

For neurodegenerative diseases such as Alzheimer's, no curative treatments are available. Depending on the nature of the disease, however, certain drugs can in some instances delay or prevent further deterioration for extended periods.

Cranial injury

Based on the type of injury, the doctor may perform surgery (to drain excess blood from the brain, for example) or send the patient for rehabilitation.

Brain tumour

Treatment involves surgery to remove the tumour or radiation therapy.

Migraine headaches

Treatment depends on the individual case and diagnosis, as well as the frequency and intensity of the episodes (*see Headaches*).

Tumour of the tongue or throat

The doctor will recommend surgery to remove the tumour, or radiation therapy.

Inflammatory and infectious neurological diseases

Treatment for inflammatory diseases will depend on the nature of the illness. Infectious diseases are managed with antibiotics or antivirals.

Spinal Pain

Pain in the spinal column has different names, depending on the area affected: cervicalgia denotes neck pain, dorsalgia refers to back pain, and lumbalgia (the most common type) describes pain in the lumbar region. Ninety percent of cases are caused by mechanical disorders in the spine such as joint sprains or disc problems. Most people experience a problem in the spine at some point in their lives, but only 10% consult a doctor.

The symptoms can be difficult to interpret because of the following phenomena:
- Pain from the cervical spine often radiates to the shoulder blade.
- Back pain often radiates to the sides and the sternum.
- Lower back pain often radiates to the pelvis.
- Lumbar pain often radiates to the muscles in the buttocks and legs.
- These types of pain may partially limit movement or block it altogether.

WHAT ARE THE CAUSES?

- *Physical trauma.* Common risk factors for a herniated disc include poor physical condition, physically demanding work, violent sports, or simply improper back movement.
- *Psychological causes* such as stress and mental problems are frequently responsible for chronic pain.
- *Spinal deformity.* Scoliosis curves the spine into the shape of an S and tilts the pelvis, while kyphosis rounds the back. Both are genetic diseases with severe effects on the health of the spine.
- *Arthritis and osteoarthritis.* Osteoarthritis is part of the normal aging process of joints, while arthritis is an inflammatory joint disease.
- *Infections and tumours* are serious problems, but fortunately quite rare.

PRACTICAL ADVICE

Apply cold treatment for the first 48 hours. Apply ice to the sore area for as long as possible, several times a day. Heat is not recommended during this period as it will increase inflammation.

Rest the affected area. Avoid moving the painful area as much as you can, but do not take to your bed. Studies have shown that staying in bed for longer than two days is not beneficial. Non-prescription painkillers and anti-inflammatories can help ease the pain. Take one or two acetaminophen tablets (325 mg to 500 mg) four times a day, never exceeding four grams daily. If taking anti-inflammatories, follow the manufacturer's dosage recommendations. Take both medications if the pain is difficult to control.

Apply heat or cold after the first 48 hours. Apply a hot or cold compress to ease the pain. Consult your doctor if there is no improvement.

Consult your doctor early on. Be sure you have a clear diagnosis before beginning a series of treatments.

Beware of friendly advice. People around you are probably more than happy to give you advice on how to sit, lie down, position your computer monitor, and so on, but only do what the doctor orders. Remember that everyone is different and what is good for some may be harmful for others. Get an accurate diagnosis.

Spend your money wisely. There are various types of chairs, mattresses, pillows, electromagnetic soles, cervical collars, lumbar supports, and back support cushions on the market. They are of varying suitability and some can even aggravate your condition, so unless your physician has recommended the product, save your money.

WHEN TO CONSULT?

► The pain lasts more than 48 hours.
► You are unable to resume your regular activities.
► The symptoms have worsened and now include pain and swelling in the legs or arms.

WHAT HAPPENS DURING THE EXAM?

The doctor performs a complete exam, identifies the origin of the pain, and informs the patient.

WHAT IS THE TREATMENT?

Treatment for pain due to mechanical troubles (sprain, hernia, disc problems) begins with patient education on the nature of the problem and how to improve it.

Tips for people with frequent back pain

Do not stay in the same position for an extended period of time. If you are sedentary at work, make an effort to get up and walk around often. A few simple exercises can also help you manage your back pain:

1. Standing up, bend slightly forward with your legs apart. Raise your left arm and lean gently to the right, stretching the left side. Hold this position for seven seconds, then repeat on the other side. Repeat seven times.
2. Standing with your legs apart, bend slightly forward, then to the left and right.
3. Standing with your back against the wall, grab your right knee with your hand and gently bring it up to your stomach. Repeat twice with each leg. This exercise can also be done lying on your back.

Check your posture at work. Do you have an appropriate chair? Is your computer screen well-positioned?

Wear comfortable shoes. Although there is no scientific proof, it is generally believed that high-heeled shoes (over 5 cm) cause tension in the back of the spinal column.

Does smoking play a role? One theory says that nicotine contracts the small arteries that nourish the discs and vertebrae, impeding circulation. This hypothesis has not yet been proven.

Physical medicine: manual or mechanical techniques
This type of treatment includes lumbar traction, mobilization and manipulation.

Lumbar traction is the manual or mechanical extension of the spine to diminish pressure on the vertebrae or discs in between.

Mobilization is similar to manipulation, without extending the spine's normal range of movement.

Manipulation involves applying tension and extending the spine to enable movement beyond its normal range. It may create a cracking sound in the back.

Current literature discusses the relative benefits of these techniques. Treatment usually results in improvement after five sessions and should not extend over months or years.

Health professionals employ several other methods to reduce pain or induce relaxation, including ultrasound or laser therapy, balms, acupuncture, TENS (transcutaneous electrical nerve stimulation), massage, and biofeedback. These techniques do not directly address mechanical problems.

Medication
Doctors can prescribe anti-inflammatories, painkillers and cortisone injections. Cortisone is a powerful anti-inflammatory that does not modify the mechanical problem.

Surgery
Surgery is a last resort.

Exercise programmes
Mechanical back troubles caused by osteoarthritis or disc problems are best treated with regular physical exercise over the long term. A good exercise program has three essential elements: aerobics, muscle-building and stretching. Patients should exercise at least three times a week.

Stress

Stress is an emotional state reflecting the body's response to some form of stimulus or pressure. It is most often a nervous or psychological reaction to an intense, unpleasant emotion, but can sometimes act as a motivating force, for example, when a pending exam forces a student to study harder.

Whether the stress is physical, chemical, organic or nervous in origin, it can bring about many somatic disturbances, from gastrointestinal upset, to headaches and back pain. It can also intensify already existing physical symptoms. Some individuals are more tolerant to stress than others.

There are different types of stress:

Stress associated with a psychological crisis
► Sadness, insomnia, loss of appetite or bulimia.
► Difficulty thinking rationally.
► Tendency to withdraw socially.
This type of stress does not last more than three months.

Stress associated with adjustment problems
► Emotional disruption, anxiety, depression.
► Behavioural disruption, irritability at work or in the family.
This type occurs within three months of a clearly identifiable crisis and can last as long as the stress factor remains. If the symptoms are still pronounced after six months, this is considered a major depression; if the symptoms diminish but still fluctuate according to circumstance after a year, the condition may be chronic.

Post-traumatic stress
► Panic attacks, brought on by situations reminiscent of the traumatic event, characterized by intense anxiety, palpitations, perspiration and tremors, sometimes accompanied by a feeling of choking or being in a stranglehold and nausea.

- ► Can manifest as a depressive state involving insomnia, weight and appetite loss, lack of concentration and psychomotor slowness.
- ► Occurs within weeks and months of a very traumatic event.
- ► Avoidance reaction or strong sense of fear or impotence when faced with the stressful situation.
- ► The traumatic event is relived in nightmares, intrusive memories and flashbacks.
- ► Between 10 and 15% of individuals develop post-traumatic stress within weeks and months of a highly distressing event.

WHAT ARE THE CAUSES?
Stress associated with a psychological crisis
- ► *Difficult lifecycle events,* such as adolescence and menopause.
- ► *Emotional or psychological upsets,* such as job loss, career change, or relationship problems.
- ► *Loss or mourning* of a loved one after a separation or death.
- ► *Social and family factors* can affect an individual's vulnerability to stress.

Stress associated with adjustment problems
- ► *Inability to cope,* such as the fear of not being able to adjust to a new job or routine (e.g., in the case of parents who must deal with a child's chronic illness).
- ► *Negative social factors,* such as rejection because of one's sexual orientation or religion.

Post-traumatic stress
- ► *Unusual shock or attack,* such as rape, physical assault, a car accident, death threats, etc.

PRACTICAL ADVICE
Analyze the situation. Studies show that individuals manage pressure better if they analyze the stressful situation instead of panicking or reacting instinctively.

Stay in touch with people. Speaking openly about problems will help ease nervous tension. Above all, do not isolate yourself, as solitude will only heighten your anxiety. If the stress is too intense, do not hesitate to seek the help of a relative, friend or health professional.

Adopt a positive and flexible attitude. Remain hopeful by telling yourself there is light at the end of the tunnel and things will eventually improve. View times of stress as opportunities for personal growth. Do not try to overcome all obstacles at once, setting reasonable daily objectives to tackle difficult situations. Moreover, do not impose restrictions on yourself or paint yourself into a corner by saying things like "I could never do that sort of work." Always be prepared to make compromises.

Learn to relax. During stressful situations, it is essential to relax more. Allow yourself a weekend away from home, for example, to leave your problems behind and make it easier to tackle them when you return. If you cannot get away, reserve some time during the day to listen to soft music, do yoga or meditate. Imagine yourself on a beach doing nothing but listening to the soothing sound of the waves. Such moments of reprieve will allow you to get back on track.

Practice relaxation techniques. Breathe slowly and deeply to reduce anxiety and nervousness. Take deep cleansing breaths, filling your stomach with air as you inhale and relaxing it slowly as you exhale. This will regulate the pulse, which accelerates under stress. Enjoy a neck or back rub to release the muscle tension caused by the secretion of adrenaline in a stressful situation.

Exercise. A simple walk can reduce the tension of a stressful meeting or lovers' quarrel. The body is ready for action under pressure, a phenomenon known as the "fight or flight" reflex inherited from our ancestors. Physical exercise burns the chemical substances produced by tension; the resulting fatigue relaxes the muscles.

Maintain a healthy lifestyle. Take care not to consume alcohol or coffee in excess (more than one or two cups a day, for example). Do not take drugs or medicines unless they are essential to your health.

WHEN TO CONSULT?

► You have been irritable, aggressive or silent for a month. This change in character may be accompanied by gastrointestinal upset, insomnia, muscle pain, dizziness or headaches.

► You feel depressed for at least a month.

► Your anguish persists despite relaxation and externalization efforts.

► You are consistently revisited by painful images of a traumatic event experienced more than three months ago.

WHAT HAPPENS DURING THE EXAM?

The doctor will investigate the causes of the stress and evaluate the patient's defence mechanisms in the face of difficulty. He or she will interview the patient to determine the level of distress, asking questions about sleep patterns, appetite, the level of depression and/or apathy, fatigue, agitation, ability to concentrate, self-esteem, and suicidal thoughts. A blood work-up may also be ordered to make sure that no disease (such as hyperthyroidism) is responsible for the anxiety. If necessary, the doctor will refer the patient to a psychologist or psychiatrist.

WHAT IS THE TREATMENT?

Whatever the type of stress, treatment usually involves the formulation of a strategy to relieve it, such as setting objectives to find another job, face a divorce or overcome a mourning period.

Stress associated with a psychological crisis

This type may sometimes require psychotherapy, which draws on the individual's previously successful coping strategies. If a fishing trip has relieved stress in the past, for example, the practitioner will recommend it as a solution for the current problem.

The doctor may also resort to cognitive-behavioural therapy in an attempt to change the way the individual thinks and reacts to unforeseen events. In some cases, tranquilizers may be prescribed to reduce anxiety, or antidepressants to improve concentration and the ability to sleep.

Stress associated with adjustment problems

If difficulty adjusting persists, the doctor may recommend a specified rest period, prescribe drugs to temporarily lower stress levels, or refer the individual to a psychologist or psychiatrist.

Post-traumatic stress

Someone who has lived through a traumatic event often benefits from exposure therapy, which employs positive reinforcement strategies to enable him or her to face and overcome the situation.

Drug therapy is the last resort after the individual's usual defence mechanisms fail to bring relief. If sleep is no longer restorative, for example, anxiety is pervasive, and avoidance is interfering with daily functioning, the doctor will prescribe anti-anxiety drugs, such as benzodiazepines, to reduce stress levels. These drugs will be prescribed only for a limited time to avoid dependency. Hypnotics are sometimes required for insomnia. Antidepressants should be considered when there is appetite or weight loss, lack of concentration and psychomotor slowness.

Swollen Lymph Nodes

The lymph nodes (or lymph glands) are small accumulations of cells that form part of the lymphatic system, a complex network of vessels through which lymphatic fluid circulates, transporting immune system cells and "cleaning" the body.

Located all over the body, lymph nodes are most easily felt in the neck, groin and armpits. They play an important role in the body's defenses, purifying lymphatic fluid and acting as a barrier against disease. As soon as the nodes encounter a concentration of infection in their filtering process, they begin producing antibodies to fight the invader. They then rapidly swell, and if working particularly hard, become painful. Painful lymph nodes, therefore, are a sign of serious infection. In rare cases, gradual and painless swelling may point to the presence of a malignant tumour. Heat sensation and redness occasionally accompany swelling.

WHAT ARE THE CAUSES?

► *Infections* are by far the most common cause. Mononucleosis and throat or ear infections, for example, affect the nodes in the neck. An infected insect bite on the arm may cause the nodes in the armpit to swell. Sexually transmitted diseases can lead to swelling in the nodes in the groin, and HIV is often accompanied by generalized lymph node hypertrophy, depending on the stage of the infection.

► *Cancerous tumours.* In some cases, such as Hodgkin's disease, the cancer is located in the lymph nodes themselves. In others, it originates in an organ and spreads cancerous cells through the lymphatic fluid to the lymph nodes. The nodes automatically filter out these cells, which may then continue to develop in the glands. This is why doctors treating breast cancer test the lymph nodes in the armpit to determine whether the disease has spread. While the lymph nodes gradually swell in all cases of cancer, they are not painful.

► *Certain immune disorders,* such as allergies, systemic lupus erythematosus, and rheumatoid arthritis, among others.

PRACTICAL ADVICE

Wait and do not worry. A swollen lymph node is most commonly caused by an infection. If the body can fight the infection off, the swelling will disappear on its own after a few days or weeks. If it persists, medical treatment is required. Of course, consult your doctor at any time if the swelling worries you.

Do not underestimate your condition. If you are experiencing lymph node hypertrophy but no infection is apparent, keep a close watch and consult your doctor.

Take analgesics. Acetaminophen will relieve the pain. Take one or two tablets (325 mg to 500 mg) four times a day, up to a maximum of 4 grams a day. Do not take anti-inflammatories as they only treat inflammation and do nothing to combat infection.

WHEN TO CONSULT?

► The swelling in your lymph nodes has still not gone down after three weeks.
► Your lymph nodes are red, hot and sensitive to the touch.
► You notice swelling in a node behind your ear. (This may be worrying because it is near the meninges.)
► One or more lymph nodes are swelling gradually, for no apparent reason.
► The infection is worrying you.

WHAT HAPPENS DURING THE EXAM?

The doctor will take a history and perform a complete physical examination. The doctor will palpate the lymph nodes, inspect the ears and throat, perform pulmonary ausculation, and examine the abdominal area. Blood tests and a sample from the swollen lymph node are sometimes required for diagnosis.

WHAT IS THE TREATMENT?

Infections
Antibiotics are used to fight off bacterial infection. If the cause is viral, the swelling will disappear on its own with time.

Cancerous tumours

If an underlying tumour is causing the swelling, appropriate treatment includes surgery, radiation therapy, or chemotherapy.

Immunity disorders

Treatment varies according to the specific disorder.

Testicular Pain and Swelling

Pain or swelling in the testicles is a common reason for medical visits. This is benign in many cases, but immediate medical attention is occasionally required to preserve sexual or reproductive function. Although rare, testicular cancer is the most common cancer in men between 15 and 35 years of age.

Acute pain

► In cases of testicular torsion (torsion of the spermatic cord), the pain is sudden and intense, sometimes accompanied by nausea. Neither movement nor rest can provide relief.

► Those who have had a vasectomy may suffer a rupture of the sperm reservoir, which causes sudden sharp pain, concentrated in one area.

► In cases of infection, the pain develops over a few days and the testicles swell. The man may also have a fever. It is easier to tolerate the pain in a seated position or if the scrotum is raised.

► In cases of trauma, the pain appears suddenly and the scrotum may become bluish in colour.

Chronic pain

► The pain persists for weeks, months or years.

► The man has a sensation of malaise and/or heaviness in the testicles.

► The scrotum may increase in size.

► Testicular pain is occasionally accompanied by back pain.

► In most cases, pain is the only symptom.

Lump or induration in the testicle

► Relatively hard lump.

► May be accompanied by pain.

WHAT ARE THE CAUSES?

Acute pain

► *Testicular torsion.* This very painful condition affects men of all ages, but is most common in boys. It is an emergency situation that must be treated within six hours to avoid permanent damage.

► *Congestion in epididymis (reservoir) in men with vasectomies.* This is neither serious nor urgent.

► *Infection of the testicle or epididymis.* Sexually transmitted infections (most common in young people with many partners) or other bacteria may lead to testicular infection (epididymitis), which affects the epididymis, a kind of reservoir for sperm. This is an emergency.

► *Trauma.* This is particularly urgent if the scrotum becomes bluish in colour, possibly indicating a tear in the inner lining of the testicle. The man must be treated within twelve hours—the sooner medical intervention is sought, the better the chances of preserving fertility.

► *Mumps* sometimes causes inflammation of the testicles.

Chronic pain

► *Spermatoceles,* the medical term for cysts on the epididymis.

► *Hydroceles,* the medical term for clear fluid collecting in a sac around the testicles.

► *Varicoceles,* or varicose veins in the testicles, which impede blood circulation. This results in decreased vascularization (fewer veins) in the testicles and diminished sperm production.

► *Abdominal hernia.* For example, the intestine may protrude into the scrotum.

► *Herniated disc or pinched nerve in the spinal column* may cause pain that radiates to the testicle.

Lump or induration in the testicle

► *Testicular cancer* (rare). The lump that forms in the testicles usually does not cause any pain. It appears on only one side of the scrotum (the sac containing the testicles).

PRACTICAL ADVICE

Examine yourself carefully. Whatever your age, self-examination may help to detect testicular cancer, a hydrocele or a varicocele. If possible, the exam should be performed in the shower because the scrotum is most flexible under water. Roll each testicle between the thumb and fingers, looking for lumps, indurations, or irregularities (learn to recognize the epididymis). Regular self-exams are particularly important if you had surgery for undescended testicles at a young age, as the chance of developing testicular cancer in this case is 20 times higher than average.

For chronic pain only

Take hot baths. This will ease the pain and stimulate blood circulation.

Wear a jock strap. Doctors sometimes recommend wearing athletic supports (special underwear that supports the testicles), which are available in pharmacies. A supportive pair of underwear made of strong material may also help.

Consult immediately if you feel sudden and intense pain. The healthy function of your testicles depends on it.

Enjoy your sex life. Chronic testicular pain does not require any modifications to your sexual practices.

WHEN TO CONSULT?

► You (or your son) experience sudden and intense pain in the testicles.
► You feel a sensation of malaise or heaviness in the testicles.
► You feel a lump, induration or swelling in or around the testicle.
► You experience chronic pain in the testicles.

WHAT HAPPENS DURING THE EXAM?

Acute pain

The doctor performs a clinical exam of the scrotum and testicles. If a torsion is suspected, an ultrasound or Doppler is ordered to check the vascularization of the testicle. In cases of trauma, an ultrasound will detect a rupture of the membrane lining the inner testicle. A urine analysis screens for infection.

Chronic pain
The doctor performs a clinical exam of the external organs. He or she may also recommend an ultrasound as well as a neurological or orthopedic examination.

WHAT IS THE TREATMENT?
Acute pain
Testicular torsion
The doctor will attempt to replace the testicle manually, although this procedure is rarely successful since the patient is in too much pain. Surgery is usually necessary.

Pain in men who have had a vasectomy
The doctor will prescribe a scrotal support and painkillers. Everything should go back to normal after a few days or weeks with no serious consequences.

Infection
This is treated with antibiotics.

Trauma
Surgery may be necessary to repair or, in some cases, remove the testicle. This does not generally affect fertility.

Mumps
There is no medical treatment available for this infectious disease. Testicular pain will dissipate as the mumps go away.

Chronic pain
Caused by cysts on the epididymis, spermatic cord cysts, and hydroceles. These conditions are benign and usually do not require treatment.

For greater comfort, excessively large cysts may be surgically removed and hydroceles drained or excised.

Varicoceles

Ligation surgery is performed if varicoceles cause significant discomfort and disrupt the patient's daily life. Varicoceles may be determined as the cause of infertility if the man has been infertile for one year and three separate sperm counts have shown decreased production. Ligation surgery is performed and, in many cases, the man regains fertility.

Abdominal hernia

Hernias are repaired surgically, although this does not always alleviate the pain. While doctors are generally unwilling to perform surgery on the testicles of young children because it is likely to cause infertility, they will do so in the case of a hernia.

Pinched nerve or herniated disc

Since the testicles generally appear normal in the exam and spinal examinations usually prove inconclusive, all the doctor can do is reassure the patient and prescribe painkillers to provide temporary relief.

Lump or induration in the testicle

If the tumour is cancerous the testicle is removed surgically. The prognosis is excellent if the disease is detected early.

Thirst

Water makes up 60% of the human body. When the volume drops below a certain threshold level, the brain releases a fluid-balancing hormone known as vasopressin, which triggers an alarm signal—thirst—to alert the body of its need for water.

WHAT ARE THE CAUSES?

- *Dehydration.* Heat, sunstroke, excessive physical activity, fever, diarrhea and vomiting can all cause dehydration, which manifests as dryness of the mouth, lips and throat. Failure to drink at this stage can produce more intense thirst, fatigue, weakness and even fainting.
- *Drugs.* Diuretics to promote urinary secretion cause water loss, inducing thirst.
- *Diabetes.* All diabetics (type 1 and type 2) produce excess glucose (sugar) and urinate frequently to eliminate it from their systems, causing thirst.
- *Diabetes insipidus* is a disorder caused by a deficiency or absence of vasopressin. Unable to maintain its fluid balance, the body sends an alarm signal in the form of constant thirst.
- *Psychiatric disorders.* Some mental health problems like schizophrenia can disturb the thirst centre in the brain, giving rise to potomania. In afflicted persons, potomania manifests as an abnormal craving to drink, especially water.

PRACTICAL ADVICE

Make sure to drink enough. To maintain proper hydration, dietitians recommend 6 to 8 glasses of liquids daily, including 4 glasses of water.

Replace fluids. Fluids lost through fever, diarrhea or vomiting must be replaced. Water, juice, flat 7Up or a commercial electrolyte preparation, such as Pedialyte or Gastrolyte, are recommended. The following home remedy is also effective:

- ► 1 litre of boiled water
- ► 5 mL of salt
- ► 50 mL of sodium bicarbonate
- ► 20 mL of sugar
- ► 120 mL of sugar
- ► 120 mL of apple or orange juice

Note that beverages like Gatorade, intended for athletes, are not recommended for diabetics and persons with hypertension because of the sugar and salt content. Consult a doctor before consumption.

Replace fluids during physical activity. The body needs to replenish its water supply before the warning signals are triggered, so it is important to drink often when exercising. Drink a glass of water 15 minutes before starting an activity, every 15 minutes while exercising, and once during cool down.

Use visual cues. The sensation of thirst diminishes with age. It is therefore especially important for the elderly to have something to drink regularly. They should post notes in various locations (on the refrigerator door, for example) reminding them to drink more often in hot weather, or just keep fresh bottled water handy.

Pay attention to urine colour. Clear urine indicates proper hydration, except in the morning, or in the case of pregnant women, when it is normally more concentrated.

WHEN TO CONSULT?

- ► You are always thirsty, even at night.
- ► You urinate often, regardless of your water intake, and are always hungry.
- ► Your skin, mouth and lips are abnormally parched.
- ► You have recurrent infections and wounds that do not heal.
- ► You are unable to determine the reason for your thirst.
- ► You have had a fever, diarrhea, or been vomiting non-stop for over 24 hours.

WHAT HAPPENS DURING THE EXAM?

The doctor will take a history, perform a physical examination and test your blood and urine. Other tests may be performed if necessary.

WHAT IS THE TREATMENT?

Dehydration

Serious dehydration may require hospitalization, though drinking lots of water usually corrects the problem. If fatigue is a factor, rest will also be prescribed.

Drugs

If your medication is making you thirsty, your doctor will change the dose or the prescription itself.

Diabetes

Treatment will be specific to the type of diabetes you have and usually entails the administration of a balanced diet, exercise program and, if need be, insulin or oral glucose-lowering agents.

Diabetes insipidus

The doctor may prescribe a synthetic hormone to replace vasopressin.

Psychiatric disorders

Treatment for the illness will have to be undertaken. Drugs alone are often enough to eliminate the thirst.

Tics and Tremors

Tics and tremors are both uncontrollable body movements, but should not be confused with each other.

Tics are brief, automatic and repeated gestures with no functional purpose. Often appearing in childhood, they are hereditary in 30% to 50% of cases. They may take the form of blinking, head turning, or shrugging, for a few examples. Tremors, on the other hand, are abnormal muscle movements that manifest as rapid, continuous, and involuntary oscillations. They can affect the hands, fingers, head, or torso and are more common in people over 40 years of age.

There are different types of tics and tremors.

Tics
Normal or iatrogenic tics (triggered by medication)
► Temporary movements related to a specific period in one's life.
► Affect approximately 10% of children during their development.
► May become more intensified during puberty but generally gradually diminish into adulthood.
► May develop in some adults subsequent to a highly charged emotional or stressful situation.

Pathological tics
► Tics triggered by a disease

Gilles de la Tourette Syndrome
► Defined by the number and severity of tics.
► Starts in childhood and primarily affects boys.
► Can encompass various complex movements such as jumping, continuous arm thrusting and repetitive touching. Whistling, uttering obscenities and making obscene gestures are also features.
► May include an obsessional tendency to repeat gestures or words.
► Is often accompanied by an attention disorder and hyperactivity.

Tremors
Normal or iatrogenic tremors (triggered by medication)
► Mild and intermittent.

Pathological tremors
► Triggered by a disease

Familial or Essential Tremors
► Develop in adulthood during the thirties or forties.
► Characterized by slight jerky movements of the hands that may be predominant on one side (tremors in one hand or arm). In some cases, they develop in both sides of the body.
► Although benign, writing or raising a glass to drink, for example, can become problematic.
► Intensify with age, eventually affecting the neck, head, and voice.

Parkinson's Disease
► Occurs between 50 and 60 years of age, affecting 1% of the population over 55.
► Movements are slower and more wide-ranging than familial tremors.
► Often affects only one side of the body and occurs only when the muscle is at rest.
► Begins with an uncontrollable tremor that involves rubbing the thumb and forefinger together as if rolling an imaginary pill (pill-rolling tremor).
► Idiopathic Parkinson's describes stiffness and loss of dexterity for rapid movement.
► Speech difficulties, in severe cases.

WHAT ARE THE CAUSES?
Tics
Normal or iatrogenic tics
► **Stress and anxiety, fatigue and emotional overload.** Tics sometimes reappear in adulthood and during stressful or depressing circumstances.

► *Overuse of stimulants or medications.* Stimulants such as coffee, tea or tobacco can cause certain neurotransmitters (adrenaline and dopamine) to become hyperactive, triggering tics in those with a predisposition. Certain medication, such as the amphetamine derivatives found in certain decongestants and broncho-dilators (for asthma treatment), can have the same effect. Ritalin, a drug used in the management of hyperactivity disorders, may cause temporary tics in children.

Pathological tics

► *Endocrine disorders.* Hyperthyroidism and pheochromocytoma, for only two examples, increase the release of dopamine and adrenaline, possibly leading to tics.
► *Certain rare disorders of the central nervous system* such as Huntingdon's chorea and schizophrenia may trigger tics.

Gilles de la Tourette Syndrome

► *Neurological disease of unknown cause.*
► *Socioaffective problems may intensify tics.*
► *At puberty, tics are often triggered by the production of hormones, especially in boys.*

Tremors

Normal or iatrogenic tremors

► *Physiological response to stress,* extreme fatigue, or stimulants such as coffee, tea, tobacco, or illicit drugs (such as cocaine or ecstasy).
► *Medications,* particularly broncho-dilators and decongestants. Certain psychotropic agents (mood medications) such as antidepressants, lithium and neuroleptic drugs may cause tremors similar to the familial variety. Some high blood pressure drugs also cause mild but very rapid tremors. These medications stimulate the release of dopamine and adrenaline, neurotransmitters that may provoke tremors in people who are already predisposed.

Pathological tremors

▶ ***Certain diseases,*** including endocrine disorders such as hyperthyroidism, or neurological diseases like schizophrenia may be accompanied by tremors. These disorders increase the amount of dopamine and adrenaline released.

Familial or essential tremors

▶ ***Heredity.*** Some tremors run in the family and are not associated with any other neurological symptoms.

Parkinson's Disease

▶ ***Chronic neurological disease.*** This common disease (affecting 1% to 2% of the population) leads to nerve cell degeneration and an insufficient supply of dopamine, the hormone in the brain that regulates movement.

PRACTICAL ADVICE

Tics

Avoid stimulants. Consume tea or coffee in moderate amounts or not at all.

Avoid refined sugar. Refined sugar seems to aggravate tics, especially in children, so eliminate it from snacks.

Avoid the use of nasal decongestants. Cold and nasal decongestant medicines are stimulants.

Practice relaxation techniques. Before prescribing any drug, a doctor will recommend that you practice relaxation techniques such as yoga to help control the tics.

Follow an exercise program. Swim, run, walk or work out regularly. At least 20 minutes per session, three times a week, will reduce the frequency of tics.

Tremors

Be careful of alcohol. Even if it can lessen an essential tremor, the effect is only temporary and will be followed by an increase in tics.

Relax your muscles. If you are tense, relaxing your muscles can alleviate tremors. Ask your doctor to recommend someone who can teach you biofeedback, in conjunction with other relaxation techniques.

Get enough sleep. Sleep will rest your muscles. Most people need at least 7 to 8 hours a night on a regular schedule.

Make a list of your medications. Over-the-counter cold and flu medicines, as well as prescription asthma medications, contain decongestants like pseudoephedrine that can also cause tremors. Ask your doctor or pharmacist if any of the medicine you are taking can increase tremors.

Use special cutlery. Heavy cutlery (knives, forks and spoons) can make mealtime easier, as the weight of the utensils helps control tremors. There are also plates available with raised lips or edges to prevent food from sliding (these can be ordered from a medical or surgical supply house). It may also be helpful to fill your glasses or cups only half way to avoid spilling.

Tire out your muscles. Before the execution of a task, sit in a chair or armchair and let your arms hang down at your sides. Grab the seat of the chair or the armrests with the palms of your hands and, with your shoulders straight, press your hands gently down against the chair for two minutes. This exercise will tire out the muscles and give you a short break from the tremors.

WHEN TO CONSULT?

► You have been having tics for over six months.
► The seriousness and number of tics have an impact on your lifestyle and professional life.

- ► You have tremors.
- ► You are over 50 and one of your hands trembles even when at rest.
- ► You have Parkinson's disease.

WHAT HAPPENS DURING THE EXAM?

For both tics and tremors, the diagnosis is simple and based on a personal and family history. The examination will include a blood work-up to check certain biological parameters (notably thyroid function).

In rare cases where the tics and tremors are accompanied by symptoms that suggest a neurological disorder, a brain scan (computed axial tomography, or CAT-scan) will be administered.

WHAT IS THE TREATMENT?

Tics

Normal or iatrogenic tics

The benign tics of a child, as well as those associated with nervousness or fatigue, do not require treatment, as they disappear or become manageable by adulthood in most cases. If necessary, the doctor can prescribe benzodiazepines such as Valium or Rivotril.

Tics triggered by an excess of stimulants or medication disappear if consumption is reduced or the prescription modified. Likewise, tics induced by Ritalin in children go away once the dose is reduced.

Pathological tics

Treating or managing the underlying disorder usually eliminates the tics.

Gilles de la Tourette syndrome

Treatment entails relaxation techniques and neuroleptic drugs, especially new-generation neuroleptics, such as risperidone, which have fewer adverse side effects.

Tremors

Normal or iatrogenic tremors

If caused by medication, the tremors disappear once the pharmacological treatment is stopped.

Pathological tremors
If a disease is responsible, treating or controlling the underlying problem usually eliminates the tremors.

Familial tremors
Two types of drugs are usually prescribed: propranolol (Inderal) and primidone (Mysoline). They do not, however, prevent disease progression and have adverse side effects. Although propranolol can cause dizziness when standing up after lying down, it does control tremors relatively well. Primidone is a sedative that can make the patient weak at the outset of treatment.

Parkinson's disease
Treatment involves replacing dopamine (a hormone deficient in persons with Parkinson's disease) with levodopa, its precursor or forerunner. Available drugs include Sinemet and Prolopa. The doctor may also prescribe a drug that imitates dopamine by acting on its receptors. Such agents are called dopamine agonists and there are a number of varieties, including Parlodel, Permax, Requip and Mirapex.

Dopamine agonists can produce such adverse effects as dizziness upon waking, nausea and vomiting. At high doses, they can cause overexcitement, hallucinations and even a state of paranoia.

Treatment of unilateral Parkinsonian tremors (on one side of the body) can involve a surgical procedure that uses an electrode to destroy or stimulate the area of the brain responsible for the tremors.

Tinnitus

Tinnitus is an internally produced auditory sensation that only the sufferer can hear. The generally high-pitched sound occurs regularly and is of moderate volume. Although easily drowned out by other sounds, it can become bothersome in silent environments, for example, at bedtime. Loud noises cause the volume to increase.

Tinnitus sufferers hear two types of sound: subjective and objective. The first is only an impression of sound, while the second is real, produced by the body itself.

The sound may be perceived in both ears or only one. In some cases, the sufferer cannot tell if one particular side is affected and may think the sound is emanating from the centre of the cranium.

It is believed that tinnitus is the result of malfunctioning neurotransmitters. These "messengers" transport nervous impulses along the auditory nerve and can become defective for various reasons.

Rarely so severe as to be unbearable, tinnitus can nevertheless decrease the sufferer's quality of life by directly affecting his or her mood and, consequently, relationships with others. It may also be accompanied by episodes of vertigo and loss of balance or hearing.

This problem affects half the population at some point in their life, and 5% of the elderly permanently.

The types of sounds heard vary:

Subjective sounds
- Ringing bells.
- A human voice.
- Murmuring.
- Crackling.
- Buzzing.
- Whistling.

Objective sounds
- The sound of rushing blood or contracting muscles

WHAT ARE THE CAUSES?

Inner ear problems

► *Age.* Aging and the hardening of arteries frequently bring about presbyacusia, which is a loss of higher frequency hearing, often associated with tinnitus.

► *Atherosclerosis.* The hardening of the arteries is caused by cholesterol plaque deposits.

► *Ménière's disease.* An increase in pressure of the endolymph, the naturally occurring liquid of the inner ear, results in sudden and regular attacks of vertigo, accompanied by a buzzing in the ear and deafness.

► *Sound trauma.* Exposure to loud noise, such as high volume music on headphones (on a portable tape or compact disc player, for example) or through daily work in a very noisy environment, can damage the inner ear.

► *Cerebrovascular accident (stroke).*

► *Auditory nerve tumour.*

► *Skull fracture.*

Middle ear problems

► *Otitis media (middle ear infection).* This inflammation partially blocks the auditory canal.

► *Perforated eardrum.* An extremely loud noise, a middle ear infection or a blow to the ear can perforate the eardrum.

► *Ostospongiosis.* Also known as ostosclerosis, ostospongiosis is a hereditary condition that reduces the mobility of the stapes, one of the three auditory ossicles in the middle ear that transmit sound vibrations to the inner ear. If left untreated, this disease leads to deafness.

Outer ear problems

► *Impacted cerumen (wax build-up).* Earwax build-up can block the external auditory canal.

PRACTICAL ADVICE

Avoid excessively loud noise. It is very important to protect your ears from extremely loud noises that can cause tinnitus or worsen an existing condition. If using headphones, listen at a reasonable volume. Wear ear plugs or some other ear protection if you work in a noisy area or go hunting.

Get some sleep. The auditory sensations caused by tinnitus are more noticeable in silence. If this prevents you from falling asleep, try playing soft relaxing music to mask the sound.

Try some relaxation techniques. Stress does not cause tinnitus, but there does appear to be a relationship between the two and learning to relax can help decrease the symptoms. Ask your doctor to recommend a psychologist. The therapist will use electronic sensors to measure the stress reactions of your heart, muscles and breathing, and teach you relaxation techniques specifically adapted to your needs.

Try electronic masking methods. Audioprosthetists sell devices that produce white noise, a sound covering a wide range of frequencies, which can mask the sound of tinnitus when set at low volume. These devices can be used whenever it is convenient. This method, however, works for only a small number of sufferers. Consult your doctor.

Change medications. Aspirin can sensitize the auditory nerve. If this was the original cause of the condition, avoiding this medication can alleviate or even stop the tinnitus. Taking acetaminophen or nonsteroidal anti-inflammatories is recommended instead.

Prevent wax build-up from developing. Using cotton swabs (Q-tips) to clean your ears pushes wax deeper into the external ear canal, leading to build-up. Use the corner of a damp facecloth instead and always avoid penetrating the ear canal. If your glands secrete large amounts of cerumen, place a hot (but not boiling) water bottle on your ears from time to time. This will soften the wax and allow it to drain more easily. Drops to soften the wax are also sold over-the-counter in drugstores.

Get support. The Canadian Hearing Society can provide support and advice.

Avoid stimulants. Nicotine, alcohol and caffeine stimulate the auditory nerve of the inner ear and increase tinnitus.

WHEN TO CONSULT?

► You frequently hear noises in the absence of external stimulus.

WHAT HAPPENS DURING THE EXAM?

The doctor will take a history and perform a complete physical examination. If necessary, he or she will ask you to take a hearing test (audiometry) to evaluate your auditory responses. In most cases, this assessment is enough to make a diagnosis.

WHAT IS THE TREATMENT?

Inner ear problems

Tinnitus is frequently chronic, especially when caused by aging, sound trauma, stroke, tumour, or skull fracture. In these cases, the sufferer must simply find a way to live with the condition and learn to decrease tension with relaxation techniques such as listening to soft music. Medications that dilate the blood vessels (such as peripheral vasodilators) may help control the symptoms, but their effectiveness is limited. In very severe cases, the doctor may prescribe cortisone to relieve some of the congestion in the inner ear.

Treating high cholesterol by changing certain dietary habits and taking medication may help decrease the symptoms of tinnitus.

Certain treatments for Ménière's disease (also a chronic condition) are sometimes able to control auditory sensations. A salt-free diet and diuretics can be used to regulate endolymphatic pressure. If these measures are insufficient, the doctor may administer gentamicin (a type of antibiotic) via injection through the eardrum, draining the endolymph and, hopefully, decreasing the symptoms. This treatment is quite common, easily tolerated by the patient, and usually performed under local anesthesia.

Middle ear problems

Tinnitus disappears with the appropriate treatment. Otitis media can be quickly and easily treated with antibiotics.

Perforated eardrums heal on their own in most cases, though surgical intervention is sometimes necessary. The procedure involves attaching a thin, sterile paper (resembling a small piece of cigarette rolling paper) over the perforation to hold the skin together so that proper healing can occur.

Ostospongiosis can also be treated surgically. The minor surgery involves cutting the ligament attached to the stapes to restore mobility.

Outer ear problems

The doctor simply removes the cerumen build-up obstructing the auditory canal. This is done by curettage (using a curette to remove the wax) or by irrigating the ear with water using a syringe.

Upset Stomach

All ingested food goes to the stomach first. With a volume of approximately two litres, it provides an acidic environment to prepare food for digestion, a process that takes an average of two to three hours.

Poor digestion can cause three types of stomach upset: heartburn, when gastric juices rise from the stomach to the esophagus (gastroesophageal reflux); cramps, caused by muscle dilations; and eructation (burping), when swallowed air is expelled (sometimes noisily!).

An upset stomach may be accompanied by the following symptoms:

Heartburn

► May be associated with slow digestion.
► May be accompanied by abdominal cramps, nausea, chest pain and in some cases, weight loss.
► Regurgitation may leave an acidic taste in the mouth, as well as cause hoarseness, coughing, difficulty swallowing (dysphagia), or pain with swallowing (odynphagia).

Stomach cramps

► Discomfort in the upper abdomen.
► May be accompanied by diarrhea, constipation or bloating.
► May occur intermittently or chronically (ulcer).

Eructation (burping)

► Harmless common phenomenon that may nevertheless cause discomfort.
► May be associated with heartburn.

WHAT ARE THE CAUSES?

Heartburn

► *Gastroesophageal reflux* occurs when the valve or sphincter separating the stomach and esophagus malfunctions and can no longer close properly, allowing acid to enter and irritate the mucous membranes of the esophagus.

► **Acidity.** Acid can create a hole in the stomach lining, also known as an ulcer. The acid in vomitus can also cause certain types of asthma (because of its proximity to the lungs), dental problems (destroying enamel) and esophagitis.

► **Medications.** A number of medications cause heartburn, including calcium channel blockers (used to treat hypertension and heart disease), nitrates (for heart failure), progesterone (a hormone found in birth control pills), most anti-inflammatories, and aspirin.

► **Unhealthy lifestyle.** Smoking, overeating, excessively fatty or rich diets, and irregular meal times can be linked to heartburn.

► **Hiatal hernia.** This occurs when abdominal pressure pushes the stomach above the diaphragm, inhibiting normal function of the sphincter between the stomach and esophagus and leading to reflux and heartburn.

► **Stress.** Stress can stimulate the production of gastric acid and cause heartburn.

Stomach cramps

► **Unhealthy dietary habits.** The most common causes of stomach cramps are eating too quickly and ingesting overly spicy or acidic food.

► **Stomach (peptic) ulcers.** Stomach discomfort or pain that disappears shortly after a meal suggests the presence of an acid problem and stomach ulcer. Ulcers are caused by anti-inflammatories or aspirin consumption, or by the *Helicobacter pylori* bacteria.

► **Food poisoning** causes involuntary contractions of the stomach muscles in reaction to a virus, bacteria or toxin.

► **Stomach motility disturbances** affect the ability of the stomach muscles to move food along the digestive tract. The sufferer experiences discomfort after meals, along with slow digestion, premature fullness, nausea, and abdominal bloating.

Eructation (burping)

► **Aerophagia** is a bad habit or tic causing a person to swallow too much air while eating or drinking. Too much air in the intestine leads to bloating, gas, and burping. Chewing gum stimulates salivation and encourages the swallowing of air.

► *Beer and soft drinks.* Most bubbly or sparkling drinks cause burping as the stomach tries to get rid of the air in the bubbles.

PRACTICAL ADVICE

Heartburn

Modify your diet. Eat several small meals a day to avoid getting too full. Pay attention to what you eat and try to determine which foods cause heartburn. The causes may vary from person to person, although particularly common triggers include fried and fatty food, chocolate, mint, tea, soft drinks, milk, beer, wine, tomatoes, and spicy food. Consume these items in moderation.

Avoid late meals. Eat at least three hours before going to bed to avoid producing gastric juices that will move up toward the esophagus when you lie down. Eating smaller meals is also a good way to control the amount of stomach acid produced.

The esophagus and heartburn

The esophageal sphincter is a valve that separates the esophagus from the stomach. Generally closed, the valve opens to allow food and liquid to pass when you swallow, returning to a closed position immediately afterwards. In some cases, however, the valve cannot perform properly. It may become lax due to a weakened muscle or malfunction, or shift out of place (if the stomach has moved towards the rib cage, for example, as can happen in cases of obesity). This allows liquid containing acid and other substances necessary for digestion to move up to the esophagus. While the stomach is well protected against the acid it produces, the esophagus is not, which explains why a burning sensation accompanies gastroesophageal reflux.

Use antacids. Over-the-counter antacids or so-called "anti-H_2" medications neutralize or diminish the secretion of gastric juices, providing temporary relief. If the problem persists, see a doctor.

Raise the head of the bed. Raising your head about twelve centimetres while you sleep will diminish gastroesophageal reflux. To be sure your upper body is raised evenly, put a piece of wood or bricks under the feet at the head of the bed. Sleeping with extra pillows is not effective, as they can flatten, move out of position or fall to the floor.

Lose weight. Obesity creates abdominal pressure that can cause heartburn. Losing a few kilos might solve your problem.

Loosen your belt while you eat. It will prevent or ease symptoms.

Beware of aspirin and anti-inflammatories. Research has shown that large doses of aspirin can cause stomach bleeding and heartburn. Two aspirins a week for the occasional headache is a safe dose. If you take it every day, speak to your doctor about alternative solutions, or take acetaminophen instead.

Quit smoking. Nicotine and other chemical products found in cigarettes can increase acid secretions in the stomach, causing or aggravating gastroesophageal reflux. Ask your doctor to recommend techniques for quitting smoking.

Learn how to manage stress. The negative effects of stress can be mitigated. Exercise, eat a balanced diet, sleep well, avoid alcohol or cigarettes, establish a realistic work schedule, and set aside time to do your favourite things. Above all, take one day at a time.

Stomach cramps
Pay attention to food and stress levels. Eat a healthy and balanced diet. Avoid irritants like coffee, cola, chocolate, alcohol, and fatty food, which can disturb stomach motility. Avoid excessively spicy food.

Get in tune with your body. Before seeing a doctor, try to figure out what is causing your cramps. Note their intensity, frequency and duration, as well as the time they occur, their location, whether they radiate to another part of the body and what, if anything, brings relief. This will help the doctor reach a diagnosis.

Food poisoning: drink plenty of water. Drink small amounts of water at regular intervals and increase the amount gradually.

Eructation (burping)
Avoid certain beverages. Beer, soft drinks, and any other sparkling or carbonated beverages create bubbles in the stomach. Drink water or juice instead. Never use a straw, as this increases the amount of air absorbed with the liquid.

Never chew gum. Chewing gum increases the amount of saliva in the mouth. When you swallow this saliva, you also swallow a great deal of air.

Why does the stomach gurgle?

Stomach gurgles are strange noises produced by intestinal movements and ingested air and liquid in the stomach.

Most of the time, the phenomenon is completely harmless and has the following causes:
- Aerophagia (swallowing air while eating).
- Empty stomach (particularly in the morning).
- Intolerance to food that ferments in the stomach (for example, vegetables such as cabbage, cauliflower, and corn).
- Lactose or sorbitol intolerance. Sorbitol is an artificial sweetener.

If, however, stomach gurgling is accompanied by cramps that disappear when you eat, you may be suffering from stomach ulcers and should consult a doctor.

Chew slowly with your mouth closed. You will avoid swallowing air and encourage proper digestion. Drink only after the meal.

Be calm. Some people burp when they get nervous. If this happens to you, try to relax.

WHEN TO CONSULT?
- ► You have changed your habits, but your heartburn persists.
- ► Antacids do not help.
- ► You have lost weight.
- ► You have trouble swallowing.
- ► You have persistent and bothersome cramps and are worried.

WHAT HAPPENS DURING THE EXAM?
The doctor takes a history and performs a complete physical examination, including palpating the abdomen. In some cases, he or she orders blood tests, X-rays, or a gastroscopy (internal examination of the stomach and esophagus with a camera).

WHAT IS THE TREATMENT?
Heartburn
If lifestyle changes and antacids are ineffective, the doctor prescribes proton pump inhibitors to prevent acid production. If medications are responsible for the heartburn, the prescription may be modified. Surgery is rarely required.

Stomach cramps
If cramps persist despite a change in dietary habits, the doctor will attempt to determine the underlying disorder and prescribe treatment accordingly. For example, ulcers may be treated with proton pump inhibitors. If the doctor suspects that *Helicobacter pylori* bacteria is responsible, he or she will prescribe antibiotics as well. Severe food poisoning may require intravenous rehydration, as well as intravenously or intramuscularly administered medication.

In cases of stomach motility disturbances, the doctor may prescribe medications to modify the contractions of the digestive tract.

Eructation (burping)

There is no medication to help with eructation. The only solution is to reduce aerophagia.

Urinary Incontinence

Urinary incontinence describes any degree of bladder control failure, which is largely a function of the brain. Some types of incontinence occur in both sexes, while others primarily affect women. These problems have a tendency to worsen with age.

There are three main types of incontinence:

Stress incontinence
► Involuntary loss of urine, often with increased abdominal pressure, such as when the sufferer coughs or sneezes.
► Occurs almost exclusively in women, although sometimes also in men who have undergone prostate surgery.

Urge incontinence (spastic bladder)
► Urgent need to urinate.
► Occurs in both men and women.

Overflow incontinence
► Can be caused by obstruction: difficulty urinating; flow diminished to drops.
► Obstruction primarily affects men, but not exclusively.
► Can be caused by the inability of the bladder to contract and void properly: continuous, involuntary loss of urine.
► Occurs in both men and women.

WHAT ARE THE CAUSES?
► *Fallen bladder.* This problem affects women almost exclusively. The pelvic floor is composed of muscles that support the bladder, intestines and uterus. Factors such as obesity, childbirth, and lowered estrogen levels after menopause cause these muscles to lose tone. The bladder descends, causing stress or urge incontinence. In some cases, the urethra also descends and projects outside the body. The condition is occasionally accompanied by anal incontinence. Approximately 30% of

women over the age of 65 are affected. The problem worsens with age.

► **Internal sphincter deficiency.** In women, the deficiency may be primary (caused by a weakened pelvic floor) or secondary to trauma (accident, rape). It may also result from stiffness caused by surgery or radiation therapy. The sphincter cannot contract to retain urine, causing stress or urge incontinence.

► **Hypertrophy of the prostate.** Initially the size of a walnut, the prostate gland begins to enlarge after the age of thirty. In 25% of men, the gland becomes so large it obstructs the urethra and prevents normal voiding. The sufferer may experience overflow symptoms (due to obstruction) or urge incontinence.

► **Urethral obstruction.** Obstruction of the urethra can also be caused by foreign bodies in the bladder (stone or other object), trauma to the urinary tract or pelvic region (due to surgery, catheter, bicycle or motorcycle accident), or even psychological problems. The sufferer may experience overflow symptoms (due to obstruction) or urge incontinence.

► **Neurological disorders.** Parkinson's disease, Alzheimer's disease, multiple sclerosis, cerebral palsy, and spinal cord injury (among others) can adversely affect the nerve pathways responsible for continence, causing neurogenic (of neurological origin) urge or overflow incontinence (due to lack of bladder contraction).

► **Medication.** Antidepressants and antipsychotics can inhibit normal bladder contraction, creating what is called a "lazy bladder" which leads to overflow incontinence.

► **Infections.** Cystitis (bladder infection) and sexually transmitted infections can irritate the urethra, leading to urge incontinence.

► **Chronic constipation** can cause urge incontinence, particularly in children. Scientists believe that the dilation of the rectum stretches the nerves of the bladder, triggering a reflex contraction.

PRACTICAL ADVICE

Consult a doctor. If left untreated, the pressure in the bladder created by obstruction can lead to the flooding of the kidneys, impeding their normal function and possibly leading to kidney failure in the long term.

Continue drinking plenty of liquids. Decreasing fluid intake will not solve the problem. It is important to maintain proper hydration.

Avoid coffee and alcohol. These substances are diuretics, stimulating the bladder and causing it to eliminate more liquid. People with idiopathic (of unknown origin) incontinence should avoid them, as they will only aggravate the problem.

Re-train your bladder. Sufferers of idiopathic urge incontinence can use biofeedback techniques to re-educate the bladder to contract at the desired time. Go to the bathroom at set times (for example, every three hours) and refrain from urinating in between. Empty your bladder completely (stand up, sit back down, and try again, to be sure).

Perform Kegel exercises. These simple and discreet exercises can improve stress incontinence within ten weeks. Contract the pelvic and sphincter muscles (those that control defecation and urination) for ten seconds, then release. Repeat three series of ten contractions as often as possible during the day (even while urinating).

Prevent accidents. If you need to cough, sneeze, or bend over, contract your pelvic and sphincter muscles first. Drugstores sell protective underpants and pads to control accidents caused by urinary incontinence. Keep a chamber pot by your bed.

Help your child be regular. Children should eat a healthy, balanced, and high-fibre diet to prevent constipation.

Prevent prostate problems. Many physicians believe that all men should have annual prostate exams after the age of fifty.

Strengthen the pelvic floor. After giving birth, women should have at least three sessions of perineal rehabilitation with a specialized physiotherapist. The exercises taught in hospital are usually not enough to maintain muscle tone in the pelvic floor.

Maintain a healthy weight. If menopausal, discuss your options with your doctor.

WHEN TO CONSULT?

► It is especially important to consult if you are a man, as it may indicate benign hypertrophy of the prostate.
► You have neurological problems.
► There is blood in your urine.
► The symptoms are very bothersome.

WHAT HAPPENS DURING THE EXAM?

The doctor interviews the patient, performs a physical exam, and orders a urine analysis and cytology (analysis of the cells in your urine). In some cases, an endoscopic (internal) examination of the urinary tract is necessary.

For men, a digital rectal exam is required to assess the size of the prostate. The doctor may also order urinary dynamic flow testing to measure the amount of urine eliminated over a given period of time and the leftover residue. A small amount eliminated over a long period of time suggests prostate-induced bladder obstruction.

WHAT IS THE TREATMENT?

Fallen bladder and internal sphincter incompetence.

Perineal rehabilitation exercises with a physiotherapist can usually provide some improvement. One particularly effective treatment involves the stimulation of the pelvic and sphincter muscles with mild electrical currents (entirely painless). This procedure improves the situation for 60% to 70% of pre-menopausal women because they still produce estrogen, which helps maintain muscle tone. Treatment is generally less successful for menopausal women, unless they are undergoing hormone replacement therapy.

In some cases, the doctor recommends surgery to raise the bladder whereby muscle from the thigh or stomach is transplanted to the area below the bladder or internal sphincter. Collagen injections can tighten the urethra, and in extreme cases, an artificial sphincter can be created.

Hypertrophy of the prostate

Surgical removal of the hypertrophied (swollen) section of the gland (or of the tissue around the urethra to eliminate the obstruction) is the most common treatment. The doctor may also administer thermal therapy (through a catheter) to burn away the swollen part of the prostate, cryotherapy to freeze it, or laser treatment to destroy it.

In younger men, the prostate may continue to grow. Thirty percent of men who have had a part of their prostate removed must undergo the same treatment later in life.

Certain medications reduce the size of the prostate, while others relax the muscles in the area of the gland to allow for normal urination (contracted muscles shrink the urinary passage). Patients should be aware that this treatment requires lifelong drug therapy.

Urethral obstruction

A foreign body in the bladder must be removed surgically. Trauma to the urinary tract or the pelvic area requires endoscopic surgery to repair the damage or plastic surgery to rebuild the urethra. Psychological problems require professional support. In most cases, incontinence problems can be successfully resolved.

Neurological problems

In cases of neurological urge incontinence, the doctor may prescribe medications to relax the bladder (anti-cholinergics and anti-spasmodics). If the patient is suffering from overflow incontinence, a catheter can void the bladder at regular intervals (every four hours, for example). Patients install and remove the catheter themselves, as needed.

Medications

The prescription is modified.

Infections

Antibiotics will clear up the infection and eliminate incontinence.

Chronic constipation

Chronic constipation in children is usually cleared up with diet modification. A consultation with a dietician may be necessary.

Vaginal Problems

Vaginal discharge, unpleasant odour, abnormal spotting, redness, irritation, genital itching, and pain during sexual intercourse are symptoms of "vaginitis". These symptoms, particularly if they are recurrent, may also be caused by other disorders.

WHAT ARE THE CAUSES?

Infections

► *Yeast or candida vaginitis ("yeast infection")* is characterized by redness, irritation and itchiness of the vulva, as well as abnormally thick, sticky, and possibly strong-smelling discharge. Antibiotics or uncontrolled diabetes are common causes, although most of the time the origin is unknown. It is not a sexually transmitted infection and the woman's partner does not require treatment. Recurring vaginitis indicates that the immune system of the vagina (but not of the body as a whole) is compromised.

► *Bacterial vaginosis* is the most common vaginal infection. Its characteristic fish-like odour intensifies after sexual intercourse, when the woman may also develop vaginal irritation. Bacterial vaginosis is not a sexually transmitted infection and is not contagious, so there is no treatment the woman's partner can undergo to reduce the infection's recurrence.

Other possible causes

► *Lack of lubrication during sexual penetration.*
► *Over-zealous hygiene and/or irritating drying soaps.*
► *Skin disorders (sclerous lichen, lichen planus, eczema, etc.).* These can cause redness, itching, and a burning sensation during urination.
► *Fissure at the vaginal opening.* The cause is usually unknown, but often due to an injury that causes the skin in the area to tear rather than stretch.
► *Local sores or lesions* caused by herpes, cancer or certain sexually transmitted infections such as condyloma (genital warts) and molluscum contagiosum (a small, benign skin tumour).

- *Vulvodynia* (burning irritation or raw skin of the vulva). The cause is unknown, although researchers believe it may result from nerve damage in the area. Sexual intercourse is painful and sometimes impossible. It may also cause a burning sensation with urination.
- *Vestibulitis.* This is a complex condition that may be caused by excess amounts of oxalic acid (found in foods such as rhubarb, plums and peaches) in vaginal secretions. It causes the vaginal opening to become painfully sensitive to the touch, creating a burning sensation with contact.
- *Desquamative inflammatory vaginitis* is a rare condition resulting from a disturbance of the vaginal flora that causes serious inflammation. It manifests in abundant, odourless yellowish or greenish discharge, as well as intense, constant itchiness that is aggravated by urination. This condition may become chronic, seriously impeding the woman's ability to have sexual intercourse and possibly affecting her daily activities. Although the exact cause is still unknown, it is believed to originate in an abnormal immune response that attacks the vaginal tissues as though they were foreign to the body.

Vaginal discharge: normal or abnormal?

Normal vaginal discharge is ivory- or cream-coloured, odourless, and does not cause itching or burning. Women who do not take oral contraceptives have clear, almost egg-white discharge in the middle of their cycle, whereas that of women on the pill remains the same throughout the month.

Yellowish, greenish, or bloody discharge is considered to be abnormal, as well as discharge that has a fish-like odour, particularly if it becomes stronger after sexual intercourse.

It is normal for discharge to appear yellowish on white underwear.

PRACTICAL ADVICE

Get a clear diagnosis. There are a number of different vulvar and vaginal disorders that cause similar symptoms. Be sure your doctor performs thorough tests before determining the diagnosis.

Soothe the itch until you receive your diagnosis. Apply cold compresses to the genital organs or dissolve baking soda in your bath water. Avoid soap, panty-liners, tight clothes, or other irritants.

Use a lubricant if needed. Be sure the vagina is well lubricated before sexual penetration. K-Y Jelly (available in pharmacies) is effective, although it may lead to further dryness if sexual intercourse is prolonged. Use Astroglide (available in specialty shops) or K-Y Liquid instead. Vaginal moisturizers that last for about three days (such as Replens or long-acting K-Y) are also available in biodegradable applicators.

Avoid experimenting with products or medications. Using leftover creams or antibiotics can make it more difficult for the doctor to reach a precise diagnosis. Avoid over-the-counter medicated creams, as they may not be appropriate to your condition. Get a clear medical diagnosis before using any products.

Do not use irritating soaps or vaginal douches. Although douches may momentarily soothe the discomfort, they contain chemical products that can actually aggravate the symptoms and prevent the vaginal flora from returning to its normal levels. Even so-called "mild" soaps can be irritating. If you still feel compelled to use soap, buy gentle unscented cleansers like Cetaphil or SpectroJel.

Continue taking the birth control pill. Unreliable medical studies from the past have led many women to blame their oral contraceptive for vaginitis. More recent and rigorous studies, however, show no link between the two.

Condoms prevent sexually transmitted infections, but do not cure vaginitis. Women with vaginitis may believe they have a sexually transmitted infection and ask their partner to wear a condom. Note, however, that sexually transmitted infections rarely cause the same symptoms as vaginitis and sexual intercourse, particularly with a male condom, aggravates its symptoms. Female condoms, on the other hand, may in fact reduce the irritation. Women with new sexual partners should use condoms until they have been tested for sexually transmitted infections.

Spermicides? Gel or foam spermicides are 80% effective when used alone and many couples combine them with condoms for greater contraceptive protection. There are drawbacks, however: spermicides can alter the bacterial balance of the vagina, leading to vaginitis, vaginosis, or irritation. When used without a condom, furthermore, they provide no protection whatsoever from sexually transmitted infection and may actually encourage the transmission of the HIV/AIDS virus, which can more easily penetrate vaginal mucous membranes when they are irritated.

Lactobacillus supplements? These products contain the bacteria Lactobacillus acidophilus (also contained in certain types of yogurt), which is not the same as the lactobacillus found in the vagina. They do not help re-establish the proper balance of the vaginal flora.

There is a cure. Some women feel guilty or ashamed when they have a condition that causes genital symptoms. This may cause them to become wary of sexual intercourse in general, leading to anxiety, depression, and possibly the loss of any desire for sexual intimacy. This state of anxiety may develop into vaginismus, the involuntary and painful contraction of the muscles of the vagina during sexual penetration. It is very important to remember that there is no reason to feel badly, as your symptoms can be cured.

WHEN TO CONSULT?

▶ Your vagina is irritated and red and the condition is very bothersome.

► You have abnormal vaginal discharge.
► Your vaginal secretions are abundant or have an abnormal odour or appearance.
► You feel pain during sexual intercourse.
► There are fissures or lesions on your genitalia.
► Treatment diminishes the symptoms but does not make them disappear.
► Treatment eliminates the symptoms for only a few days, or your symptoms recur more than three times a year.

WHAT HAPPENS DURING THE EXAM?

The doctor takes a thorough history of the symptoms and performs a physical examination. He or she asks the patient about her sex life, method of contraception, and what products she uses that might be causing the irritation. The doctor then examines the vulva, vagina, and cervix, looks at the woman's vaginal secretions under a microscope, and takes a few samples for microbiological testing.

WHAT IS THE TREATMENT?

Yeast or candida vaginitis (yeast infection)
Antifungal medications are administered orally or by vaginal applicators or suppositories. If the condition is recurrent, the doctor may prescribe long-term preventive oral therapy. There are no permanent cures.

Bacterial vaginosis
The doctor will prescribe pill-form, gel, or cream antibiotics, depending on the symptoms. There is no treatment that can permanently stabilize the vaginal flora.

Skin disease (sclerous lichen, lichen planus, eczema, etc.)
The specific treatment depends on the disease. The doctor will usually prescribe an oral antihistamine to soothe the itching and local cortisone to heal the lesions.

Fissure at the vaginal opening

Initial treatment involves physiotherapy or sex therapy to teach the patient desensitization techniques. A female condom—a small bag inserted in the vagina, with the edges covering the vulva—may help some women have painless sexual intercourse. Female condoms are available in pharmacies and certain specialty condom shops. If the fissure does not heal, some doctors recommend a surgical procedure known as vestibuloplasty (rebuilding the vestibule, i.e., the vaginal opening).

Local sores or lesions

Condyloma or molluscum contagiosum lesions can be removed with liquid nitrogen or laser treatments as well as vestibuloplasty. In cases of lesions due to genital herpes, the doctor will prescribe oral (not gel or cream) antiviral medication.

Vulvodynia

The patient can apply a cold (not frozen) compress to the vulva. The doctor may prescribe the antidepressant amitriptyline (Elavil) for its analgesic properties. Physiotherapy, acupuncture, or other chronic pain management treatments may also be recommended.

Vestibulitis

This complex condition involves a number of different treatments. The doctor may prescribe calcium citrate supplements (up to six a day) and a low-oxalate diet, which eliminates foods like rhubarb, plums, peaches, spinach, cacao, peanuts, peppers, beans, beets, celery, parsley, strawberries, zucchini, grapes, and tea. Antidepressants, physiotherapy, or acupuncture may also be recommended and sex therapy may be undertaken to complete the treatment. If the patient sees no results after six months of treatment, the doctor may recommend vestibuloplasty.

Desquamative inflammatory vaginitis

This requires long-term treatment with antibiotics or a cortisone-based medication.

Vertigo

Vertigo and dizziness are sometimes hard to distinguish. While vertigo describes the sensation of whirling about as if on a merry-go-round, or feeling like objects are whirling around you, dizziness describes a feeling of imbalance, as if the floor is moving beneath you and you are about to fall (similar to the sensation of standing in a rowboat).

Vertigo can be a symptom of many diseases although it is usually caused by mild damage to the inner ear, where the body's balance centre is located. In 80 to 90% of cases, the damage is caused by an inner ear disease.

Generally speaking, vertigo comes on suddenly and recurs several times throughout the day. Bouts of vertigo are accompanied by nausea, loss of balance, falls and sometimes vomiting. In the case of an ear disease, the sufferer may experience diminished hearing, pain or ringing in the ears.

WHAT ARE THE CAUSES?

Ear diseases

- ► **Benign paroxysmal positional vertigo (BPPV).** This is the most common ear disorder and occurs when abnormal pressure impedes the flow of the inner ear liquid. BPPV is a benign problem triggered by activities such as scuba diving, merry-go-round rides, playing on a seesaw, etc.
- ► **Viral infections.** Labyrinthitis, or inflammation of the inner ear (also called otitis interna), and vestibular neuritis (inflammation of the inner ear nerve) also cause fever, sore throat and sometimes diminished vision.
- ► **Ménière's disease.** This condition is characterized by congestion and water retention in the inner ear. It is a rare chronic disease that results in three main symptoms: recurrent spells of severe vertigo that last up to one hour and occur without moving the head, sudden deafness, and tinnitus (noise or ringing in the ears). Nausea and vomiting may also be present.

Other causes

► *Brain disorders.* Cerebrovascular accident (CVA or stroke), multiple sclerosis, some types of epilepsy, brain malformations and tumours cause a disruption in the electrical current that transmits information from the ear to the brain.

► *Diseases.* While the reasons are not well known, viral infections (mononucleosis, influenza, etc.), colds, high blood pressure problems, hypoglycemia, diabetes, malnutrition, allergies and heart disease can all cause vertigo.

► *Psychological problems* such as anxiety, panic, hyperventilation and severe nervous breakdowns. Persons with psychological disorders are likely to be more acutely aware of normal body fluctuations and misinterpret some of them as vertigo or dizziness.

► *Drugs.* Sedatives, antidepressants, tranquilizers and arthritis drugs seem to affect the autonomous nervous system (the part of the brain responsible for maintaining vital functions).

► *Aging.* Elderly persons suffering from vision problems (blurry, unreliable vision) and cervical spondylosis (degeneration of the joints) often experience vertigo accompanied by dizziness and loss of balance. For this particular group, vertigo is exacerbated by anti-hypertensives (drugs for high blood pressure), which upset elderly persons' autonomous nervous system, and/or anti-inflammatories, which can lower their blood pressure and disturb the centre of balance.

► *Alcohol.* The liquid in the ear's balance centre absorbs alcohol, thereby causing abnormal pressure that results in vertigo and balance loss.

► *Allergies.* Although quite rare, vertigo may indicate an allergy to pollen, animal dander or some foods. Other symptoms may include red stinging eyes, a runny nose, and a sensation of heaviness or burning in the ears.

PRACTICAL ADVICE

Do not be unduly alarmed. Vertigo often goes away as quickly as it occurs. If no other symptoms are present, there is nothing to worry about.

Slow the pace. To prevent it from getting worse and causing vomiting, it is very important to walk slowly and avoid sudden movements during a bout of vertigo. Slow down and, if possible, sit or lie down. Avoid walking on unsteady terrain to prevent falls.

Close your eyes. Reducing ocular movement helps control vertigo.

Get comfortable. Find a comfortable position to help reduce the anxiety caused by the vertigo.

Drink water. Although there is no explanation, it seems that inadequate hydration increases the number and intensity of vertigo spells. Make sure you drink 6 to 8 glasses of water a day. If you feel nauseous, take small sips only to avoid stimulating the stomach and vomiting.

Get up slowly. If you are prone to vertigo, get into the habit of standing up slowly. In the morning, for example, sit on the edge of the bed for a few seconds before gently standing up.

Do special exercises. If you experience vertigo when simply getting up or walking, the following exercise may help. Four or five times a day, get up slowly, take a few steps, and sit down when the vertigo starts. You may initially only be able to take three or four steps before the onset of vertigo, but this will gradually improve considerably.

Do not drive. If you have had a temporary bout of vertigo, it is best to wait two or three hours before driving to be certain the episode will not recur. If you experience vertigo regularly, as in the case of an ear disease, consult your doctor before driving.

Make lifestyle changes. Reduce your consumption of stimulants that increase vertigo episodes like tobacco, alcohol and caffeine (tea, coffee, carbonated drinks, chocolate). Also eliminate or reduce your salt intake as salt causes water retention and can disrupt the balance mechanism of the inner ear.

Practice relaxation techniques. If anxiety is the cause of your vertigo, practice relaxation techniques like yoga or meditation. Simply engaging in an activity you enjoy will also help manage the problem.

Rest if you have the flu. The flu can cause vertigo so be sure to rest and drink plenty of fluids. To ease the pain, take one or two acetaminophen tablets (325 mg to 500 mg) four times a day, not exceeding four grams daily. Your vertigo should go away quickly.

Avoid strict diets. Calorie-poor diets (500 calories a day) cause rapid weight loss that can be accompanied by vertigo, dizziness and even fainting. If you want to diet, consult your doctor first.

Be active. Staying physically fit helps you maintain a healthy musculoskeletal system, train and stimulate your equilibrium system, and avoid certain illnesses (infections, diabetes, etc.).

WHEN TO CONSULT?

► The vertigo is significant and lasts for two or three weeks.
► Vertigo is accompanied by fever, headaches or deafness (partial or total).
► Your vision changes.
► You have trouble speaking or walking.
► You experience numbness affecting the extremities and the mouth.
► Vertigo runs in your family.

WHAT HAPPENS DURING THE EXAM?

The doctor will perform a thorough examination to detect signs such as arrhythmia (abnormal heart beat rhythm), a drop in blood pressure, perspiration, pallor, inflammation of the oropharynx (back of the throat), fever and stiffness in the nape of the neck, which may indicate a disease other than an ear disorder.

If the doctor finds none of these signs, he or she will administer auditory and visual tests, as well as perform oculo-vestibular movements designed to induce vertigo. Neurological tests may sometimes be necessary.

WHAT IS THE TREATMENT?
Ear Diseases
BPPV
The doctor will recommend that you avoid any vertigo-inducing activities and may also prescribe medication for nausea or anti-vertigo drugs, if the symptoms are severe.

Viral infections
Treatment simply consists of acetaminophen, rest and good hydration. Anti-vertigo drugs may also be prescribed. In the vast majority of cases, the symptoms go away on their own after about 10 days. In some cases, auditory reconditioning exercises will be required. These are simple exercises that can easily be done at home.

Ménière's disease
When the doctor prescribes a drug for Ménière's disease, he or she will explain how it works and the side effects. This disease requires regular medical follow-up.

Other Causes
Treatment depends on the underlying problem and may entail anything from a change in prescription or diet, to the management of allergy and flu symptoms, to prescription tranquilizers and therapy for persons with anxiety.

Brain disorders and aging
If someone with vertigo has risk factors for cerebrovascular disease (i.e., is over 60, a diabetic, smoker, obese, or has heart disease or hypertension), the doctor may recommend an aspirin a day in addition to a prescription for anti-vertigo medication.

The doctor may also recommend mild physical activity for elderly vertigo sufferers to improve joint flexibility and strengthen their musculature.

Vision Problems

It is normal for vision to change with age. Once most people reach their forties, they start to experience blurred vision and see less well at close range and in the dark. It is often at this age that people start wearing glasses.

Myopia (poor distance vision), presbyopia (poor close-range vision) and hyperopia (poor vision both near and far) are not diseases of the eye per se, but irregularities caused by heredity or the aging process. There are, however, diseases that affect one's sight, causing loss of vision that is gradual or sudden, partial or total, and sometimes accompanied by eye pain or headaches.

WHAT ARE THE CAUSES?
Gradual Vision Failure

► *Cataracts.* The crystalline lens (a small lens inside the eye) gradually becomes opaque (less transparent), resulting in blurred vision akin to seeing through fog or mist. Although cataracts can develop at any time (even at birth), diabetics and individuals over the age of 70 are particularly susceptible. Long-term, unprotected exposure to sunlight is also a possible cause.

► *Diabetic retinopathy.* In diabetics, small blood vessels burst at the back of the eye (an area known as the fundus) and are no longer able to nourish the retina, resulting in gradually failing vision.

► *Glaucoma.* For reasons yet unknown, the canals through which the eye's watery fluid (aqueous humour) is drained become narrow and blocked. Consequently, inner pressure begins to build, risking damage to the optic fibres and eventually to vision. There are different types of glaucoma. Chronic glaucoma involves a very subtle degeneration, initially only affecting the peripheral (side) vision, which the sufferer does not even generally notice. According to statistics, chronic glaucoma affects 4% of persons over the age of 40 and is often hereditary. Acute glaucoma is much more rare, causing severe eye pain and the perception of halos around lights. A form of congenital glaucoma also exists, but is extremely rare.

► *Macular degeneration.* The macula (commonly known as the "yellow spot") is located a few millimetres behind the retina and ensures acute vision and colour distinction. With age, it can gradually degenerate, causing loss of visual acuity, i.e., the ability to read, thread a needle or make out fine details. Macular degeneration results in blurred vision interspersed with wavy lines and affects one in three persons over the age of 70 to some degree. Sometimes the damage can be sudden and complete, caused by a burn resulting from looking directly into the sun or a partial solar eclipse.

Sudden Failing Vision
► *Vascular diseases.* The eye is nourished by tiny vessels known as capillaries that can become blocked as a result of a venous or arterial thrombosis. It is rare for both eyes to be simultaneously affected by this sudden, partial or complete loss of vision.
► *Detached retina.* In myopic (nearsighted) people, the retina may detach because the curvature of the eye is too broad. In diabetics, it may detach because of vascularization problems in the eye. This condition may also occur in elderly people as their eye tissue loses tone, or in individuals with eye damage from cataract surgery. A detached retina causes sudden partial loss of vision.
► *Eye injuries* can cause, among other problems, cataracts, glaucoma or a detached retina. Loss of vision can be gradual or sudden, partial or total.

PRACTICAL ADVICE
Find ways to make your life easier. Once a doctor identifies the problem, there are things you can do to improve your quality of life. For example, wear glasses or use a magnifying glass/sheet to read (a yellow sheet will make your vision even clearer). Read large-print books, use a large-button phone, and increase the light in your environment. Do not be afraid to watch television at a closer more comfortable range. Contrary to popular belief, it does not emit radiation and causes no harm to the eyes.

Protect your eyes from the sun. Wear sunglasses with UV/infrared protection and frames that protect the sides of the eyes as well. Wearing a cap or wide-brimmed hat will also help protect you from the sun's reflective rays.

Make sure children have a preventive eye examination. People should have their eyes checked throughout their lifetimes, beginning when they are preschoolers. Because glaucoma is hereditary, eye exams are all the more crucial if this disease runs in the family.

Wear protective eye gear. Always wear protective eye gear when doing woodwork or home repairs and, obviously, if your occupation (carpentry, mechanics, welding, etc.) exposes your eyes to risk.

Do not smoke. Smoking increases the risk of a vascular accident.

Test your own vision. You can easily see if you are suffering failing vision by closing or covering one eye with your hand and trying to read the small print in the phone book. Do the same with the other eye.

WHEN TO CONSULT?
► You experience unusual failing vision.
► You lose your vision suddenly.

WHAT HAPPENS DURING THE EXAM?
The doctor will conduct a thorough eye exam and prescribe additional tests, as necessary. The earlier the problem is assessed, the better the chances of recovering normal vision, or at the very least, preventing any further degeneration.

WHAT IS THE TREATMENT?
Gradual vision failure
Cataracts
Cataracts require a surgical intervention known as phacoemulsification. The procedure involves making a very small incision in the

eye, crushing the diseased crystalline lens, removing it by aspiration, and replacing it with an artificial one. The operation is usually a day surgery, thereby allowing for a quick resumption of regular activities. Contrary to popular belief, cataract removal does not involve laser surgery. Anti-inflammatory and antibiotic drops are prescribed for three to six weeks after surgery to facilitate healing. Colours will seem brighter after the surgery, but otherwise vision will return to normal.

Diabetic retinopathy
Laser surgery is the pre-eminent treatment choice. It stops the bleeding by destroying the damaged vessels. While lost vision cannot be recovered because nerve tissue does not regenerate, the procedure will halt any further progression of the disease.

Glaucoma
Several types of drugs are available to treat chronic glaucoma, including hypotensive drops and beta-blockers. These medications lower the internal pressure of the eye and must be used permanently. If drug treatment is unsuccessful, laser surgery can unblock the drainage canals and facilitate circulation of the watery fluid, halting the progression of the disease, even if it does not restore lost vision. In the case of acute glaucoma, laser surgery often restores perfect vision because the internal pressure has not had enough time to destroy the optic fibres.

Sudden Failing vision
Vascular diseases
Surgery sometimes helps restore vision to some extent.

Macular degeneration
Visudyne is a new pharmacological treatment for so-called "wet" macular degeneration. There are no specific treatments for other forms of the condition. Vitamin supplements (vitamin A, selenium, copper and zinc) may sometimes be recommended as some studies show they slow down the degenerative process. These are, however,

experimental and controversial treatments. If the loss of vision occurs after directly looking into the sun or an eclipse, there is a chance vision may be restored shortly afterwards, depending on the severity of the burn.

Detached retina
A detached retina is repaired surgically. The quality of restored sight depends on the time lapse between the detachment and medical consultation.

Vomiting

Vomiting is the expulsion of the contents of the stomach through the mouth. It occurs in response to the stimulation of an area called the vomiting centre, which is located in the medulla oblongata.

Once stimulated, the vomiting centre triggers a complex process to expel the stomach's contents beginning with a contraction of the abdominal muscles and diaphragm that compresses the stomach. This causes the pylorus (one of the two stomach openings that transports food to the intestines) to close, and the cardia (which transports food to the mouth) to open. The contents of the stomach then only have one means of expulsion: the mouth.

Vomiting is generally preceded by nausea, but may also be accompanied by stomach pain, abdominal cramps, hypersalivation, heart palpitations, migraines (a rare occurrence), stiffness in the nape of the neck, fever, dizziness, and even fainting.

The duration and intensity of these associated symptoms vary on a case-by-case basis and should be taken more seriously in the elderly and young children. It should also be noted that vomiting can sometimes cause complications serious enough for hospitalization. Although rare, for example, if the glottis does not close properly, the vomited matter (vomitus) can be inhaled into the respiratory airways and later cause aspiration pneumonia.

WHAT ARE THE CAUSES?

- ► *Myocardial infarction.* Onset is often characterized by nausea and stomach pains that progress to vomiting.
- ► *Pregnancy* is a frequent cause of nausea and vomiting, especially in the first 14 to 16 weeks. See chapter on Nausea and Vomiting of Pregnancy.
- ► *Motion sickness* is caused by stimulation of the balance centre in the ear, producing stomach motility disorders that cause nausea and vomiting.
- ► *Digestive disorders,* such as gastroduodenal ulcer, biliary duct ("liver attacks") or pancreas diseases, gallbladder stones, appen-

dicitis, intestinal blockage, alcohol abuse, certain foods, or smoking.
- ► *Psychic disorders,* such as anorexia, bulimia, fear and stress.
- ► *Viruses,* such as gastroenteritis or viral hepatitis.
- ► *Bacteria,* as in the case of food poisoning or meningitis.
- ► *Some drugs and treatment* like antibiotics (erythromycin), chemotherapy or morphine.

PRACTICAL ADVICE

Take preventive action. If you have an illness that can make you dizzy, discuss the matter with your doctor to become more familiar with your disease and avoid triggering the vomiting reflex.

Lie down and rest. Vomiting is often enough to eliminate other symptoms. If the vomiting does not recur, you will probably feel fine again within a few hours.

Settle your stomach and drink plenty of liquids after vomiting. Eat light meals and only drink fluids like broth, water and flat soft drinks, re-introducing solids into your diet gradually. Until you have completely recovered, avoid fatty meals, alcohol, coffee, fried foods, cured meats or spicy foods. Eat red meat, rice, bread, rusks (soda biscuits, crackers, etc.) and cereals or grains. Make sure to drink plenty of water since vomiting can be dehydrating. Other hydration solutions are available in pharmacies.

Avoid dairy products. As they are not easily digested and slow recovery.

Try to keep track of when you vomited. This can be helpful in determining the cause. Perhaps you overindulged in food or wine or started a new medication, for example. Two medications that frequently cause vomiting are Lanoxin, a drug used in the treatment of heart failure, and theophylline (Theo-Dur), a bronchodilator used in the management of asthma.

Prevent motion sickness. If you are prone to motion sickness, take an anti-nausea drug a few hours before your trip. Gravol and scopolamine patches are available in pharmacies without prescription.

Check with others. See if your friends or work colleagues have the same symptoms to rule out the possibility that you have contracted an infection. Do the same if you have just come back from a trip or shared a meal with friends, since it could be a case of food poisoning. Lastly, if you are taking a new drug, consult your pharmacist to find out if it could be the cause.

WHEN TO CONSULT?

The following situations warrant immediate medical attention:
► You suspect the vomiting is caused by a heart problem.
► A child or elderly person has five bouts of vomiting in the same day.
► You vomit more than 10 times in a single day or the frequency of vomiting increases and continues for more than 48 hours.
► You are vomiting blood.
► Your vomit contains matter similar in colour to coffee or feces.

WHAT HAPPENS DURING THE EXAM?

The doctor will take a thorough history and perform a complete physical examination to determine the origin of the problem. This will generally include a blood pressure reading, blood work, and basic abdominal and neurological assessment. The doctor may then decide to perform more exhaustive testing involving X-rays, echography and endoscopy.

WHAT IS THE TREATMENT?

If an underlying illness is responsible for the vomiting, the doctor will first treat the illness and then manage the vomiting as necessary.

Gravol (available in pharmacies without a prescription) can keep vomiting and the nausea associated with it in check. If taken a few hours before departure, it is also effective against motion sickness. It can, however, cause drowsiness and should not be taken if you have to drive. Scopolamine patches (available over the counter) are also effective against motion sickness-induced nausea and vomiting. Their possible side effects include dry mouth, drowsiness and accelerated heart rate. Scopolamine is not recommended for children and persons with glaucoma or prostatism (bladder outlet obstruction). Metoclopramide (Maxeran) is an anti-nausea drug available by prescription only.

Acute vomiting may require hospitalization for intravenous rehydration. Hospitalization will also be required for aspiration pneumonia.

If the vomiting is caused by appendicitis or an intestinal obstruction, surgery is required.

Psychotherapy combined with drug therapy may be of some help for vomiting related to a psychological disorder.

Water Retention (Edema)

Water retention, or to use the medical term, edema, is defined as an excessive accumulation of liquid in the body or one part of the body.

The body makes a constant effort—primarily regulated by the kidneys—to balance the amount of water lost (through urine, stool, and perspiration) and taken in (through drinking or eating). Water retention occurs when the body stores up more water than it eliminates. It is also caused by blood vessel dilation, which expels water from the vessels which is then absorbed by tissues. The force of gravity generally makes water retention more apparent in the lower parts of the body, which is why complaints of swollen feet and ankles at the end of the day are so common.

WHAT ARE THE CAUSES?

- *Prolonged or frequent standing.*
- *Heat* dilates the blood vessels.
- *Hormonal fluctuations* (estrogen and aldosterone). Many women experience water retention in the breasts and abdomen during their premenstrual period.
- *Pregnancy.* During the final weeks of pregnancy, the fetus exerts pressure on the veins returning blood to the heart, reducing circulation and causing the blood vessels to dilate.
- *Salt-rich diet.* Salt increases water retention.
- *Medications.* Certain high blood pressure drugs (calcium channel blockers), corticosteroids and hormone replacement therapy can contribute to edema.
- *Varicose veins.* These bluish dilated veins diminish circulation.
- *Acute thrombophlebitis.* This term describes the inflammation of a vein and the formation of a blood clot, causing pain and swelling in the lower limb's affected area.
- *Kidney failure.* One of the kidney's primary functions is to ensure the elimination of water. If it is not functioning properly, the body retains liquid. Certain kidney diseases are associated with a protein deficiency that also causes edema.

- *Liver disease and cirrhosis.* The liver is the body's blood filtration system. Any malfunction in this organ increases pressure in the veins, leading to vasodilation and edema.
- *Heart failure.* The heart acts like a hydraulic pump. If the left ventricle is unable to pump blood out to the body properly, the blood accumulates and overloads the right ventricle, impeding its ability to pump the blood coming in. This accumulation causes very high blood pressure in these vessels, which then dilate and cause edema.
- *Severe hypothyroidism* causes the entire body to slow down. The heart beats more slowly and impedes efficient pumping and circulation, leading to dilated blood vessels and edema.

PRACTICAL ADVICE

See a doctor. It is not normal to retain water and you should always visit a doctor if the cause is unknown. Some cases may be serious and require medical treatment.

Drink an appropriate amount of liquid. The doctor may recommend a reduction in the amount of liquid you ingest, depending on the cause of the edema. Liquid, of course, refers not only to water, but also to juice, soup, coffee, etc., as well as to the water contained in foods such as lettuce and celery.

Be cautious with diuretics. The doctor may prescribe diuretics, again depending on the root of the problem. This medication acts on the kidneys to facilitate the elimination of water and salt in the urine. It should not be used to lose weight and should only be taken on a doctor's recommendation.

Put your feet up. Raise your legs above hip-level and rest them on a chair or some pillows. Sit in this position several times a day for at least five minutes at a time.

Discuss your medications with your doctor. Tell him or her about any prescription or over-the-counter medications you are taking to determine whether they might be causing the edema.

Eat less salt. Very salty foods increase water retention. If necessary, consult a dietician to find out what foods contain the most salt. Cut down on salted French fries, cold cuts, and salty dishes. Read labels carefully before making a purchase. The higher up on the list of ingredients salt appears, the more the product contains.

Avoid exposure to heat. If you tend to retain water, remember that exposure to hot temperatures aggravates the symptoms. If edema bothers you, try to stay in cool environments.

Be patient. Follow the advice given here and any doctor's recommendations to help control water retention. It may take a few days or weeks to reduce the edema.

WHEN TO CONSULT?

► You have persistent and unexplained edema. Pressing on your skin with a finger leaves a mark. Consult immediately.

WHAT HAPPENS DURING THE EXAM?

The doctor takes a history of the problem and performs a complete physical examination, including taking the blood pressure. He or she may also recommend blood tests or a urine analysis.

WHAT IS THE TREATMENT?

Varicose veins

The doctor will recommend wearing support stockings (available in pharmacies or medical supply stores) to ease the symptoms. They prevent blood from accumulating in the small vessels near the surface of the skin by pushing it to a depth where it can be more easily pumped toward the heart.

Acute thrombophlebitis

The doctor will prescribe anticoagulant medications and recommend support stockings.

Kidney failure
Treatment involves diuretics and a salt-free diet.

Liver disease
Treatment varies according to the type of liver disease. Specific medications are required and the patient is strongly advised to abstain from alcohol and salt.

Heart failure
The doctor will prescribe heart tonics, diuretics, and a salt-free diet.

Index